Pediatric Emergency Medicine

Chief Complaints and Differential Diagnosis

T0179889

Pediatric Emergency Medicine

Chief Complaints and Differential Diagnosis

Edited by

Rebecca Jeanmonod
St. Luke's University Health Network, Bethlehem, PA, USA

Shellie Asher
Albany Medical Center, Albany, NY, USA

Blake Spirko
Baystate Medical Center, Springfield, MA, USA

Denis R. Pauzé
Albany Medical Center, Albany, NY, USA

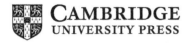

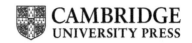

Shaftesbury Road, Cambridge CB2 8EA, United Kingdom

One Liberty Plaza, 20th Floor, New York, NY 10006, USA

477 Williamstown Road, Port Melbourne, VIC 3207, Australia

314–321, 3rd Floor, Plot 3, Splendor Forum, Jasola District Centre,
New Delhi – 110025, India

103 Penang Road, #05–06/07, Visioncrest Commercial, Singapore 238467

Cambridge University Press is part of Cambridge University Press & Assessment,
a department of the University of Cambridge.

We share the University's mission to contribute to society through the pursuit of
education, learning and research at the highest international levels of excellence.

www.cambridge.org
Information on this title: www.cambridge.org/9781316608869

DOI: 10.1017/9781316652923

First published 2018 (version 7, January 2024)

Printed in Great Britain by Ashford Colour Press Ltd., January 2024

A catalogue record for this publication is available from the British Library

ISBN 978-1-316-60886-9 Paperback

. . . .

Contents

List of Contributors   *page* viii
Preface   xi
List of Abbreviations   xiii
Reference Values   xv

1 **A Statement**   1
Denis R. Pauzé

2 **Resuscitation**   3
Case 1   3
Contributing Author: Erica Escarcega
Case 2   7
Contributing Author: Michael Leonard
Case 3   10
Contributing Author: Donald Jeanmonod
Case 4   16
Contributing Authors: Denis R. Pauzé
and William H. Hauda
Case 5   19
Contributing Authors: John Tran and
Rebecca Jeanmonod
Case 6   23
Contributing Authors: Ryan Fulton and
Melanie K. Prusakowski
Case 7   26
Contributing Author: Edwin Layng
Case 8   29
Contributing Author: Erica Escarcega
Case 9   32
Contributing Author: Sean Zwiebel
Case 10   35
Contributing Author: Sean Zwiebel
Case 11   38
Contributing Author: Ben Church

3 **Breathing Complaints**   42
Case 1   42
Contributing Author: Lauren Snyder
Case 2   45
Contributing Author: Natalie Moore
Case 3   47
Contributing Author: Dorka M. Jiménez
Almonte

Case 4   49
Contributing Author: Amanda Shorette
Case 5   52
Contributing Author: M. Bryan Dalla
Betta
Case 6   55
Contributing Authors: Daniel K. Pauzé
and Denis R. Pauzé
Case 7   59
Contributing Authors: Ben Church and
Rebecca Jeanmonod
Case 8   64
Contributing Authors: Natalie Moore and
Rebecca Jeanmonod

4 **Fever**   68
Case 1   68
Contributing Author: Rebecca Jeanmonod
Case 2   71
Contributing Author: Shellie Asher
Case 3   73
Contributing Authors: David H. Long and
Janet Young
Case 4   76
Contributing Author: Shellie Asher
Case 5   78
Contributing Authors: Kristine Marie J.
Casal and Melanie K. Prusakowski
Case 6   81
Contributing Author: Taylor R. Spencer
Case 7   85
Contributing Author: Sarah Hudgins
Case 8   88
Contributing Author: Rebecca Jeanmonod
Case 9   91
Contributing Authors: Keel Coleman and
Khalief Hamden

5 **Eye, Ear, Nose, and Throat Complaints** 95

Case 1   95
Contributing Authors: Jason Schwaber,
Taylor R. Spencer, and Rebecca Jeanmonod
Case 2   98
Contributing Author: Edwin Layng
Case 3   102
Contributing Author: Shellie Asher
Case 4   104
Contributing Author: Tom Dittrich
Case 5   106
Contributing Authors: Jonathan R.
Morgan and Melanie K. Prusakowski
Case 6   109
Contributing Authors: Denis R. Pauzé
and Daniel K. Pauzé
Case 7   112
Contributing Authors: Dorota
Pazdrowska and Melanie K. Prusakowski
Case 8   114
Contributing Author: Rebecca Jeanmonod
Case 9   117
Contributing Author: Khalief Hamden

6 **Extremity Complaints** 121

Case 1   121
Contributing Author: Rebecca Jeanmonod
Case 2   123
Contributing Author: Lauren Snyder
Case 3   126
Contributing Author: Melanie K.
Prusakowski
Case 4   129
Contributing Author: Dorka M. Jiménez
Almonte
Case 5   133
Contributing Author: Rachel A. Patterson
Case 6   135
Contributing Author: Benjamin Kitt
Case 7   138
Contributing Author: M. Bryan Dalla
Betta
Case 8   141
Contributing Author: Rebecca Jeanmonod
Case 9   144
Contributing Author: Rebecca Jeanmonod

7 **Vomiting** 147

Case 1   147
Contributing Author: Rebecca Jeanmonod

Case 2   150
Contributing Author: Erica Escarcega
Case 3   152
Contributing Author: Kinsey Leonard
Case 4   155
Contributing Authors: Angela
Mastantuono and Melanie K. Prusakowski
Case 5   157
Contributing Author: Rebecca Jeanmonod
Case 6   160
Contributing Author: Jason Black
Case 7   163
Contributing Author: Kinsey Leonard
Case 8   165
Contributing Author: Sarah Hudgins
Case 9   168
Contributing Author: Erica Escarcega
Case 10   170
Contributing Author: Kinsey Leonard

8 **Abdominal and Chest Pain** 173

Case 1   173
Contributing Authors: Jonathan Nogueira
and Janet Young
Case 2   176
Contributing Author: Michelle Clinton
Case 3   180
Contributing Authors: Alyssa Milano and
Sadé McKenzie
Case 4   183
Contributing Authors: Holly Stankewicz
and Rebecca Jeanmonod
Case 5   187
Contributing Author: Sadé McKenzie
Case 6   189
Contributing Author: Brian Kelly
Case 7   192
Contributing Authors: Cara V. Tillotson,
Melanie K. Prusakowski, and Rebecca
Jeanmonod
Case 8   195
Contributing Author: Donald Jeanmonod

9 **Altered Mental Status** 201

Case 1   201
Contributing Author: Rebecca Jeanmonod
Case 2   203
Contributing Author: Abhishek
Chaturvedi

Case 3 206
Contributing Author: Denis R. Pauzé
Case 4 209
Contributing Author: Rebecca Jeanmonod
Case 5 211
Contributing Authors: Tom Williams,
Emily Miller, and Denis R. Pauzé
Case 6 215
Contributing Author: Rebecca Jeanmonod
Case 7 219
Contributing Author: Kinsey Leonard
Case 8 221
Contributing Author: Kinsey Leonard

10 **Head and Neck Pain** 224
Case 1 224
Contributing Author: Sonika Raj
Case 2 226
Contributing Author: Rebecca Jeanmonod
Case 3 230
Contributing Authors: Tom Dittrich,
Denis R. Pauzé, and Matthew Adamo
Case 4 234
Contributing Authors: Anst Gelin and
Janet Young
Case 5 236
Contributing Authors: Christine M.
George and Melanie K. Prusakowski
Case 6 240
Contributing Author: Carl Daniel
Case 7 243
Contributing Authors: Michael Leonard
and Rebecca Jeanmonod
Case 8 247
Contributing Author: Jason Schwaber
Case 9 249
Contributing Authors: Jamaine Ortiz Jr.,
Rebecca Jeanmonod, Carl Daniel, Denis
R. Pauzé, and Matthew Adamo

11 **Genitourinary Complaints** 253
Case 1 253
Contributing Author: Shellie Asher

Case 2 255
Contributing Author: Shellie Asher
Case 3 257
Contributing Author: Abhishek
Chaturvedi
Case 4 260
Contributing Author: Jennifer Pelesz
Case 5 263
Contributing Author: Pamela Young
Case 6 266
Contributing Author: Leah A. Perez
Case 7 269
Contributing Authors: Shellie Asher and
Rebecca Jeanmonod

12 **Skin Complaints** 273
Case 1 273
Contributing Author: Efrat Rosenthal
Case 2 276
Contributing Author: Efrat Rosenthal
Case 3 278
Contributing Authors: Sundeep M.
Shukla and Rebecca Jeanmonod
Case 4 282
Contributing Author: Amanda Shorette
Case 5 286
Contributing Author: Benjamin Kitt
Case 6 288
Contributing Author: Rebecca Jeanmonod
Case 7 291
Contributing Author: Dorka M. Jiménez
Almonte

Case Key 295
Index 296

*Color plates are to be found between pages 152 and
153*

Contributors

Matthew Adamo
Albany Medical Center, Albany, NY

Dorka M. Jiménez Almonte
Baystate Medical Center, Springfield, MA

Shellie Asher
Albany Medical Center, Albany, NY

M. Bryan Dalla Betta
Baystate Medical Center, Springfield, MA

Jason Black
St. Luke's University Health Network, Bethlehem, PA

Kristine Marie J. Casal
Carilion Clinic, Roanoke, VA

Abhishek Chaturvedi
Pt. B.D. Sharma PGIMS, Rohtak, India

Ben Church
Baystate Medical Center, Springfield, MA

Michelle Clinton
Carilion Clinic, Roanoke, VA

Keel Coleman
Carilion Clinic, Roanoke, VA

Carl Daniel
Albany Medical Center, Albany, NY

Tom Dittrich
Roper St. Francis Hospital, Mount Pleasant, SC

Erica Escarcega
St. Luke's University Health Network, Bethlehem, PA

Ryan Fulton
Carilion Clinic, Roanoke, VA

Anst Gelin
Carilion Clinic, Roanoke, VA

Christine M. George
Carilion Clinic, Roanoke, VA

Khalief Hamden
Carilion Clinic, Roanoke, VA

William H. Hauda
Inova Fairfax Hospital, Falls Church, VA

Sarah Hudgins
St. Luke's University Health Network, Bethlehem, PA

Donald Jeanmonod
St. Luke's University Health Network, Bethlehem, PA

Rebecca Jeanmonod
St. Luke's University Health Network, Bethlehem, PA

Brian Kelly
St. Luke's University Health Network, Bethlehem, PA

Benjamin Kitt
Baystate Medical Center, Springfield, MA

Edwin Layng
St. Luke's University Health Network, Bethlehem, PA

Kinsey Leonard
Baystate Medical Center, Springfield, MA

Michael Leonard
St. Luke's University Health Network, Bethlehem, PA

David H. Long
Carilion Clinic, Roanoke, VA

Angela Mastantuono
Carilion Clinic, Roanoke, VA

Sadé McKenzie
Albany Medical Center, Albany, NY

Alyssa Milano
St. Luke's University Health Network, Bethlehem, PA

Emily Miller
Albany Medical Center, Albany, NY

Natalie Moore
Baystate Medical Center, Springfield, MA

Jonathan R. Morgan
Carilion Clinic, Roanoke, VA

Jonathan Nogueira
Carilion Clinic, Roanoke, VA

Jamaine Ortiz Jr.
St. Luke's University Health Network, Bethlehem, PA

Rachel A. Patterson
St. Luke's University Health Network, Bethlehem, PA

Daniel K. Pauzé
Albany Medical Center, Albany, NY

Denis R. Pauzé
Albany Medical Center, Albany, NY

Dorota Pazdrowska
Carilion Clinic, Roanoke, VA

Jennifer Pelesz
Albany Medical Center, Albany, NY

Leah A. Perez
Albany Medical Center, Albany, NY

Melanie K. Prusakowski
Carilion Clinic, Roanoke, VA

Sonika Raj
Albany Medical Center, Albany, NY

Efrat Rosenthal
Baystate Medical Center, Springfield, MA

Jason Schwaber
Ellis Hospital, Schenectady, NY

Amanda Shorette
Baystate Medical Center, Springfield, MA

Sundeep M. Shukla
Baystate Medical Center, Springfield, MA

Lauren Snyder
Baystate Medical Center, Springfield, MA

Taylor R. Spencer
Ellis Hospital, Schenectady, NY

Holly Stankewicz
St. Luke's University Health Network, Bethlehem, PA

Cara V. Tillotson
Carilion Clinic, Roanoke, VA

John Tran
St. Luke's University Health Network, Bethlehem, PA

Tom Williams
Albany Medical Center, Albany, NY

Janet Young
Carilion Clinic, Roanoke, VA

Pamela Young
Albany Medical Center, Albany, NY

Sean Zwiebel
St. Luke's University Health Network, Bethlehem, PA

Preface

Textbooks abound, electronic resources are ubiquitous, and there is an app for everything. Where does this book fit, as you struggle to "learn" clinical medicine?

The issue is always application. Most physicians, physicians-in-training, and physician assistants can take a test. They know how to look at a question with a list of closed possibilities and choose the right choice. If given four possibilities, the correct answer is often obvious, or at least recognizable. Question banks and question books are designed to help learners with this, and they work well.

Textbooks are generally, almost universally, organized by organ system. This is a very rational way to write a text book. It is straightforward from a writing perspective, and allows the learner to get in-depth information about everything in a given organ system in a step-by-step fashion. When you haven't learned about gastrointestinal physiology, let alone gastrointestinal pathophysiology, this makes sense, as well.

But the practice of medicine isn't really like either of these things. Not really. Patients come in with *complaints*. Their complaints don't come with a closed list of answers to choose from, and they don't come with their organ-system chapter. A complaint may seem to be referable to a specific organ system, but ultimately may be multifactorial. Take, for instance, the complaint of "shortness of breath." Your brain wants you to think about the lungs and the airway as the source of the problem. But maybe it's symptomatic anemia. Maybe it's cardiac. Maybe it's acidosis from an ingestion. Maybe it's renal failure with fluid overload. Maybe it's a foreign body. Maybe it's traumatic, even with no history of trauma. It happens.

But most written resources do not invoke the model of the patient as a mystery, the disease as an unknown. They presuppose you know it's a GI problem because the complaint is vomiting, or that it's a toxin because every teenager is honest about substance use. But we know better.

This book strives to fill the gap between traditional textbooks and bedside medicine. Instead of being organized by organ system, this book is organized by chief complaint, based on published frequencies of the most common pediatric chief complaints seen in emergency departments. Each chapter represents a chief complaint. Each case is presented as an unknown, with a historical vignette and an examination and ancillary tests, after which we have provided questions for thought. The reader should stop and consider the case and really think about these questions, the next steps, the dilemmas that are real, presented by these patients that are real, written by the physicians who actually cared for them. This is followed by the diagnosis, and a discussion of the disease as well as the other diseases that you should have considered, and how to distinguish them from one another.

You can use this book on your own, or you can use it with a friend. The book can easily be used for case-based teaching for clerkships, residencies, or small group learning.

What you won't find is a chapter on "staph scalded skin syndrome," or a chapter on "new onset diabetes." You will, however, learn when to worry about a rash, how to resuscitate a baby, which seizure patient needs labs and what your differential diagnosis should be, and basically, how to think about illness in children.

If you happen to find yourself wanting to read about a specific disease without the mystery of the case, we do provide a key at the back of the book to "cheat" and find a discussion on intussusception, or reading on intracranial tumors. And it's ok to do that, but remember that human tradition was based on stories, handed down through generations by the telling and remembering. You will learn better from stories than from tables and graphs. You will retain information when you care about the outcome, and the providers who wrote these cases want you to care the way they do. If you use this book as it's intended, you will have broader differential diagnoses. You will be less tempted to close your differential prematurely. You will be less likely to short-cut your examination or skip the important questions on your history. And you will be a better doctor and take better care of our most vulnerable population. And what could be better than that?

Abbreviations

AAP	American Academy of Pediatrics		CSF	cerebrospinal fluid
ABC	airway, breathing, and circulation		c-spine	cervical spine
ABG	arterial blood gas		CT	computed tomography
ACE inhibitor	angiotensin-converting-enzyme inhibitor		CTA	clear to auscultation
			CVC	central venous catheter
ACLS	Advanced Cardiac Life Support		CXR	chest X-ray
ALL	acute lymphoblastic leukemia		DKA	diabetic ketoacidosis
ALT	alanine transaminase		EBV	Epstein–Barr virus
ALTE	apparent life-threatening event		ECMO	extracorporeal membrane oxygenation
AML	acute myeloid leukemia			
ARDS	acute respiratory distress syndrome		ED	emergency department
AST	aspartate transaminase		EEG	electroencephalogram
ATLS	Advanced Trauma Life Support		EKG	electrocardiogram
BiPAP	bilevel positive airway pressure		ELISA	enzyme-linked immunosorbent assay
BLEEP	bedside-limited echocardiogram by emergency physician			
			EM	emergency medicine
BNP	B-type natriuretic peptide		EMS	emergency medical services
BP	blood pressure (in millimeters of mercury [mmHg])		ENT	otolaryngology
			EPO	erythropoietin
BRUE	brief resolved unexplained event		ESR	erythrocyte sedimentation rate
BUN	blood urea nitrogen		ET tube	endotracheal tube
CBC	complete blood count		FAST	focused assessment with sonography for trauma
c-collar	cervical spine immobilization collar			
CHALICE	Children's Head Injury Algorithm for the Prediction of Important Clinical Events		FEV1	forced expiratory volume in 1 second
			FVC	forced vital capacity
			GCS	Glasgow Coma Scale
CHD	congenital heart disease		GERD	gastroesophageal reflux disease
CDC	Centers for Disease Control and Prevention		GI	gastrointestinal
			Hb	hemoglobin
CHF	congestive heart failure		β-hCG	beta-human chorionic gonadotropin
CI	confidence interval		HCT	hematocrit
Cl	chloride		HEENT	head, ears, eyes, nose, and throat
cm	centimeter		HIV	human immunodeficiency virus
CMV	cytomegalovirus		HR	heart rate (in beats per minute)
CNS	central nervous system		HSV	herpes simplex virus
CPAP	continuous positive airway pressure		ICU	intensive care unit
CPR	cardiopulmonary resuscitation		IgG	immunoglobulin G
Cr	creatinine		IgM	immunoglobulin M
CRP	C-reactive protein		IM	intramuscular
c-section	caesarean section		INR	international normalized ratio

IO	intraosseous
IU	international units
IV	intravenous
JVD	jugular venous distension
K	potassium
kg	kilogram
LDH	lactate dehydrogenase
LFT	liver function test
LP	lumbar puncture
LSD	lysergic acid diethylamide
M/R/G	murmurs, rubs, gallops
mcg	microgram
MCHC	mean corpuscular hemoglobin concentration
MCV	mean corpuscular volume
mEq	milliequivalents
MIGB	metaiodobenzylguanidine
mL	milliliter
μL	microliter
mmHg	millimeters of mercury
MRI	magnetic resonance imaging
MRSA	methicillin-resistant *Staphylococcus aureus*
MSSA	methicillin-sensitive *Staphylococcus aureus*
Na	sodium
NEXUS	National Emergency X-radiography Utilization Study
NICU	neonatal intensive care unit
NKDA	no known drug allergies
NMDA	N-methyl-D-aspartate
NMS	neuroleptic malignant syndrome
NPO	nothing per os (do not feed)
NSAIDs	non-steroidal anti-inflammatory drugs
O_2 sat	oxygen saturation
OR	operating room
$PaCO_2$	partial pressure of carbon dioxide in arterial blood

PCP	primary care provider
PCR	polymerase chain reaction
PECARN	Pediatric Emergency Care Applied Research Network
PEEP	positive end expiratory pressure
PERRL	pupils equally round and reactive to light
PGE1	prostaglandin E1
PICC	peripherally inserted central catheter
PICU	pediatric intensive care unit
Plt	platelets
PO	per os, or by mouth
PTLD	post-transplant lymphoproliferative disease
RBC	red blood cells
RICE	rest, ice, compression, elevation
RR	respiratory rate (in breaths per minute)
RSV	respiratory syncytial virus
SIDS	sudden infant death syndrome
SIRS	systemic inflammatory response syndrome
T	temperature
TBI	traumatic brain injury
TBSA	total body surface area
TIBC	total iron binding capacity
U/A	urinalysis
U/S	ultrasound
URI	upper respiratory infection
USA	United States of America
UTD	up to date
UTI	urinary tract infection
UTO	unable to obtain
VBG	venous blood gas
W/R/R	wheezes, rales, rhonchi
WBC	white blood cells
WHO	World Health Organization

Reference Values

Pediatric normal laboratory values

Test	Value	Unit	Age
Complete blood count (CBC)			
White blood cells (WBC)	5,000–30,000	cells/µL	0–30 days
	5,000–19,000	cells/µL	1–6 months
	6,000–17,500	cells/µL	6–12 months
	4,500–14,500	cells/µL	1–16 years
Hemoglobin (Hb)	15.0–22.0	g/dL	0–30 days
	9.5–15.0	g/dL	>30 days
Hematocrit (HCT)	44–70	%	0–30 days
	29–45	%	>30 days
Mean corpuscular hemoglobin concentration (MCHC)	28–36	g/dL	
Mean corpuscular volume (MCV)	86–115	fL	0–30 days
	72–100	fL	>30 days
Platelets (Plt)	150,000–450,500	platelets/µL	
Serum chemistries			
Alanine aminotransferase (ALT)	6–50	U/L	
Albumin	2.9–5.5	g/dL	
Alkaline phosphatase	110–400	U/L	
Ammonia	47–94	µmol/L	0–30 days
	15–48	µmol/L	30 days–16 years
	9–26	µmol/L	>16 years
Amylase	30–115	U/L	
Aspartate aminotransferase (AST)	35–140	U/L	0–5 days
	20–60	U/L	>5 days
Bilirubin	1–14	mg/dL	0–5 days
	0.2–1.0	mg/dL	> 5 days
Blood urea nitrogen (BUN)	5–28	mg/dL	
Calcium	8.0–10.7	mg/dL	
Chloride	95–105	mEq/dL	
C-reactive protein (CRP)	<1.0	mg/mL	
Creatine phosphokinase (CPK)	60–365	U/L	
Creatinine (Cr)	0.12–1.06	mg/dL	
Erythrocyte sedimentation rate (ESR)	0–20	mm/hour	
Ferritin	36–391	ng/ml	0–6 months
	36–100		7 months–5 years
	36–311		>5 years
Glucose	30–80	mg/dL	0–3 days
	70–110		>3 days
Iron	55–150	µg/dL	
Iron (transferrin) saturation	56–74	%	0–10 days
	17–44		>10 days
Lactate	0.2–2.0	mmol/L	
Lactate dehydrogenase (LDH)	934–2,150	U/L	0–5 days
	420–900		5 days–9 years
	313–750		>9 years
Lipase	15–300	U/L	
Magnesium	1.2–2.6	mg/dL	

Test	Value	Unit	Age
Phosphorus	2.3–8.0	mg/dL	
Potassium (K)	4.5–7.0	mEq/L	0–30 days
	4.0–5.5		>30 days
Sodium (Na)	132–145	mEq/L	
Total iron binding capacity (TIBC)	100–400	µg/dL	0–11 months
	250–425		>11 months
Transferrin	200–360	mg/dL	
Arterial blood gas (ABG)			
pH	7.33–7.43	pH	
Partial pressure of carbon dioxide ($PaCO_2$)	26–41	mmHg	0–12 months
	33–46		>12 months
Partial pressure of oxygen (PaO_2)	65–76	mmHg	0–12 months
	88–105		>12 months
Cerebrospinal fluid (CSF)			
Glucose	50–70	% of serum glucose	
Protein	<100	mg/dL	0–30 days
	14–45		>30 days
Red blood cells (RBC)	<10	cells/µL	
White blood cells (WBC)	<30	cells/µL	0–12 months
	<20	cells/µL	1–4 years
	<10	cells/µL	>4 years
Coagulation studies			
Prothrombin time (PT)	12.2–15.5	seconds	
International normalized ratio (INR)	0.8–1.2		
Partial thromboplastin time (PTT)	26.5–35.5	seconds	
Urine			
Specific gravity	1.001–1.035		
pH	4–9		
Bilirubin	None		
Glucose	<30	mg/dL	
Ketones	None		
Protein	None		
Urobilinogen	<2.0		
White blood cells (WBC)	0–4	cells/high-powered field	
Red blood cells (RBC)	0–4	cells/high-powered field	
Epithelial cells	0–4	cells/high-powered field	

Reference: *Gregory's Pediatric Anesthesia*, 5th edition. Gregory G, Andropoulos D (eds). Wiley-Blackwell, 2011.

A Statement

Denis R. Pauzé

A 3-year-old boy with a bead stuck up his nose. A helpless 4-month-old girl with a devastating traumatic brain injury…from abuse. A 15-year-old with four months of persistent headaches, countless healthcare visits…and today…diagnosed with a brain tumor.

Kids are unique. They are different. And most certainly…they are incredibly special.

Kids represent our future.

As clinicians, we are entrusted with someone's most valuable possession, their child. We are entrusted to take care of them, to fix them, to cure them. Sometimes, it may be as simple as removing a nasal foreign body or reducing a nursemaid's elbow. Very easy, yet incredibly satisfying. But for other children, the situation and consequences are much more dire. In critical situations, we are asked to save them, *to save their lives.* A child on a bicycle hit by a car…An infant in cardiogenic shock from a critical coarctation…Or a teenager with anaphylaxis from a peanut ingestion. We are there to save their lives.

We who take care of children must be ready for these dramatic and life-threatening encounters. But we must also be prepared for the less obvious, the less dramatic, the "subtle" presentation. A fussy 4-month-old infant with abusive head trauma may harbor only one small diagnostic clue, such as a small scalp bruise, which the astute physician must discover. Failure to identify equates to further abuse. A wheezing 4-month-old infant during RSV season may actually harbor an undiagnosed cardiomyopathy. Can we pick out that needle in the haystack? That child with a persistent headache, could it be a brain tumor, carbon monoxide poisoning, or just a simple migraine headache? And the ever so common sore throat that you see day in and day out in Fast Track, will your next encounter be Lemierre's syndrome?

Just think how vastly the care of the pediatric patient has evolved in the past 75 years. In the middle of the last century, antibiotics were rarely used,

we didn't have vaccines for measles or *Haemophilus influenzae* or *Streptococcus pneumoniae*, bacterial meningitis was common and deadly, and the care of the pediatric trauma patient was similar to that of the dark ages. As an example, in 1946, Caffey described a series of pediatric patients with subdural hematomas and long-bone fractures. He writes, "For many years we have been puzzled by the roentgen disclosure of fresh, healing and healed multiple fractures in the long bones of infants whose principal disease was chronic subdural hematoma." At the time, we still hadn't heard of the term "child abuse." Several years later, in 1962, Kempe and colleagues introduced the term "The Battered Child Syndrome" in a landmark *JAMA* article.[1] Today, hundreds of articles, conferences, and teaching seminars discuss non-accidental trauma.

Technology has also changed pediatric care. Seventy-five years ago we struggled to interpret low-quality X-rays. Today, we have pediatric X-ray technicians and pediatric radiologists. The CT scan was not invented until 1972! Today, low-dose CT, clinical indications for CT, PECARN traumatic brain injury prediction rules, and "pan-scan" are ever so common medical vernacular for the pediatric patient. Imagine a shift in the ED without a CT scan machine?! And of course there is ultrasound, first used for clinical purposes in the 1950s. Today, not only is there three- and four-dimensional ultrasound, but also pediatric emergency medicine physicians who perform point of care emergency ultrasound and make life-saving treatment decisions based upon these immediate bedside images.

In this book, the authors present dozens of interesting pediatric case vignettes. A pediatric story is followed by thought-provoking clinical questions, many very "cool" images, and subsequently an engaging discussion of the diagnostic topic. The authors discuss a wide range of clinical situations, such as trauma, toxicology, resuscitation, orthopedics, and infectious disease. There are simple "bread-and-butter" cases described, things we see and do everyday. A nurse-maid's elbow, a lodged foreign body, appendicitis, and pharyngitis. The reader will also experience critical scenarios, cases in shock, respiratory failure, and multi-trauma. These are unique situations where seconds count to save a young one's life.

As you read through this book, remember, you are the safety net for our children.

Kids are unique, kids are special.

Kids represent our future.

Reference

1. Kempe CH, Silverman FN, Steele BF, et al. The battered-child syndrome. *JAMA* 1962; 181: 1–24.

Resuscitation

Chapter 2

Case 1

Contributing Author: Erica Escarcega

History

The patient is a 10-year-old male brought in by EMS as a trauma alert after his bicycle was struck by a car at low speed. According to bystanders, the front wheel of the bicycle was struck by the front end of the car while the child was attempting to cross an intersection. The child fell forward over the handlebars and then landed on the street. The child was unhelmeted. There was a loss of consciousness at the scene for approximately 1 minute. He sustained significant facial injury, with soft-tissue swelling, and is unable to speak. He occasionally spits out a moderate amount of blood, but is able to handle his secretions and does not appear to be in respiratory distress. He was unable to ambulate at the scene and cries in pain with every touch.

Past Medical History

- None. He sees his pediatrician regularly and is UTD on vaccinations.

Medications

- None.

Allergies

- NKDA.

Physical Examination and Ancillary Studies

- *Vital signs*: T 98.6 °F, HR 114, BP 110/68, RR 20, O_2 sat 100% on room air.
- *General*: The patient is distressed, anxious, and crying. However, he is able to cooperate with examination.

Table 2.1 Glasgow Coma Scale. A score of 15 is normal. A score of 8 is considered comatose. A score of 3 is entirely unresponsive. In children < 4 years of age, modified verbal response includes 5 - smiles/coos, 4 - cries and is consolable, 3 - cries inappropriately or persistently, 2 - grunting or moaning, agitation, and 1 - no response.

Eyes open	Voice response	Motor response
• 4: spontaneous	• 5: coherent speech	• 6: follows commands
• 3: voice	• 4: confused	• 5: purposeful/ localizes
• 2: pain	• 3: inappropriate words	• 4: withdraws to pain
• 1: no opening	• 2: incomprehensible sounds	• 3: decorticate
	• 1: no speech	• 2: decerebrate
		• 1: no movement

- *Primary survey*:
  - *Airway*: Child with swollen bleeding tongue, but able to spit. No pooling secretions.
  - *Breathing*: Good air entry, adequate effort and oxygenation.
  - *Circulation*: Tachycardic, good central and peripheral pulses.
  - *Disability*: GCS 12 (eyes open spontaneously: 4, verbal is incomprehensible: 2, motor able to follow commands: 6) (see Table 2.1).
  - *Exposure*: Multiple abrasions and contusions.
- *Secondary survey*:
  - *HEENT*: PERRL. Mucous membranes are moist. There is significant swelling to the right mandible with abrasions over the right cheek, chin, and forehead. A 2-cm laceration is present to the left side of the tongue, with moderate active bleeding. Patient is currently in a c-collar and cries with palpation of the posterior c-spine. Trachea is midline.
  - *Cardiovascular*: He is tachycardic, with normal rhythm and no M/R/G. Peripheral pulses are normal. Capillary refill < 3 seconds.

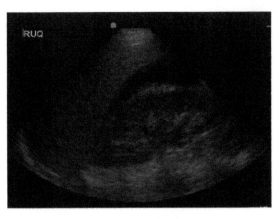

Figure 2.1 FAST examination with free fluid.

- *Lungs*: CTA bilaterally, with no W/R/R. No chest-wall tenderness.
- *Abdomen*: The patient's abdomen is diffusely tender; however, soft and non-distended without rebound or guarding. There are no palpable masses on examination.
- *Extremities and skin*: There are multiple abrasions including a large abrasion over the right flank, right arm, bilateral palms, bilateral knees, and shins. Abrasions are dirty, impregnated with asphalt, and have minimal venous oozing at the time of examination. There is tenderness to palpation over the right hip. The patient is unable to tolerate range of motion of the right leg secondary to pain. He has tenderness over the left knee and cries with attempts at range of motion. He has full range of motion of bilateral upper extremities.
- *Neurologic*: He has tenderness over the c-spine. No thoracic or lumbar spine tenderness. No step-offs present on palpation of the spine.
- *Ancillary studies*: FAST examination with free fluid (Figure 2.1).

Questions for Thought

- What steps should be taken to evaluate and stabilize a pediatric trauma victim?
- How do pediatric trauma patients differ from adult trauma patients?
- What injuries are common in children who have been victims of severe trauma?
- How much blood volume can a child lose prior to becoming hypotensive?

Diagnosis

- Multiple trauma.

Discussion

- *Epidemiology*: It is estimated that 12,175 children die every year in the USA due to traumatic injuries, with the largest percentage of fatal injuries related to motor vehicle accidents.[1] Of motor vehicle-related fatalities, an average of 3,724 children die each year as occupants of the vehicle, 724 of annual fatalities are pedestrians, and 162 children are struck by a vehicle while riding their bicycles.[1] Seatbelt and bicycle helmet laws are measures that have been taken to attempt to reduce the number of childhood fatalities; however, pediatric trauma continues to be a major concern for public health, both in the USA and internationally.[2]
- *Pathophysiology*: Trauma presents a different disease spectrum in children as compared to adults. The bones of children are generally more pliable than those of the more calcified adult skeleton; therefore, fractures are often sustained in the setting of higher force mechanisms and internal injuries may occur despite an absence of fractures.[2,3] The proportionally larger and softer skull in small children results in an increased risk of traumatic brain injuries as well as facial injuries. Additionally, the ligaments of the child's c-spine have an increased laxity, which may increase the risk of c-spine injury that may not be seen on radiography. In regards to the circulatory system, a child's heart has a fixed stroke volume, which results in a reliance on an increase in heart rate in order to improve cardiac output. The low cardiopulmonary reserve in small children may result in a rapid, precipitous progression into shock. Hypothermia may also occur more quickly in children due to their higher relative body surface area.
- *Presentation*: Children are often unable to provide history and may not be able to cooperate with examination, which makes evaluation for the

extent of injuries challenging. Significant injuries may exist despite an inability to elicit tenderness on physical examination, especially in the setting of a decreased mental status. Indeed, the most common cause of pediatric trauma mortality is in fact head injury, and specific decision rules exist to guide the clinician in determining when neuroimaging is indicated. This is covered in Case 2 in this chapter.

Neck and spine injuries can be devastating, but are relatively uncommon in children. Children are more likely to have a ligamentous injury than a c-spine fracture. Decision rules exist for neuroimaging in neck injury, as well, and this is covered in Case 3 in this chapter.

The most common intrathoracic injury in significant blunt trauma is pulmonary contusion and the most common immediately life-threatening injury in children is tension pneumothorax.[4] Children may also sustain rib fractures, simple pneumothorax, hemothorax, pneumomediastinum, as well as injuries to the heart, aorta, and diaphragm in the setting of blunt trauma. Children may have significant intrathoracic trauma in the absence of rib fractures.

Abdominal injuries are common after severe blunt trauma with highest risk of injury to the liver and spleen.[5] Be wary of signs of injury related to seatbelts (such as abdominal bruising) as this may be an indication of significant underlying injury.[3,4] Fractures of the lumbar spine (Chance fracture) are caused by a flexion-distraction injury associated with lap belts and are often accompanied by GI injuries. Children presenting with femur fractures may also have concomitant intra-abdominal and intrathoracic injuries as these fractures are generally associated with a high impact mechanism.[3]

- *Diagnosis*: Many decision rules have been formulated with the goal of reducing radiation exposure in children. Although as many as 58 percent of intra-abdominal injuries present with abdominal pain, significant injuries may be missed due to the unreliability of the patient's examination; therefore, providers should have a low threshold for CT of the abdomen in patients with significant mechanism, especially in the setting of hypotension and laboratory abnormalities, including decreased HCT,

hematuria, and elevated liver enzymes.[5] Signs which should increase suspicion for intrathoracic injuries include hypotension, tachypnea, abnormal mental status, and abnormal lung sounds on auscultation and should prompt the performance of CXR.[4] CXR, however, may miss up to 40 percent of intrathoracic injuries and if suspicion remains high despite negative CXR, further studies should be considered such as chest CT.[4] FAST examinations are often performed quickly at the bedside to evaluate for the presence of free fluid in the abdomen as well as around the heart; however, a negative FAST does not obviate the need for further imaging.

- *Treatment*: Cases of severe trauma are ideally managed by a multidisciplinary team consisting of emergency providers, surgeons, nurses, respiratory therapists, intensivists, radiologists, and subspecialists. Treatment of all pediatric traumas should begin with a primary survey and stabilization, as taught in ATLS courses, and should follow the ABCDE mnemonic (*Airway, Breathing, Circulation, Disability, Exposure*).[3] This algorithm applies to all causes of shock, not just shock related to trauma. In traumatized patients, the c-spine should remain immobilized until the child has been completely assessed.

Airway: orotracheal intubation is the preferred method of securing the airway in the absence of facial or laryngeal trauma if there are signs of respiratory distress, apnea, airway obstruction, or decreased mental status resulting in an inability to protect the airway.[3] In the rare cases where orotracheal intubation is contraindicated or unable to be established, a surgical airway is necessary. Needle cricothyroidotomy is a temporizing measure which can be used in young children. Standard cricothyroidotomy may be performed in children over the age of 12 in which the cricothyroid membrane can be palpated.[3] Nasotracheal intubation is not recommended in children. Hoarseness or crepitus may suggest a laryngeal injury that is best managed in consultation with ENT. In these cases, cricothyroidotomy may worsen the patient's injury, and stabilization of the airway in an operating suite may be required.

Breathing: The patient should be evaluated for bilateral breath sounds, the absence of which should prompt immediate intervention with placement of chest tubes to relieve suspected pneumothorax or hemothorax.[3] The most common cause of cardiac arrest in children is hypoxia, so it is vital to establish appropriate ventilation in pediatric trauma victims using weight-based lung volumes and titrating to oxygenation and end-tidal carbon dioxide or using serial ABGs.

Circulation: Evaluation of the circulation of a child is best performed by assessing peripheral perfusion (capillary refill and quality of peripheral pulses) as patients may lose more than 25 percent of their blood volume before becoming hypotensive.[3] Crystalloid fluid boluses of 20 mL/kg (preferably warmed) should be given initially, followed by boluses of 10 mL/kg of blood if needed. IV access in small children can be challenging, and IO access should be obtained if peripheral access cannot be obtained after two attempts.[3]

Disability: The disability portion of the ABCDE mnemonic refers to the patient's neurologic status. The Glasgow Coma Scale (GCS), which is commonly used in adult trauma, may also be used in the evaluation of mental status in pediatric trauma with modification of the verbal score in children under the age of 4. This score contributes to imaging decisions in the head-injured patient.

Exposure: Be sure to fully expose and inspect the patient for external signs of injury. Palpate for deformity, swelling, and crepitus. During the assessment, care should also be taken to keep the child as warm as possible to avoid hypothermia, which can worsen coagulopathy and acidosis. If the child's condition worsens at any point during the assessment, the primary survey should be repeated, beginning with reassessment of the patient's airway.

Once the primary survey is complete and the child is stable, a careful head-to-toe examination, called the secondary survey, takes place. Every inch of the child should be examined to avoid missing injuries.

Imaging should be performed in a stabilized patient after the primary survey as directed by findings during examination of the child. Children with multiple severe injuries may need to be managed in a staged approach, addressing the most life-threatening injuries first followed by further stabilization prior to subsequent interventions.[6]

- *Disposition*: Children presenting to a center without PICU capabilities, who are seriously injured, should be stabilized and transferred to a trauma center. It is appropriate for EMS to bypass a non-trauma center to bring children who are hemodynamically stable to the appropriate nearest trauma facility.

Historical clues	Physical findings	Ancillary studies
• High impact mechanism • Loss of consciousness	• Tachycardia • External signs of trauma (abrasions, contusions, lacerations, crepitus, deformities) • Tenderness to abdomen, spine, and lower extremities	• Positive FAST

Follow-Up

Although the patient had a positive FAST, he was hemodynamically stable to undergo CT scanning to further assess his injuries. CT chest, abdomen, and pelvis performed with IV contrast showed a grade III splenic laceration without active extravasation. CT facial bones revealed a non-displaced mandibular fracture. CT head showed no intracranial hemorrhage or skull fractures and CT c-spine was negative for fractures or dislocations. An X-ray of his left knee showed a non-displaced patellar fracture. The tongue laceration was sutured and his jaw was banded shut by ENT. The patient was admitted to the PICU for airway monitoring as his tongue had swollen significantly and there was concern of potential airway compromise. He also underwent serial abdominal examinations and hemodynamic monitoring for his splenic laceration. His patellar fracture was managed conservatively by orthopedics with splinting. The bands for his mandibular fracture were exchanged for wires when the swelling resolved. After an uneventful stay in the ICU, he was eventually discharged home with ENT, general surgery, and orthopedics follow-up.

References

1. Borse N, Gilchrist J, Dellinger A, et al. CDC Childhood Injury Report: Patterns of Unintentional Injuries among 0–19 Year Olds in the United States, 2000–2006. Atlanta (GA): Centers for Disease Control and Prevention, National Center for Injury Prevention and Control, 2008.

2. Sharar S. The ongoing and worldwide challenge of pediatric trauma. *Int J Crit Illn Ing Sci* 2012; 2: 111–13.

3. American College of Surgeons. Pediatric trauma. In *Advanced Trauma Life Support Student Course Manual*, 9th edition. Chicago, IL: American College of Surgeons, 2012, pp. 246–70.

4. Homes J, Sokolove P, Brant W, et al. A clinical decision rule for identifying children with thoracic injuries after blunt torso trauma. *Ann Emerg Med* 2002; 39: 492–9.

5. Homes J, Sokolove P, Brant W, et al. Identification of children with intra-abdominal injuries after blunt trauma. *Ann Emerg Med* 2002; 39: 500–9.

6. Wetzel R and Burns C. Multiple trauma in children: Critical care overview. *Crit Care Med* 2002; 30: S468–77.

Case 2

Contributing Author: Michael Leonard

History

A 5-year-old male presents to the ED after being struck by a bicycle ridden by another child. The child had been playing on the sidewalk. The child struck his head on the pavement. Bystanders rushed to the scene and EMS was contacted immediately, who note the patient was briefly unconscious. Upon arrival, abrasion is noted to the right parietal area, and the child is confused and agitated. He does not follow commands but appears to be moving all extremities.

Past Medical History

- Full-term birth with no complications, developmentally normal, immunizations are UTD.

Medications

- None.

Allergies

- Strawberries.

Physical Examination and Ancillary Studies

- *Vital signs*: T 98.6 °F, HR 115, RR 18, BP 100/60, O_2 sat 100% on room air.
- *General*: Confused and agitated, resisting any effort to examine him.
- *Primary survey*:
  - *Airway*: Patent, no pooling secretions.
  - *Breathing*: Clear and equal breath sounds.
  - *Circulation*: Intact central and peripheral pulses.
  - *Disability*: GCS 13 (eyes = 4, speech = 4, motor = 5), non-focal.
  - *Exposure*: Bleeding laceration to right parietal area, with palpable bony depression and numerous facial abrasions. Abrasion to right elbow. No bony deformity. Bleeding is controlled.
- *Secondary survey*:
  - *HEENT*: Lacerations and abrasions as noted. Normal ear examination without evidence of hemotypanum or periauricular ecchymosis. Normal funduscopic examination without evidence of hyphema and with apparently normal extraocular movements from a limited examination due to patient cooperation.
  - *Neck*: Non-tender, child spontaneously ranging neck, with no apparent pain.
  - *Cardiovascular*: Heart with regular rate and rhythm, no M/R/G, good capillary refill.
  - *Lungs*: CTA bilaterally, with no W/R/R.
  - *Abdomen*: Soft, no tenderness, no rebound or guarding, no masses.
  - *Extremities*: No deformity. Abrasion on elbow as noted. Normal range of motion.
  - *Axial skeleton*: No back tenderness or step-offs, pelvis stable to rock and compression.
  - *Neurologic*: Confused, disoriented, and uncooperative. Examination appears non-focal and symmetric.

Questions for Thought

- What is the differential diagnosis of pediatric head injuries?
- What additional testing or imaging would be useful in this patient?
- What instructions should be given to the parents of children with less severe injuries?

Diagnosis

- Fall with depressed parietal skull fracture, dural tear with surrounding brain edema but without evidence of intracranial hemorrhage.

Discussion

- *Epidemiology*: The incidence of ED visits for TBI-related issues has been increasing over the last several years with the highest incidence (1,889 visits/100,000 person-years) occurring in children less than 3 years old.[1] Fortunately, the vast majority of pediatric head trauma is benign and the resultant rate of TBI-related deaths is lowest in the 0–4 year (4.3/100,000) and 5–14 year (1.9/100,000) age groups.[2] Hence, the challenge for the EM provider relates to identifying the rare cases of a potentially devastating condition within an exceedingly common presenting complaint.
- *Pathophysiology*: The majority of pediatric head injuries are due to blunt traumatic mechanisms. Significant injuries are rare but can result in skull fractures or intracranial injuries, including epidural, subdural, or subarachnoid hemorrhages. Additionally, the increasing emphasis on the long-term effects of concussion has contributed to the increasing number of ED visits. The pathophysiology of concussions or mild TBI is complex and incompletely understood and remains an area of evolving research.
- *Presentation*: Key components of the history include details of the mechanism of injury, any reported loss of consciousness, vomiting, or headache following the incident, and any change in behavior. In the case of a motor vehicle accident, acquire details from EMS or witnesses about the location of the child in the car, the extent and location of damage to the vehicle, whether the child was restrained and secured appropriately in a car seat, and any history of vehicular ejection. If the child fell, obtain information about the height of the fall or if the fall was from standing. If the child was on a bicycle, identify whether a helmet was worn at the time of the incident. Any history that seems implausible or does not fit with the injury pattern demonstrated on physical examination raises the possibility of abuse. Whenever practical, query the patient directly about mechanism, headache,

or nausea. Elicit further details from the patient's parents regarding whether the child is acting normally and at his or her baseline.

Initial assessment of the child should be focused on the ABC algorithm instituted with ATLS training to identify and intervene upon any potentially life-threatening conditions. An initial neurologic assessment of the child must account for age-specific variation in relation to expected findings. Following primary assessment, the secondary survey, including a head-to-toe examination, should be completed. Specific focus on scalp examination for any hematoma, lacerations, or other signs of trauma should be performed. Hemotympanum, posterior auricular ecchymosis (Battle's sign), or periocular ecchymoses that spare the tarsal plates (Raccoon eyes) are potential signs of a basilar skull fracture that, although rare, should be promptly evaluated by a trauma surgeon. Funduscopic examination, including evaluation for retinal hemorrhages, and complete eye examination, assessing for hyphema, globe rupture, and corneal injury, should be completed; if there is concern for non-accidental trauma, a formal examination by an ophthalmologist should be performed to assess for retinal hemorrhages.

- *Diagnosis*: Although ultrasound has been evaluated for the diagnosis of skull fractures, intracranial evaluation typically requires CT imaging, and recent efforts have been focused on limiting the exposure to ionizing radiation, particularly in the pediatric population.[3] To this extent, identifying which children are most at risk becomes a critical component of the evaluation and diagnosis of a potentially serious injury while limiting the risks from testing. Several decision aids have been developed and when compared in prospective trials, the PECARN clinical decision rules were found to be superior to other guidelines.[4] The PECARN consortium evaluated 42,412 children (less than 18 years old) presenting to 25 North American EDs, to develop a set of highly sensitive clinical decision aids that predict which children are at risk for intracranial injury and may benefit from imaging.[5] The decision aids include separate algorithms for children less than 2 years old and for older children. Each algorithm stratifies patients into three distinct groups:

Table 2.2 PECARN high- and intermediate-risk definitions for children with head injury[5]

	Children less than 2 years old	Children greater than 2 years old
High risk (CT recommended)	Palpable skull fracture	Signs of basilar skull fracture
	GCS $\leq$ 14 including any signs of altered mental status (agitation, somnolence, repetitive questioning, or slow responses to verbal communication)	
Intermediate risk (observation versus CT)	Loss of consciousness greater than 5 seconds Occipital, parietal, or temporal scalp hematoma Not acting normally per parent	Loss of consciousness any period History of vomiting Severe headache
	Severe mechanism of injury, including: a motor vehicle collision where the patient was ejected, the collision involved the death of another passenger, or a rollover; the patient was a pedestrian or a bicyclist without helmet and was struck by a motor vehicle; or the patient's head was struck by a high-impact object	
	Fall > 3 feet	Fall > 5 feet

- *High-risk patients* warranting immediate imaging, with a greater than 4 percent risk of clinically important TBI (ciTBI).
- *Intermediate-risk patients* who may be observed or may warrant imaging based upon additional factors (approximately 1 percent risk of ciTBI).
- *Low-risk patients* who are unlikely to benefit from imaging (<0.05 percent risk of ciTBI).

Low-risk patients are those who do not meet any criteria for high or intermediate risk. Based upon the high sensitivity demonstrated in multiple validation studies, the risk of clinically significant TBI is exceedingly low in these patients, and the risks of imaging likely outweigh any benefit. The different risk categories are shown in Table 2.2.

For those children in the intermediate-risk group, the decision whether to observe or perform imaging on the patient should be considered in consultation with the child's parents and in accordance with the physician's experience and comfort. Observation allows the opportunity to assess for symptom evolution, which might warrant a change in care. Ultimately, like any decision aid, the use of the PECARN algorithm is meant to be a guideline and should not supersede clinician judgment.

- *Treatment*: After initial resuscitation of a patient with a traumatic head injury, the identification of any clinically significant TBI warrants immediate consultation with an appropriately trained neurosurgeon or transfer to a center capable of managing these injuries. Additional interventions, such as the use of osmotic agents (including hypertonic saline and mannitol) and seizure prophylaxis, may be warranted based upon the severity of the injury and the potential for worsening due to evolution of the initial injury. These agents should be given in consultation with a neurosurgeon, and in cases where a child shows evidence of increased intracranial pressure (hypertension, bradycardia, worsening of mental status), osmotic agents may be life-saving. These agents, though, are only temporizing, and definitive care is surgical. There is further discussion of these topics in Chapter 10, Case 3.

- *Disposition*: The majority of pediatric patients presenting to the ED can be safely discharged home. Any patient identified as an intermediate risk, who is not undergoing imaging, should be observed in the ED for several hours and reassessed throughout that period and prior to discharge. All patients and their parents should be given detailed return instructions for repetitive vomiting, worsening pain, or alterations in mental status. It is also critical to educate patients and families on injury prevention, focusing on the inciting event. In particular, seatbelt and helmet safety should be addressed.

For patients diagnosed with a concussion, the current evidence supports a limited period of rest (1–2 days) with stepwise return to activity.[6] Due to the developing arena of concussion management and the potential for long-term monitoring, the patient should be referred to a physician specially trained in this area, such as a sports medicine physician.

Historical clues	Physical findings	Ancillary studies
• High-risk mechanism • Loss of consciousness	• Altered mental status/GCS • Palpable skull fracture	• Child warrants CT

Follow-Up

The child underwent CT scanning and, due to dural violation, had operative elevation of his depressed skull fracture. He was hospitalized for 10 days and then transferred to a rehabilitation center, where he has recovered with no deficits.

References

1. Marin JR, Weaver MD, Yealy DM, et al. Trends in visits for traumatic brain injury to emergency departments in the United States. *JAMA* 2014; 311: 1917–19.

2. Centers for Disease Control and Prevention, Traumatic brain injury & concussion. See http://www.cdc.gov/traumaticbraininjury/data/ (accessed June 22, 2016).

3. Rabiner JE, Friedman LM, Khine H, et al. Accuracy of point-of-care ultrasound for diagnosis of skull fractures in children. *Pediatrics* 2013; 131: e1757–64.

4. Easter JS, Bakes K, Dhaliwal J, et al. Comparison of PECARN, CATCH, and CHALICE rules for children with minor head injury: A prospective cohort study. *Ann Emerg Med* 2014; 64: 145–52.

5. Kuppermann N, Holmes JF, Dayan PS, et al. Identification of children at very low risk of clinically-important brain injuries after head trauma: A prospective cohort study. *Lancet* 2009; 374: 1160–70.

6. Thomas DG, Apps JN, Hoffman RG, et al. Benefits of strict rest after acute concussion: A randomized controlled trial. *Pediatrics* 2015; 135: 213–23.

Case 3

Contributing Author: Donald Jeanmonod

History

A 4-year-old female presents to the trauma bay via EMS. She was the restrained passenger-side rear-seat passenger in a booster seat in a car involved in a multicar accident on the interstate at highway speeds. There was a fatality within her vehicle. It is unknown if she had loss of consciousness. EMS immobilized the child on a pediatric immobilization board and initiated IV access. Their primary survey has identified a significant scalp laceration, whose bleeding they have attempted to control with direct pressure, and an obviously deformed right femur. The child was administered 1 µg/kg of fentanyl pre-hospital.

Past Medical History

• Unknown.

Medications

• Unknown.

Allergies

• Unknown.

Physical Examination and Ancillary Studies

• *Vital signs*: T 97 °F, HR 146, RR 32, BP 96/54, O$_2$ sat 94% on room air.
• *Primary survey*:
  · *Airway*: The child is somnolent and there is blood noted at the oropharynx.
  · *Breathing*: Respirations are sonorous but present bilaterally.
  · *Circulation*: The child is tachycardic and has intact distal pulses in four extremities.
  · *Disability*: GCS is 9 (eyes = 2, speech = 3, motor = 4), and the child seems to respond to pain in all four extremities.
  · *Exposure*: Right-femur deformity, 12-cm scalp wound with venous oozing, bruising to abdomen.
• *Secondary survey*:
  · *HEENT*: 12-cm full-thickness laceration to the right parietal-occipital area with venous oozing. The skull beneath appears to be intact. No hemotympanum. Eyes open to pain. Pupils 4 mm and reactive bilaterally. Blood noted within oropharynx from an unknown source.
  · *Neck*: Neck is immobilized in a c-collar. Trachea is midline, without subcutaneous emphysema appreciated.
  · *Chest*: Clavicles intact, but ecchymosis noted over the right shoulder. Lungs are rhonchorous bilaterally. Chest wall is stable without subcutaneous emphysema.
  · *Heart*: Tachycardic and regular.
  · *Abdomen*: Non-distended and soft, without apparent tenderness. There is an ecchymosis over the lower abdomen.
  · *Pelvis*: Stable to rock and compression. No perineal hematoma.
  · *Extremities*: There is deformity of the right femur with moderate thigh hematoma. The

remainder of the extremities are unremarkable. Back is without step-offs.

· *Neurologic*: GCS is 9 and the child withdraws all four extremities to painful stimuli.

Questions for Thought

- What are the appropriate steps in the initial stabilization of this child?
- In evaluating this child for traumatic injury, what are the appropriate imaging studies to obtain and why? Are there risks to obtaining these studies?
- If the child has negative imaging studies but remains obtunded, can the c-collar be removed?

Diagnosis

C-spine dislocation, femur fracture, cerebral contusion.

Discussion

- *Epidemiology*: Spinal injury in children is relatively rare. In 2009, the estimated incidence of spinal injury of all kinds was 170 per 1 million population less than 21 years of age and the incidence of spinal cord injury was 24 per 1 million population.[1] In the very youngest of patients (0–2 years) the majority of injuries are to the c-spine, while older children more commonly injure the lumbar spine. C-spine injuries are relatively rare in children, occurring in less than 1 percent of children who were imaged for injury in the NEXUS study[2] and in less than 2 percent of seriously injured children in trauma databases.[3] The mortality rate for children with c-spine injury has been reported to be between 13 percent and 28 percent, likely reflecting the association with head injury, rather than significant mortality from the spine injuries.[4]

  Most commonly, injuries are simple fractures without spinal cord involvement. However, because of the anatomic differences noted below, dislocations of the pediatric spine are also relatively common, accounting for approximately 15–25 percent of injuries in patients less than 12 years of age.[1] As well, because of the relatively increased flexibility of the pediatric spine, spinal cord injury without radiographic abnormality (SCIWORA) is responsible for approximately 5–20 percent of injuries in those less than 21 years of age, being increasingly common with decreasing age. Luckily, spinal cord injury is fairly uncommon, representing 5–7 percent of all injuries. The majority of pediatric c-spine injuries are the result of motor vehicle accidents, followed by falls.

- *Pathophysiology*: There are a number of anatomic features of the pediatric c-spine that result in unique injury patterns. To start, the pediatric head is relatively large compared to body size, and the neck musculature is proportionally underdeveloped, potentially causing greater force of motion. In younger children, the incompletely ossified c-spine is characterized by horizontally oriented facets and intervertebral joints, anterior vertebral body wedging, and ligamentous laxity, allowing for significant flexion motion of the c-spine and a propensity to dislocate. The spinal cord, however, is relatively anchored by the brachial plexus, so while the pediatric c-spine can move up to 2 inches, the spinal cord can be significantly damaged with as little as 1 cm of movement,[4,5] putting it at risk to be pinched or crushed, resulting in higher rates of SCIWORA in children. Younger pediatric patients are more likely to have higher c-spine injuries, from the base of the skull to C4, but because the developing spine reaches adult proportions by age 10, after this age, c-spine mechanics and injury patterns mirror adults.[6] Several congenital abnormalities in children, including Down's syndrome, juvenile rheumatoid arthritis, Morquio syndrome, and Grisel syndrome, predispose to increased ligamentous laxity and increased rates of injury.

- *Presentation*: As with any trauma patient, the systematic examination will help to identify any potentially life-threatening injury first, and then any injury that will potentially cause significant morbidity. Although we believe that appropriate immobilization is important to prevent progression of injury in unstable fractures and ligamentous disruptions, the data supporting these assumptions are scarce. Furthermore, because of the wide variety of sizes in children, c-spine immobilization in a hard collar can be difficult. That said, during the primary and secondary survey, spinal precautions should be maintained while rolling the child. If a child is immobilized in a c-collar, it is important to have a bolster behind the shoulders to compensate for the relatively large occiput in children, which will tend to cause neck flexion if not supported.

After the primary assessment with the ABC algorithm, assessment of mental status should be obtained. Multiple studies have demonstrated that the presence of altered mental status both precludes the ability to be able to adequately clear a c-spine, as well as potentially increases the probability that there is a fracture, because significant head injury is a well-established risk for significant neck injury. Additionally, the disability portion of the primary assessment should be able to identify if the child is moving all four extremities, identifying patients with paraplegia or quadriplegia from significant c-spine spinal cord injuries.

The secondary survey then proceeds from head to toe. Injuries to the head and face should be noted, as these are often associated with cervical injury. The significant findings pertaining to the neck include neck tenderness and the presence of injuries which might distract the

Table 2.3 NEXUS low risk criteria[7]

- Normal mentation
- No neurologic deficit
- Non-tender neck
- No distracting injury
- No alcohol intoxication

patient from appreciating significant neck tenderness. The presence and absence of ecchymosis, the presence of neck hematomas, and the position of the trachea and airway should be noted. Additionally, a detailed neurologic examination, including strength and sensation, can help to illicit any neurologic abnormalities which may be attributable to an injured c-spine.

- *Diagnosis*: In order to balance the very low risks of missing a significantly disabling condition with the risks of medical radiation-induced cancer from over-testing, a number of investigators have sought to produce c-spine clearance rules. The NEXUS criteria[7] (Table 2.3) and the Canadian C-spine Rule[8] (Figure 2.2) are large multicenter

Figure 2.2 Canadian c-spine Rule.

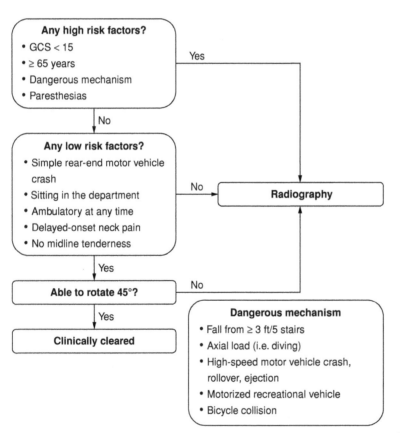

studies of adults and children that were prospectively derived and validated and demonstrate very good sensitivities (99.0 percent [95% CI 98.0–99.6%] and 100 percent sensitivity [95% CI 98–100%], respectively)[7,8] for identifying clinically significant injuries in a predominantly adult population. One of the criticisms of applying these rules in the pediatric population has been the low numbers of children with significant injuries from which to derive and validate their decision points. Nine percent ($n =$ 3,065) of the NEXUS cohort were aged less than 18, including only 88 children who were less than 2 years of age.[1] Of the NEXUS cohort of adolescents and children, there were only 30 injuries in the 3,065 included patients. Although in the pediatric subset the NEXUS criteria demonstrated an excellent sensitivity of 100 percent, the relatively small number of injuries resulted in the lower limit of the 95% CI of 87.8%.[2] A case-matched cohort study where the NEXUS criteria and the Canadian C-spine Rule were retrospectively applied to a cohort that was imaged and a cohort that was not imaged found that neither rule had adequate sensitivity, but was limited both in study design and the low numbers of clinically important injuries.[9] A similar retrospective application of NEXUS criteria to a cohort of imaged injured (all had fractures and/or ligamentous injuries) pediatric trauma patients revealed 100 percent sensitivity in the detection of fracture in 158 patients older than age 8, but only a 94 percent sensitivity in those under age 8. The American Association of Neurosurgical Surgeons have endorsed the use of NEXUS criteria in children above 9 years of age, and likely it is applicable in any communicative child when there is a low likelihood of ligamentous disruption in the proximal spine.

Several investigators have sought to clarify the appropriate way to evaluate the c-spine in younger children. The PECARN collaboration performed a retrospective case–control study which identified eight variables (Table 2.4) associated with increased risk of cervical injury in children under 16 years of age. Comparing their cohort of 540 patients with injuries with 1,060 matched controls, they found that the presence of any one of the eight criteria had a sensitivity of 98 percent (95% CI 96–99%) for any injury and 98 percent

Table 2.4 PECARN model[10]

- Altered mental status
- Focal neurologic findings
- Complaint of neck pain
- Torticollis
- Substantial torso injury
- Predisposing conditions
- Diving
- High-risk motor vehicle crash

(95% CI 95% to >99%) for any injury requiring neurosurgical intervention.[10]

Using the protocol outlined in Figure 2.3, Anderson et al.[11] prospectively evaluated 575 children aged 0–3 who were trauma activations in a level 1 trauma center, identifying 19 ligamentous injuries, 9 fractures, with 4 patients requiring stabilization. Although the protocol required plain X-ray in 100 percent of patients, there were no missed injuries in this cohort.

Although CT is more sensitive for the identification of c-spine injury, plain radiography remains the imaging modality of choice in children to minimize radiation exposure. Because children usually are not obese and do not have degenerative spine disease, plain films may be easier to interpret. The reported sensitivity of a single-view, lateral neck X-ray is 74 percent and may be higher in children older than age 8, with a reported sensitivity of 93 percent.[4] Open-mouth odontoid views may improve the ability to recognize burst fractures of C1, but are very difficult to obtain in the smallest of children. Flexion–extension views and oblique views are not routinely recommended.

Evaluation of plain radiographs in pediatric patients can be challenging due to anatomic differences in the c-spine. The most common variant seen on plain radiographs is pseudosubluxation of C2 on C3, and sometimes of C3 on C4. To differentiate pseudosubluxation from real subluxation, one should draw a line through the anterior portion of the posterior arch from C1 to C3 (Swischuk's line). In physiologic pseudosubluxation, the line should be within 1 mm of the posterior arch. A distance of ≥ 1.5 mm is concerning for true injury. In children under 8 years of age, the atlanto-dens interval (the space between the anterior portion of the dens to the posterior aspect of the anterior ring of the atlas)

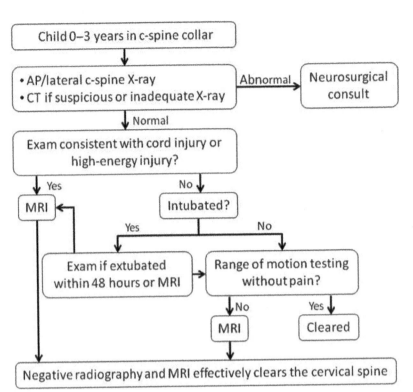

Figure 2.3 Algorithm for clearing the cervical spine in children ≤ 3 years of age.

may be up to 5 mm as opposed to 3 mm seen in older children and adults. Finally, wedging of the anterior portion of the vertebral body is common in children as the vertebral body changes shape from a more oval appearance to the classic rectangular appearance of the developed spine.[5]

When patients have severe mechanism of injury, significant head injury, or continued pain despite normal radiographs, CT can be obtained. In the youngest of patients, some recommend only scanning from the base of the skull to C3, to evaluate the areas most commonly injured.[4]

Whenever possible, it is imperative to decrease radiation exposure from unnecessary imaging. The incidence of thyroid cancer has doubled since 1985, and is not thought to be just the result of increased diagnostic yield.[12] The baseline prevalence of thyroid cancer is 5.2 in 100,000 males and 15.2 in 100,000 females and the theoretical excess relative risk of developing thyroid malignancy after plain radiographs is 0.24 percent for males and 0.51 percent for females, resulting in an absolute risk of 5.21 in 100,000 for males and 15.3 in 100,000 for females. Because

of the increased radiation exposure with CT, the risk to the thyroid is increased with a theoretical excess risk of CT of 13 percent for males and 25 percent for females. This results in an absolute risk of 5.87 in 100,000 in males and 19 in 100,000 in females.

SCIWORA is the term used to describe an acute spinal cord injury that results in sensory and/or motor deficits without radiographic abnormalities being present on plain radiographs or CT scans. SCIWORA is more common in younger children, representing as much as 20 percent of the spinal injuries in these patients. The patterns of neurologic presentation can vary and depend on which portion of the cord is injured but may include partial cord syndrome (55 percent), complete cord syndrome (27 percent), central cord syndrome, (10 percent), Brown–Sequard syndrome (5 percent), and anterior cord syndrome (3 percent).[13] If SCIWORA is suspected, the patient should undergo further imaging with an MRI while maintaining adequate cervical immobilization. Most SCIWORA will spontaneously resolve with 8 to 12 weeks of cervical immobilization.

- *Treatment*: Once an injury is identified, it is important to maintain spinal immobilization. Consultation with the appropriate specialist and transfer to a pediatric tertiary care facility with specialization in the management of pediatric cervical injuries is important to deliver the appropriate continued care for these patients. In patients with significant paralysis, continual reassessment of breathing mechanics is essential to identify possible hypoventilation. Likewise, in patients with high-up cervical injuries, loss of vascular tone may lead to neurogenic shock with associated hypotension, which requires treatment with fluid resuscitation and appropriate weight-based vasopressors like norepinephrine. Although once recommended for spinal cord injury, the most recent guidelines from the American Academy of Neurological Surgeons advise *against* use of methylprednisolone for spinal cord injury.[14]

  Although the c-spine remains the most commonly injured structure in the pediatric neck, one needs to consider injury to other structures including superior tracheal injuries and blunt vascular injuries to the carotid arteries in children who have had direct trauma to the neck from a clothes lining mechanism or inappropriately positioned shoulder portion of a seatbelt.

  Airway injury may be suggested by change in voice or significant respiratory distress. On examination, the patient may present with blood in the airway, noisy breathing, deviated trachea, or subcutaneous air in the anterior neck. In a patient with suspected airway injury or signs of significant distress, endotracheal intubation should be performed by the most experienced provider using either direct laryngoscopy or video-assisted laryngoscopy.

  Vascular injuries to the pediatric neck are exceedingly rare with a reported incidence of 0.035 percent in 57,659 pediatric blunt trauma patients. There is limited experience with CTA of the neck in pediatric patients, but the reported sensitivity of CTA is 100 percent for penetrating trauma to the neck and 50 percent for blunt trauma.[15]

- *Disposition*: Children with c-spine or cord injury should be admitted to a PICU with neurosurgery consultation.

Historical clues	Physical findings
- High-speed trauma - Death in vehicle - Cannot be cleared by NEXUS or PECARN	- Traumatic injury to head - Bruising to shoulder - Altered mental status/GCS - Cannot be cleared by NEXUS or PECARN

Follow-Up

Because of concerns of potential airway compromise given the blood at the oropharynx and the sonorous respirations, the child was intubated using video-assisted laryngoscopy and rapid sequence intubation. The child underwent trauma-bay evaluation with a CXR that demonstrated aspiration versus contusion in the right lung and a FAST examination that was negative. With IV fluid and pain medication, the post-intubation HR improved to 128.

The child underwent CT imaging of the head, neck, abdomen, and pelvis, which demonstrated a small right parietal cerebral contusion and atlanto-occipital dislocation. The abdomen and pelvis were uninjured. The child was admitted to the PICU where she was seen in consultation by neurosurgery and treated with a halo-vest. Her femur was operatively repaired.

References

1. Piatt JH. Pediatric spinal injury in the US: Epidemiology and disparities. *J Neurosurg Pediatr* 2015; 16: 463–71.

2. Viccellio P, Simon H, Pressman BD, et al. A prospective multicenter study of cervical spine injury in children. *Pediatrics* 2001; 108: E20.

3. Pieretti-Vanmarcke R, Velmahos GC, Nance ML, et al. Clinical clearance of the cervical spine in blunt trauma patients younger than 3 years: A multi-center study of the American Association for the Surgery of Trauma. *J Trauma* 2009; 67: 543–9.

4. Tat ST, Mejia MJ, Freishtat RJ. Imaging, clearance, and controversies in pediatric cervical spine trauma. *Pediatr Emer Care* 2014; 30: 911–18.

5. Jones TM, Anderson PA, Noonan KJ. Pediatric cervical spine trauma. *J Am Acad Orthop Surg* 2011; 19: 600–11.

6. Lustrin ES, Karakas SP, Ortiz AO, et al. Pediatric cervical spine: Normal anatomy, variants, and trauma. *Radiographics* 2003; 23: 539–60.

7. Hoffman JR, Mower WR, Wolfson AB, et al. Validity of a set of clinical criteria to rule out injury to the cervical spine in patients with blunt trauma. National Emergency X-Radiography Utilization Study Group. *N Engl J Med* 2000; 343: 94–9.

8. Stiell IG, Wells GA, Vandemheen KL, et al. The Canadian c-spine rule for radiography in alert and stable trauma patients. *JAMA* 2001; 286: 1841–8.

9. Ehrlich PF, Wee C, Drongowski R, et al. Canadian C-spine Rule and the National Emergency X-Radiography Utilization Low-Risk Criteria for c-spine radiography in young trauma patients. *J Pediatr Surg* 2009; 44: 987–91.

10. Leonard JC, Jaffe DM, Olsen CS, et al. Age-related differences in factors associated with cervical spine injuries in children. *Acad Emerg Med* 2015; 22: 441–6.

11. Anderson RC, Kan P, Vanaman M, et al. Utility of cervical spine clearance protocol after trauma in children between 0 and 3 years of age. *J Neurosurg Pediatr* 2010; 5: 292–6.

12. Muchow RD, Egan KR, Peppler WW, et al. Theoretical increase of thyroid cancer induction from cervical spine multidetector computed tomography in pediatric trauma patients. *J Trauma Acute Care Surg* 2012; 72: 403–9.

13. Kreykes NS, Letton RW Jr. Current issues in the diagnosis of pediatric cervical spine injury. *Semin Pediatr Surg* 2010; 19: 257–64.

14. Hurlbert RJ, Hadley MN, Walters BC, et al. Pharmacological therapy for acute spinal cord injury. *Neurosurgery* 2015; 76 Suppl 1: S71–83.

15. Hogan AR, Lineen EB, Perez EA, et al. Value of computed tomographic angiography in neck and extremity pediatric vascular trauma. *J Pediatr Surg* 2009; 44: 1236–41.

Case 4

Contributing Authors: Denis R. Pauzé and William H. Hauda

History

A 4-month-old male is brought in by his grandmother for redness of both eyes. The grandmother describes several weeks of cough and nasal congestion along with periodic breathing. There have been intermittent low-grade fevers. The infant was seen by his PCP several times during this period, as well as having a prior ED visit for these cold symptoms where he was diagnosed with a URI. The patient's mother also notes that her son's "chest makes popping sounds" over the past few weeks. Mother and grandmother both deny falls, trauma, or sick contacts.

The child has had a couple of episodes of vomiting in the past, but not recently. There has been no diarrhea or rash. The infant has been eating with good urine output. There is occasional labored breathing and cough. No reported seizures, cyanosis, or feeding difficulties.

Past Medical History

- Significant for prematurity at 35 weeks; spent 2 days in the NICU for jaundice with phototherapy treatment.

Medications

- None.

Allergies

- None.

Physical Examination and Ancillary Studies

- *Vital signs*: T 99.6 °F, HR 179, RR 48, O_2 sat 94% on room air, weight 5.3 kg.
- *General*: Infant is non-toxic and in no acute distress. Occasional crying that is consolable.
- *HEENT*: No evidence of head trauma. No facial bruising or scalp hematoma. PERRL. Right sclera has small lateral subconjunctival hemorrhage. Unable to perform adequate funduscopic examination. Oropharynx moist and normal. No lesions or signs of oral trauma.
- *Cardiovascular*: Tachycardic. S1, S2. No S3. Strong and equal distal pulses. Good capillary refill.
- *Lungs*: Decreased breath sound bilateral. Bilateral rhonchi. Otherwise good air movement. No labored breathing or accessory muscle use.
- *Abdomen*: Soft and non-distended. No hepatomegaly. No masses.
- *Skin*: Bruising on the posterior aspect of right shoulder, significant for three circular reddish and purple areas approximately 2×2 cm each, and a linear progression along the right posterior shoulder.
- *Neurologic*: Awake and alert. Interactive. Moves all four extremities. Good tone.
- *Pertinent laboratory values*: WBC 27,300, Hb 9.5, chemistry unremarkable other than AST 106 and ALT 154.
- *Pertinent radiologic studies*: CXR with scattered interstitial infiltrates and clavicle fracture. CT chest with rib fractures (Figure 2.4).

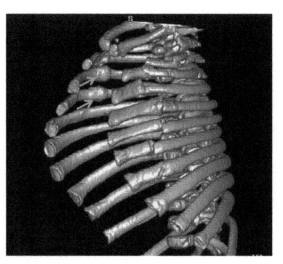

Figure 2.4 CT chest reconstruction: Lateral view showing multiple rib fractures. For the color version, please refer to the plate section.

Questions for Thought

- Does this infant need brain imaging? Which modality would be appropriate?
- Does this child need abdominal imaging? Which modality would be appropriate?
- Why do you think this infant was seen multiple times before a diagnosis was made?
- What are the risk factors for this diagnosis?
- What are some "red flags" in your history and physical examination for this diagnosis?

Diagnosis

- Non-accidental trauma.

Discussion

- *Epidemiology*: According to the National Child Abuse and Neglect Data System, over 1,500 children died in 2013 from child abuse in the USA.[1] Nearly three-quarters of these pediatric fatalities were children of 3 years of age and younger, and nearly half were less than 1 year of age.[1] This equates to four children dying every day from abuse. Not every case of non-accidental-injury-related death is diagnosed or reported, especially in cases of asphyxia or smothering deaths, so these statistics likely under-represent the extent of the problem. Abusive head trauma is the most common cause of child abuse death. According to childwelfare.gov, in 2013 parents were responsible for nearly 80 percent of child abuse fatalities.[2] Only 17 percent of fatalities were from non-parents, and in approximately 4 percent of the cases, the perpetrator was unknown.[2] There are many more children who suffer non-fatal injury every day, and up to one-third of patients with abusive head trauma are misdiagnosed at their first visit to a healthcare provider.[3]

- *Presentation*: Non-accidental trauma and abusive head trauma have many different presentations due to the severity and organs injured. Some presentations are dramatic – seizures, lethargy, respiratory distress, or apnea. These dramatic presentations are recognized by parents and cause parents to seek medical care, but may not be recognized as being caused by non-accidental injury. As a result, these symptoms often are ascribed to other medical conditions such as reflux disease, BRUE, gastroenteritis, or respiratory infections.[4,5] However, some infants with non-accidental trauma may present with common and non-specific symptoms. They often arrive looking well and in no acute distress. They may come in with a common complaint, such as vomiting, ear infection, fever, or URI. Their examination may be normal if done quickly, but a careful and detailed examination may identify seemingly minor findings which herald the presence of abuse, such as a bruise, subconjunctival hemorrhage, nosebleed, or petechiae. They may appear neurologically well, even if suffering from abusive head trauma.[3]

- *Diagnosis*: A high index of suspicion is paramount to diagnosing many cases of non-accidental trauma. The younger the age, the harder it can be to make a diagnosis. The history may be fabricated or deliberately misleading. The caregiver presenting with the child may have no knowledge of injuries caused by someone else, such as another family member or a daycare provider. Failure to diagnose non-accidental trauma allows the child to return to their dangerous environment, and repeated abuse will likely occur.[3] A detailed and thorough history and physical examination are crucial to look for red flags. Historical red flags include inconsistencies in the described mechanism and the physical findings, injuries that do not fit with the developmental stage of the child (for instance, when a child has been said to have rolled off a bed, but examination reveals that the child is developmentally unable to roll), delay to presentation for injuries, or history of repeated visits for injuries.

Red flags on physical examination include bruises on non-ambulatory children ("if you don't cruise, you don't bruise"), bruises in areas not typical for ambulatory trauma (for instance, buttock bruises or bruises to the back of legs), mouth injuries including dental injuries or frenulum tears, retinal hemorrhages, bony deformity, apnea, seizures, altered mental status, or epistaxis in children prior to fine motor control.[6,7] The physical examination can be non-specific or even normal in cases of non-accidental trauma.

Helpful diagnostic tools include neuroimaging (CT or MRI) with CT usually being done first in the ED. Evaluation for retinal hemorrhages and skeletal survey are typically part of an inpatient evaluation, but can be accomplished in the ED at times. For patients undergoing an LP, xanthochromia or fresh red blood cells may be discovered, signifying abusive head trauma. In cases of concern for abdominal trauma, CT is appropriate in the ED. Although it is important to be conscious of the untoward effects of excessive radiation exposure in infants, the risk of missed injury in an abused child is far greater than the risk of CT scanning. Unfortunately, there are no current biomarkers for abuse, although biomarkers for traumatic brain injury are being studied.

- *Treatment*: Treatment of these children varies depending upon the injuries discovered. In all cases, the provider should manage the patient's physical discomfort and ensure the child's safety.
- *Disposition*: Infants with suspected non-accidental trauma should be admitted to the hospital for both safety planning and for further diagnostic evaluation. Further studies, such as brain imaging by MRI, funduscopic evaluation by ophthalmology, and skeletal survey should be performed. CPS, social workers, and law enforcement should be involved. The infant will typically be admitted to the hospital until he or she is stabilized and a safe discharge environment is confirmed. Some children can be discharged from the ED safely if CPS is involved and

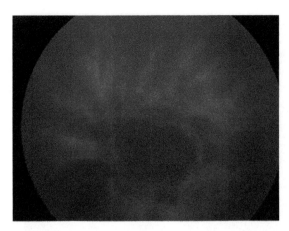

Figure 2.5 Retinal hemorrhages. For the color version, please refer to the plate section.

follow-up with a child abuse physician and CPS can be arranged.

Historical clues	Physical findings	Ancillary studies
• Numerous prior visits • Convoluted and confusing medical history	• Bruising to shoulder • Subconjunctival hemorrhage	• Elevated LFTs suggesting abdominal injury • Anemia suggesting blood loss • CXR with rib fractures

Follow-Up

The infant was admitted to the PICU after CT was performed demonstrating subdural hemorrhage. Pediatric ophthalmology assessed the child and found bilateral multilayered extensive retinal hemorrhages (Figure 2.5). Abdominal CT revealed a grade II liver laceration. A skeletal survey was performed and showed the above-mentioned chest trauma as well as metaphyseal corner fractures of the left tibia and fibula. Shortly after admission, the infant had neurologic deterioration, requiring tracheal intubation and neurosurgical evacuation of the subdural hematoma. Social workers, CPS, and the police were involved. The child was eventually discharged into foster family care.

References

1. The Children's Bureau. The National Child Abuse and Neglect Data System (NCANDS). See www.acf.hhs .gov/cb/research-data-technology/reporting-systems/ ncands (accessed November 2016).

2. The Children's Bureau. Child Abuse and Neglect Fatalities 2015: Statistics and Interventions. See www .childwelfare.gov/pubPDFs/fatality.pdf (accessed November 2016).

3. Jenny C, Hymel KP, Ritzen A, Reinert SE, Hay TC. Analysis of missed cases of abusive head trauma. *JAMA* 1999; 281: 621–6.

4. Guenther E, Powers A, Srivastava R, Bankowsky JL Abusive head trauma in children presenting with an apparent life-threatening event. *J Pediatr* 2010; 157: 821–5.

5. Altman R, Brand D, Forman S, et al. Abusive head injury as a cause of apparent life-threatening events in infancy. *Arch Pediatr Adolesc Med* 2003; 157: 1011–15.

6. Sugar NF, Taylor JA, Feldman KW. Bruises in infants and toddlers: Those who don't cruise rarely bruise. *Arch Pediatr Adolesc Med* 1999; 153: 399–403.

7. McIntosh N, Mok JY, Margerison A. Epidemiology of oronasal hemorrhage in the first 2 years of life: Implications for child protection. *Pediatrics* 2007; 120: 1074–8.

Case 5

Contributing Authors: John Tran and Rebecca Jeanmonod

History

The patient is a 4-year-old girl who is brought in to the ED by ambulance after being rescued from a burning house. While she was trying to escape from her room, her nightgown caught on fire, but was put out by one of the firefighters. En route, EMS state she was sleepy and confused. Her parents were able to escape without any significant injury. The patient arrives to the ED complaining of pain to her torso and limbs as well as difficulty breathing. She has received fentanyl for pain from EMS en route.

Past Medical History

- The child had a normal uneventful birth history and is fully immunized.

Medications

- None.

Allergies

- None.

Physical Examination and Ancillary Studies

- *Vital signs*: HR 125, BP 105/70, RR 55, O_2 sat 95% on 2 L nasal cannula, T 99.5 °F, 20 kg.
- *General*: The patient is drowsy. She opens her eyes to her name and follows commands, moving all extremities.
- *Primary survey*:
  - *Airway*: Patent airway, soot in and around the mouth, no pooling secretions.
  - *Breathing*: Rapid shallow respirations, with minimal chest-wall excursion, O_2 sat 88%, corrects to 95% with 2 L nasal cannula.
  - *Circulation*: Tachycardic, strong central and peripheral pulses.
  - *Disability*: GCS 13 (eyes = 3, verbal = 4, motor = 6), moves all four extremities.
  - *Exposure*: The child is completely exposed, revealing numerous burns. She is placed on a sterile sheet.
- *Secondary survey*:
  - *HEENT*: Cranial nerves are intact, PERRL. The child has dry mucous membranes with soot in and around her mouth. No eye involvement.
  - *Neck*: Non-tender with no signs of trauma. Trachea midline, no JVD.
  - *Cardiovascular*: Tachycardic and regular, with normal heart sounds, good pulses, and capillary refill throughout.
  - *Lungs/Chest*: Anterior chest wall with cutaneous burns. No stridor. Lungs sound clear, but with shallow rapid breaths.
  - *Abdomen*: There are cutaneous burns involving the superior region of the abdomen. The abdomen is mildly tender diffusely, with no peritoneal signs or distention. Bowel sounds are normal.
  - *Extremities*: No deformity, moves spontaneously.
  - *Skin*: There are burns involving the front of the patient's neck, her upper chest, upper back, bilateral shoulders, and right upper arm. All burn areas are erythematous, with bullous blisters both intact and unroofed. There is a small area at the sternum with a pale appearance that is non-blanching. The total burn surface area (TBSA) is approximately 22 percent.

- *Neurologic*: GCS 13, follows commands, no lateralizing findings.
- *Back and pelvis*: Non-tender, no step-offs, pelvis stable to rock and compression.
- *Pertinent laboratory values*: CBC, electrolytes, renal function, and U/A are unremarkable.
- *Radiographs*: Normal CXR.

Questions for Thought

- When is it necessary to intervene in the airway of a burn victim?
- How do you choose the volume of resuscitative fluids to deliver? How do you monitor its adequacy?
- What is the appropriate way to care for burn wounds?
- When is it necessary to transfer a patient to a burn center?

Diagnosis

- Superficial partial-thickness, deep partial-thickness, and full-thickness burns involving greater than 20 percent of the TBSA.

Discussion

- *Epidemiology*: Approximately two million burn injuries occur annually in the USA, with half of these in children.[1] Although most burns are minor, each year, 50,000 burns require admission to the hospital. There are 2,500 pediatric deaths attributable to burns annually.[1,2] Children have worse outcomes, morbidity, and mortality compared to adults with similar burns.[1] This may be due to physiologic differences, such as thinner skin, difficult vascular access, less margin for error in fluid management, and greater hesitancy for burn surgeries.

  Scald burns are more common in children younger than 5 years of age, and flame burns are usually seen in older children.[2] Most burns occur at home. Non-accidental trauma should be considered in all cases of pediatric burns, but most burns are accidental. The provider should suspect child abuse in the setting of bilateral, symmetric burn patterns, injuries to the dorsum of the hand, and burns presenting in a delayed fashion.[1,3]

- *Pathophysiology*: Depending on their depth, cutaneous burns can disrupt the function of the epidermis (whose primary function is to protect against water loss and bacterial invasion) and dermis (whose primary function is temperature regulation).[3,4] Cell damage occurs at temperatures higher than 113 °F, with the temperature, as well as time of exposure, ultimately dictating the degree of damage. In addition to local damage, extensive cutaneous burns can lead to electrolyte abnormalities, increased systemic vascular resistance, metabolic acidosis, increased blood viscosity, and depressed cardiac function.[3]

  Burns are classified as *superficial*, *superficial partial-thickness*, *deep partial-thickness*, and *full-thickness* burns. Superficial burns involve only the epidermal layer. Skin is red, painful, and tender, but without blisters, similar to a sunburn. Superficial partial-thickness burns involve the epidermis and superficial dermis. Skin is painful and has blisters with a moist/erythematous base. Both superficial and superficial partial-thickness burns typically heal without scarring, and are treated with resuscitation and pain control. These are *medically managed*.

  Deep partial-thickness burns involve the deep dermis, with resulting damage to hair follicles, sweat and sebaceous glands, and nerves. Blisters may form, and the dermis is pale white to yellow without blanching, and with absent pain sensation. Full-thickness burns involve the entire dermal layer and may involve deeper structures (such as fat, muscle, and bone), with charred skin that is pale, painless, and leathery. Both deep partial-thickness and full-thickness burns often require *surgical intervention*.

  Systemic derangement occurs with superficial partial-thickness or deeper burns involving greater than 15 percent of the TBSA. There can be cardiovascular collapse, termed "burn shock," which occurs from fluid loss, increased capillary permeability, and vasodilation. This leads to decreased cardiac output and, without adequate fluid resuscitation, it will continue to decline. Renal function may deteriorate from vasoconstriction of the renal arteries. Metabolism is increased in burn patients, up to 150–200 percent of the normal rate. This can lead to a decrease in body weight, a negative nitrogen balance, and a decrease in energy stores.

- *Presentation*: In addition to the obvious injuries evident in burn patients, the emergency provider should consider the possibility of blunt trauma related to the burn. Some patients may have jumped from a height to escape, and sometimes there is a component of the burn injury that involves blast trauma, for instance from an exploding gas can, which causes the patient to be thrown or struck by flying objects. Therefore, the provider should be cognizant of the possibility of occult blunt and penetrating traumatic injury associated with the burn.

Additionally, the patient may present with altered mental status or respiratory compromise. Some patients are intoxicated before the burn injury takes place, but the provider should also consider the possibility of inhalational intoxicants/poisons, such as carbon monoxide and cyanide, which occur not uncommonly in burn victims in enclosed spaces. If the patient is known to have come in from an enclosed fire, a carbon monoxide level should be checked. If the patient has an unexplained lactic acidosis, the provider should consider the possibility of cyanide exposure, as well, and could consider initiating treatment.

- *Treatment*: It is important to evaluate the patient's ABCs and remove any clothing or potential sources of heat. If there is a chemical burn, decontamination should be performed immediately. If the patient appears to have airway involvement from the burn injury, such as stridorous breathing, burns involving the oral cavity, or circumferential burns of the neck, it is important to secure the airway sooner rather than later, as later swelling may preclude orotracheal intubation and require surgical airway. Continuous oxygen supplementation and monitoring is important, as well as carboxyhemoglobin levels, if appropriate. Because of fluid shifts in the burn victim, patients without airway burns may need to be intubated from ARDS, especially if the burn involves more than 30 percent of the TBSA.

IV or IO access is essential early in the initial assessment to begin fluid resuscitation. The provider should determine the depth and TBSA of the burn to guide fluid resuscitation. To calculate the TBSA in children who are close to adult size/age, the rule of 9s can be employed. For this rule, each leg counts as 18 percent, each arm counts for 9 percent, the anterior torso counts as

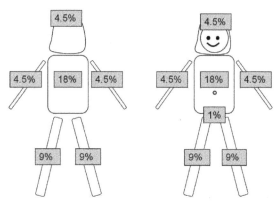

Figure 2.6 Rule of 9s for older children, depicting relative values for calculated TBSA involved in burn.

18 percent, the posterior as 18 percent, the head counts as 9 percent, and the genitalia count as 1 percent (Figure 2.6). This rule does not accurately represent the burn area in smaller children. For them, the most accurate method for TBSA burn determination is using a standardized commercial chart, such as Lund and Browder, to estimate burn area by age. If a chart is not available, a modified rule of 9s can be used (Figure 2.7). If there is greater than 15 percent TBSA burn, initial fluid resuscitation is guided by the Parkland formula (4 × TBSA burned × weight in kg). This estimates the fluid volume necessary for the first 24 hours after the burn. Half of this volume is given in the first 8 hours starting from the time of the burn, and the second half is given in the next 16 hours. This is only an approximation, and resuscitation should be titrated to adequate urine output of 1 mL/kg per hour. For infants younger than 1 year or less than 25 kg, maintenance fluids should be added to the initial 24-hour resuscitation.

Patients should have aggressive pain management, typically with narcotic analgesics. Cooling the patient and wet dressing applications must be avoided to prevent additional heat loss and vasoconstriction.

Laboratory work including electrolytes and renal function are useful to guide electrolyte replacement and resuscitation. CXR may demonstrate ARDS or inhalational injury. In electrical burns, EKG must be done. If there is concern for muscle damage or rhabdomyolysis, a myoglobin and creatine kinase level may help guide therapy.

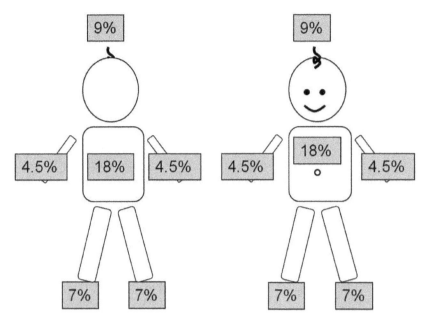

Figure 2.7 Modified rule of 9s for infants and toddlers. Subtract 1 percent from the head for each year of life over age 1 year, add 1 percent for both legs for each year of life over age 1 year.

In patients with circumferential burns, the provider should consider escharotomy to avoid compartment syndrome. This should be done in consultation with a surgeon to ensure the appropriate technique and to minimize risk.

- *Disposition*: Transfer criteria to a burn center include the following:
  - Greater than 20 percent partial-thickness burns in patients > 10 years old, and greater than 10 percent in patients < 10 years old;
  - Burns involving face, hands, feet, perineum, genitalia, major joints;
  - Circumferential burns;
  - Full-thickness burns;
  - Electrical burns and chemical burns;
  - Inhalational injury;
  - Preexisting significant comorbidities;
  - Suspected child abuse;

If a patient has minor burn wounds and does not meet the criteria for transfer to a burn center, the wound can be managed in the ED. This involves debridement of the burn wounds, after proper analgesia. This should be done with mild soap and water or dilute antiseptic solution. Scissors should be used to cut loose skin that is still attached to healthy skin. Intact blisters do not need debridement unless they overlie large joints. Topical antimicrobial should be lathered generously on the wounds. This includes bacitracin ointment or 1% silver sulfadiazine cream (except on the face). Synthetic occlusive dressings should be used to cover burned areas, followed by gauze dressings. Ideally, dressings should be changed twice a day. Some patients may require surgical intervention, which should be done at burn centers.

Discharged patients should be prescribed adequate analgesics and should follow up with a burn specialist. Antihistamines may be used for significant pruritis during the healing process. With appropriate care, most children with burns survive, even with extensive burns in smaller children.[5]

Historical clues	Physical findings
• Extricated from burning building	• Soot in mouth
	• Hypoxia and tachypnea
• Confused en route	• Burns on examination

Follow-Up

The child was intubated because of her relative hypoxia, dyspnea, tachypnea, and evidence of soot in her mouth. She was resuscitated with 1,600 mL lactated Ringer's over the next 24 hours (4 × 20 kg × 20 TBSA) and maintained adequate urinary output. Her carbon monoxide level was not significantly elevated. She had bronchoscopy, which revealed no lower-airway burns, and was ultimately extubated on hospital day 3. She has undergone skin grafting over her chest and right arm since, and has otherwise had an uneventful recovery.

References

1. Gonzalez R, Shanti C. Overview of current pediatric burn care. *Semin Pediatr Surg* 2015; 24: 47–9.

2. Kramer CB, Rivara FP, Klein MB. Variations in US pediatric burn injury hospitalization using the National Burn Repository Data. *J Burn Care Res* 2010; 31: 734–9.

3. Merz J, Schrand C, Mertens D, et al. Wound care of the pediatric burn patient. *AACN Clin Issues* 2003; 14: 429–41.

4. Reed J, Pomerantz W. Emergency management of pediatric burns. *Pediatr Emerg Care* 2005; 21: 118–29.

5. Sheridan R, Remensnyder J, Schnitzer J, et al. Current expectations for survival in pediatric burns. *Arch Pediatr Adolesc Med* 2000; 153: 245–9.

Case 6

Contributing Authors: Ryan Fulton and Melanie K. Prusakowski

History

A 2-year-old boy presents after his mother found him unconscious in the backyard swimming pool. The patient had been otherwise healthy prior to presentation. Upon EMS arrival, CPR was initiated and the patient was intubated in the field. The patient remained comatose with GCS 3 during transportation. Once the patient was attached to a monitor, asystole was discovered and CPR was continued. Initial vitals showed no discernible heart rate, hypotension, and hypothermia. Peripheral IV access was obtained and a bolus of lactated Ringer's (20 cc/kg) was administered. The patient had copious amounts of fluid suctioned from the ET tube during resuscitation efforts. Four minutes prior to arrival, following suctioning, appropriate oxygenation, and two doses of weight-based epinephrine, he had return of spontaneous circulation.

Past Medical History

- Seasonal allergies.

Medications

- Cetirizine.

Allergies

- None.

Physical Examination

- *Vital signs*: T 92 °F, HR 40, RR 5, BP 50/20, O_2 sat 80% on 100% oxygen.
- *General*: Unresponsive and intubated.
- *Primary survey*:
  - *Airway*: 4.0 uncuffed tube, 15 cm at the lip, airway confirmed with waveform capnography and auscultation. There is an air leak.
  - *Breathing*: Decreased breath sounds on the left versus the right, bilateral crackles with decreased air entry at bases.
  - *Circulation*: Bradycardia, poor capillary refill, cool extremities, thready pulses.
  - *Disability*: GCS 3.
  - *Exposure*: Wet clothing removed and patient fully exposed, no signs of trauma.

Resuscitative Measures

Based on the child's primary survey, further examination is deferred. The child's examination suggests that the ET tube is likely the wrong size, as the child has a large air leak. The examination also suggests that the tube may be placed too deeply, likely in the right mainstem bronchus. The child's bradycardia may be secondary to his hypoxia and hypothermia.

The child's ET tube is changed out for a 4.0-mm cuffed tube and a PEEP valve is attached. Consideration is given to placing an uncuffed 4.5-mm tube instead, but because of the anticipated high airway pressures, the provider recognizes that the cuff will provide a better seal for adequate PEEP. The tube is advanced to 13 cm. During this, the child is given IV 1:10,000 epinephrine at the dose recommended by the Broselow tape. The ET tube is confirmed by auscultation and waveform capnography. Rewarming is begun with heated air blankets and warmed IV saline at 20 cc/kg.

Repeat Physical Examination and Ancillary Studies

- *Vital signs*: T 93 °F, HR 110, RR 25 (bagged), BP 85/60, O_2 sat 94% on 100% oxygen.
- *Primary survey*:
  - *Airway:* Tube position confirmed, no air leak.
  - *Breathing:* Equal chest-wall excursion, equal breath sounds, bibasilar crackles, adequate oxygenation.
  - *Circulation:* Good central pulses, poor peripheral capillary refill.
  - *Disability:* GCS 3.
  - *Exposure:* Child covered with warming blanket.
- *Secondary survey*:
  - *HEENT*: No evidence of head trauma. An ET tube is taped in place. No hemotympanum. Pupils are not reactive.
  - *Neck*: No JVD. Trachea is midline, c-collar is placed.
  - *Cardiovascular:* Regular rate and rhythm, no M/R/G.
  - *Lungs:* Equal with bilateral crackles. No chest-wall crepitus or bruising.
  - *Abdomen*: Hypoactive bowel sounds, non-distended abdomen without organomegaly.
  - *Extremities*: No deformity or bruising. Pulses present throughout.
  - *Skin:* Cool to touch, no bruising or rashes.
  - *Neurologic:* No spontaneous respirations, no response to pain, pupils non-reactive.
- *Pertinent laboratory tests*: pH 7.20, $PaCO_2$ 43, bicarbonate 15, Na 135, K 3.5, Cl 110, BUN 10, Cr 0.8, glucose 110.
- *Radiographs*: CXR shows diffuse airspace infiltration, consistent with pulmonary edema.

Questions for Thought

- What concomitant illnesses or injuries must be considered in children presenting with drowning?
- What is the pathophysiology of drowning?
- What role does induced hypothermia play in post-drowning care?
- Does the liquid media in which drowning occurs affect outcome or treatment?

Diagnosis

- The patient experienced a non-fatal drowning.

Discussion

- *Epidemiology*: Drowning is defined as respiratory impairment from submersion or immersion in a liquid media.[1,2] If a patient is rescued at any point, drowning is interrupted and is considered non-fatal drowning. Older terminology includes "near drowning" and "dry drowning." In the USA, drowning is the leading cause of death among children of 1 to 4 years of age, and the second leading cause of death in children 1 to 18 years of age.[1,2] Male sex, young age, low socioeconomic status, and risky behaviors (e.g. alcohol use) are the most common risk factors associated with drowning.[1,2]
- *Pathophysiology*: The physiologic response to drowning is the same regardless of age or the media of submersion. The first response is to hold one's breath in an attempt to maintain an airway. Eventually, the drive to breathe overcomes this response and aspiration occurs. Water in the alveoli results in a significant osmotic gradient, which leads to increased permeability, fluid shifts, and electrolyte disturbances.[1,3] These electrolyte irregularities are similar in both saltwater and freshwater drowning.[3] The increased fluid in the lung also causes a wash-out effect of the surfactant in the alveoli, resulting in poor lung compliance and a mismatch between ventilated and perfused lung tissue (V/Q mismatch).[1,3] As more aspiration occurs, hypoxemia develops, leading to loss of consciousness. A typical progression of tachycardia, bradycardia, pulseless electrical activity, and asystole is documented in the literature.[1,4,5]

  The first stage of drowning is measured in seconds to minutes, but for those who drown in ice water this process can last an hour or longer.[1] Electrical and metabolic activity of the brain is reduced in the hypothermic patient, with a reduction of cerebral oxygen consumption by 5 percent for each 1.8 °F drop in body temperature.[1] Therefore, drowning in ice water is protective, and the medical provider should not terminate resuscitative efforts in an ice-water drowning victim until his or her temperature has surpassed 86 °F with no return of vital signs.[1,4-6] Warm-water drowning victims with cardiopulmonary arrest have a much more dire prognosis.

- *Presentation and diagnosis*: In any case of drowning, the medical provider must consider the context in which it occurred. Drowning is often immediately preceded by traumatic injuries, especially head and c-spine injuries. Therefore, in addition to resuscitative efforts, the provider should evaluate for multi-system trauma. Underlying seizure disorder is known to be a risk factor for drowning, and the provider should evaluate for this possibility in the right clinical circumstance (for instance, drowning in a youth who knows how to swim). Toxic ingestions are also common in the older drowning victim. Finally, the clinician should weigh the possibility of non-accidental trauma in young drowning victims.

- *Treatment*: Resuscitation of drowning victims can be described in five categories: In-water resuscitation, resuscitation on land, pre-hospital care, care in the ED, and in-hospital care. The key to in-water resuscitation is stabilization and getting the patient to safety on land. Immobilization of the c-spine is necessary only in events in which spinal injury is suspected, such as diving or accidents involving watercrafts.[1] Once on land, the patient should be evaluated for responsiveness. Since drowning is classically a respiratory arrest there may be gasping or apnea with a maintained heart rate, in which case only supported ventilation is necessary.[1] If the patient requires CPR, the traditional ABC approach of airway–breathing–circulation and not the new sequence of circulation–airway–breathing is recommended.[1,4,5] New recommendations also suggest five rescue breaths instead of the original two, due to the increased resistance found in the airway.[1,4,5]

  In nearly 86 percent of drowning cases requiring CPR, regurgitation and aspiration of stomach contents occurs.[1] This aspiration compounds the poor lung compliance and worsens oxygenation. If the patient is deteriorating or showing signs of fatigue, early intubation and mechanical ventilatory support is recommended. Due to fluid shifts across respiratory membranes, fluid may appear in the ET tube, causing oxygenation to become challenging. Due to this, a fine balance between suctioning and oxygenation must be obtained.[1] In cases of hypotension not responsive to appropriate ventilation, rapid crystalloid infusion is recommended.

  In the ED, attention to the ABCs should continue. The next steps include CXR and measurement of ABG.[1] The most common finding on ABG is a metabolic acidosis. This can be overcome by the patient's innate tachypneic response if spontaneous respirations occur. If the patient is intubated, a metabolic acidosis can be treated by increasing the ventilator rate, or with an elevation of the peak inspiratory pressure. Poor response to mechanical ventilation and typical ED care should raise concern for alternate pathology.[1] A CT scan of the head and evaluation of toxic exposure can be helpful in such a case. Electrolytes should be obtained but are minimally useful and are usually normal, regardless of the media in which drowning occurred.[1]

- *Disposition*: A patient with a history of minor submersion, no vital sign abnormalities, and normal mental status may be observed for 6–8 hours in the ED and then discharged home.[1] All others should be admitted for observation.

  People who have been stabilized and admitted to the hospital are not clear of complications. Signs and symptoms similar to ARDS are common, although recovery tends to be faster.[1,3] The literature does not support the use of broad-spectrum antibiotics, glucocorticoids, artificial surfactant, or inhaled nitric oxide in typical drowning victims.[1] While rewarming is a key goal in all cases of drowning, induced hypothermia with temperatures between 89.6 and 93.2 °F for 24 hours may be neuroprotective.[6]

- *Prevention*: Prevention is the most important step in managing victims of drowning. More than 85 percent of cases can be prevented by supervision, swimming instruction, technology, regulation, and public education.[1] Key prevention measures include: always swimming with others, use of life jackets, and swimming in areas with lifeguards. Areas that have lifeguards on duty show improved statistics on drowning outcomes. Less than

6 percent of all rescued persons need medical attention and only 0.5 percent need CPR in areas where lifeguards function.[1] New regulations on swimming pools include having a four-sided fence with a self-closing, self-latching gate. Having a fence that meets these guidelines has been shown to reduce incidence of drowning by 50–70 percent.[1]

Historical clues	Physical findings	Ancillary studies
• Found submerged • Known risks: Male, age 1–4	• Cardiorespiratory arrest • Increased secretions	• CXR with pulmonary edema • ABG with metabolic acidosis

Follow-Up

The child was admitted to the PICU with ongoing resuscitative support. He later underwent confirmatory testing and was ultimately declared brain dead. His organs were harvested for transplant.

References

1. Szpilman D, Bierens J, Handley A, et al. Drowning. *N Eng J M ed* 2012; 366: 2102–10.

2. Van Beeck EF, Branche CM, Szpilman D, et al. A new definition of drowning: Towards documentation and prevention of a global public health problem. *Bull World Health Organ* 2005; 83: 853–6.

3. Orlowski JP, Abulleil MM, Phillips JM. The hemodynamic and cardiovascular effects of near-drowning in hypotonic, isotonic, or hypertonic solutions. *Ann Emerg Med* 1989; 18: 1044–9.

4. Soar J, Perkins GD, Abbasc G, et al. European Resuscitation Council guidelines for resuscitation 2010. Section 8. Cardiac arrest in special circumstances: Electrolyte abnormalities, poisoning, drowning, accidental hypothermia, hyperthermia, asthma, anaphylaxis, cardiac surgery, trauma, pregnancy, electrocution. *Resuscitation* 2010; 81: 1400–33.

5. International Life Saving Federation Medical Committee. *Clarification Statement on Cardiopulmonary Resuscitation for Drowning*. Leuven: International Life Saving Federation, 2008.

6. Warner D, Knape J. Recommendations and consensus brain resuscitation in the drowning victim. In Bierens JJLM, ed. *Handbook on Drowning: Prevention, Rescue, and Treatment*. Berlin: Springer-Verlag, 2006, pp. 436–9.

Case 7

Contributing Author: Edwin Layng

The patient is a 4-year-old boy with a history of vomiting and diarrhea. Symptoms began 3 days ago, shortly after being picked up from daycare. The patient has had non-bloody/non-bilious vomiting about four times per day and has had eight non-bloody bowel movements per day since symptom onset. He has tried eating bland foods, such as bananas, rice, toast, as well as drinking clear liquids, but vomits shortly thereafter and has overall had very poor PO. Mom reports that he has also had a low-grade fever and cramping abdominal pain. The child states his pain is made worse by attempts to eat or drink. Of note, his older sister, who attends the same daycare, had similar symptoms before the patient began feeling ill. He denies chest pain, shortness of breath, or headache.

Past Medical History

- Otherwise healthy, immunizations are UTD.

Medications

- Acetaminophen for fever.
- Bismuth subsalicylate for nausea/vomiting.

Allergies

- Penicillin – patient gets hives.

Physical Examination and Ancillary Studies

- *Vital signs*: T 99.5 °F, HR 130, BP 75/45, RR 30, O_2 sat 100%. Per his mother, his weight at his last appointment several months ago was 28 kg, and the measured weight in the ED is 26.5 kg. Per the Broselow tape, he is in the "orange" category.
- *General*: He is awake, but drowsy. He is uncomfortable, holding his abdomen.
- *HEENT*: The patient's eyes are sunken. PERRL. Cranial nerves are intact. The patient's mucous membranes are dry. His neck is supple with a midline trachea.
- *Cardiovascular*: Tachycardic, no M/R/G. Extremities cool and pale with > 3 second capillary refill.
- *Lungs*: CTA bilaterally, without W/R/R.
- *Abdomen:* Child has hyperactive bowel sounds. His abdomen is soft with diffuse generalized tenderness to palpation, with no rebound or guarding. There are no masses.

- *Extremities and skin*: Extremities are cool. There are no rashes or skin changes.
- *Ancillary studies*: Na 145, K 3.3, Cl 90, bicarbonate 30, BUN 30, Cr 1.3, albumin 3.3, remaining LFTs normal. WBC 13,000, Hb 15.0, Plt 200,000. Lactate 2.0. U/A with elevated specific gravity, ++ ketones, negative glucose, nitrite, leukocyte esterase, and blood.

Questions for Thought

- How much and what type of fluid is indicated for treatment of this child?
- Does the fluid resuscitation process change with malnourished children?
- What is the best way to obtain IV access in patients like this?
- What therapeutic endpoints should be obtained to assess for adequate resuscitation?

Diagnosis

- Hypovolemic shock secondary to intravascular volume loss from viral gastroenteritis.

Discussion

- *Epidemiology*: Hypovolemia is the most common cause of shock in children worldwide and is broadly divided into hemorrhagic and non-hemorrhagic causes. Fluid loss from diarrhea is the leading cause of hypovolemic shock and is a major cause of infant mortality worldwide.[1] Other causes of hypovolemic shock include vomiting, inadequate fluid intake, diabetic ketoacidosis, third-space losses, and large burns. Hemorrhagic shock in children is most often the result of major trauma. Less common causes include GI bleeding, post-operative bleeding, and pulmonary hemorrhage.
- *Pathophysiology*: Shock is a physiologic state, characterized by a significant, systemic reduction in tissue perfusion, resulting in decreased tissue oxygen delivery. Although the effects of inadequate tissue perfusion are initially reversible, prolonged oxygen deprivation leads to generalized cellular hypoxia and derangement of critical biochemical processes.[2]

  Hypovolemic shock is the result of an absolute deficiency of intravascular blood volume. It is characterized by decreased preload leading to reduced stroke volume and low cardiac output. Tachycardia, increased systemic vascular resistance, and increased cardiac contractility are the main compensatory mechanisms. In addition, tachypnea is often seen once a metabolic acidosis develops.

  The shock syndrome is characterized by a continuum of physiologic stages, beginning with an initial inciting event that causes a systemic disturbance in tissue perfusion. Subsequently, shock may progress through three stages, which include compensated shock, hypotensive shock, and irreversible shock. The shock progression is often an accelerating process, and pediatric patients in particular can decompensate very quickly. While it may take hours for compensated shock to progress to hypotensive shock, it may only take minutes for hypotensive shock to progress to cardiopulmonary failure and arrest.

  During compensated shock, the body's homeostatic mechanisms are able to counteract the diminished perfusion, and systolic blood pressure is maintained within the normal range. The heart rate is initially increased. Signs of peripheral vasoconstriction, such as cool skin, decreased peripheral pulses, and oliguria can be noted as perfusion becomes further compromised.[2,3] During hypotensive shock, compensatory mechanisms are overwhelmed. Signs and symptoms of organ dysfunction, such as altered mental status, appear. Systolic blood pressure falls, although children who have lost as much as 30–35 percent of circulating blood volume can typically maintain normal systolic blood pressures. Once hypotension develops, the child's condition usually deteriorates rapidly to cardiovascular collapse and cardiac arrest. During irreversible shock, progressive end-organ dysfunction leads to irreversible organ damage and death despite resuscitative efforts.[2,3]

- *Presentation*: When patients present with hypovolemic shock, it can be anywhere on the continuum from compensated to non-compensated. For non-hemorrhagic cases, patients often present with tachycardia and are normotensive.[2] However, they can progress to hypotension quickly, if not addressed. For hemorrhagic causes, patients often present as a trauma alert and can be mildly tachycardic or unresponsive, depending on the quantity of the volume lost/severity of the inciting event.

- *Diagnosis*: When diagnosing hypovolemic shock in pediatrics, physical examination findings are critical. Common examination findings for hypovolemic shock include tachycardia, narrow pulse pressure, weak peripheral pulses, cool skin, capillary refill > 2 seconds, oliguria, and altered mental status.[2-4] Children who are hypotensive, with histories of trauma, are likely in hemorrhagic shock. They must be carefully evaluated in order to identify sources of bleeding and associated injuries.

- *Treatment*: It's important to initially do a primary assessment in a pediatric patient with shock to address airway, breathing, and circulation. If the patient is not protecting the airway, is cyanotic, or has signs of increased work of breathing and impending compromise, you should intubate the patient before proceeding with the resuscitation.[2] If active bleeding is seen, attempt to stop it with direct pressure. Fluid administration is the primary therapy for hypovolemic shock. Timely administration of fluid is key to preventing metabolic decompensation.[2-5] Children with hypovolemic shock who receive an appropriate volume of fluid within the first hour of resuscitation have the best chance for survival and recovery.

  Start fluid resuscitation for shock with 20 mL/kg of isotonic crystalloid administered as a bolus over 5 to 20 minutes.[2,3] For children in shock, IO cannulation should be performed if IV access cannot be established quickly.[2] When administering fluid boluses, it's important to use either a pressure bag, deliver aliquots using a large syringe that is refilled through a three-way stopcock ("push–pull" method), or a rapid infuser, in order to ensure adequate delivery. In a study comparing three methods of IV fluid resuscitation, delivery by gravity was measured to be 6.2 mL/kg in 5 minutes, in comparison to 20.9 mL/kg for the pressure bag and 20.2 mL/kg for the push–pull method.[5] The patient's weight or the Broselow tape should be used to decide volume and dosing of fluid and medications during resuscitation. Colloid administration may be an option for patients with decreased arterial volume related to low intravascular oncotic pressure (as in nephrotic syndrome or other

causes of hypoalbuminemia). However, randomized trials and meta-analyses have failed to consistently demonstrate a difference in clinical outcomes for adults and children receiving colloid therapy for shock when compared to crystalloid infusion. Vasoactive medications have no place in the treatment of isolated hypovolemic shock. These interventions do not address the underlying problem of inadequate circulating blood volume and may worsen tissue hypoxia.

In patients with hypovolemic shock who have a history of severe malnutrition, there is a risk that the malnutrition will cause sodium and water retention. Once resuscitation begins, there can be an over-expansion of the extracellular fluid and myocardial dysfunction. The WHO cites a risk of fluid overload, heart failure, and pulmonary edema and recommends against rapid fluid boluses of 20 mL/kg in these children.[6] Current recommendations are that severely malnourished children should receive 15 mL/kg of isotonic crystalloid fluids combined with 5% dextrose over 1 hour.[6] Further care depends upon the patient's response. A recent study in Kenya comparing resuscitation with 30 mL half-strength Darrows/5% dextrose over 2 hours to 40 mL Ringer's lactate over 2 hours found lower mortality and better response to therapy in the Ringer's lactate group that received more fluid.[7] Furthermore, there were no cases of pulmonary edema or cardiogenic failure in any of these patients. Further research needs to be conducted in order to make conclusions to optimize care for patients with severe malnutrition in hypovolemic shock.

It is important to monitor the patient's response to the fluid bolus as well as reassess endpoints to decide whether or not there is a need for additional fluid boluses. Some physical examination signs for fluid responsiveness include strong distal pulses, capillary refill less than 2 seconds, warm skin, normal mental status, urine output above 1 mL/kg per hour, correction of blood pressure with systolic at least in the 5th percentile for age, slowing of heart rate, decreased respiratory rate, and normalization of lactate. It is also important to monitor for signs of detrimental effects of fluid overload in the patient, such as pulmonary edema. If the condition does not improve or worsens after fluid boluses, try to identify the cause of shock to help determine the next interventions. Oftentimes, pediatric patients come in with shock that has a multifactorial etiology. For instance, children in septic shock may have concurrent hypovolemic shock from intravascular volume loss due to fever, diarrhea, or third-spacing.

With patients in hemorrhagic shock, blood is recommended for replacement of volume loss if the child's perfusion is inadequate despite administration of a bolus of 20 mL/kg isotonic crystalloid fluid. Administer 10 mL/kg packed red blood cells as soon as possible using a rapid infuser.

- *Disposition*: Children with hypovolemic shock warrant inpatient admission and ongoing evaluation, monitoring, and treatment. Those who have traumatic hemorrhagic shock require management by a surgical team with expertise in pediatric trauma. Use endpoints and response to treatment to guide whether or not an ICU admission is warranted.

Historical clues	Physical findings	Ancillary studies
• Prolonged vomiting and diarrhea	• Tachycardia • Dry mucous membranes • Sunken eyes • Decreased urine output	• Elevated lactate • Hypochloremic metabolic alkalosis • Acute kidney injury from dehydration

Follow-Up

This patient had hypovolemic shock secondary to intravascular volume loss from a viral gastroenteritis. After three boluses of 20 mL/kg crystalloid fluid over the course of 1 hour, the patient's vital signs normalized, urine output increased, and his lactic acid fell to a value within normal limits. His nausea resolved with administration of ondansetron and he was able to tolerate clear liquids as well as an ice pop. He was admitted to the inpatient pediatric floor to be observed overnight and was discharged to home in the morning.

References

1. Centres for Disease Control and Prevention. Global Water, Sanitation, & Hygiene (WASH). See www.cdc .gov/healthywater/global/wash_statistics.html (accessed November 11, 2016).

2. Chameides L, Samson RA, Schexnayder SM, Hazinski MF. *Pediatric Advanced Life Support Provider Manual*. Dallas, TX: American Heart Association, 2011, pp. 69–99.

3. Brierley J, Carcillo JA, Choong K, et al. Clinical practice parameters for hemodynamic support of pediatric and neonatal septic shock: 2007 update from the American College of Critical Care Medicine. *Crit Care Med* 2009; 37: 666–88.

4. Raimer PL, Han YY, Weber MS, et al. A normal capillary refill time of ≤ 2 seconds is associated with superior vena cava oxygen saturations of ≥ 70%. *J Pediatr* 2011; 158: 968–72.

5. Stoner MJ, Goodman DG, Cohen DM, *et al.* Rapid fluid resuscitation in pediatrics: Testing the American College of Critical Care Medicine guideline. *Ann Emerg Med* 2007; 50: 601–7.

6. World Heath Organization. Initial treatment of dehydration for severe acute malnutrition. See www .who.int/elena/titles/bbc/dehydration_sam/en/ (accessed November 11, 2016).

7. Akech SO, Karisa J, Nakamya P, et al. Phase II trial of isotonic fluid resuscitation in Kenyan children with severe malnutrition and hypovolaemia. *BMC Pediatr* 2010; 10: 71.

Case 8

Contributing Author: Erica Escarcega

History

The patient is a 12-year-old male brought in by his mother for evaluation of a persistent, low-grade fever and worsening weakness and fatigue over the past 2 weeks. The patient is usually very active and enjoys playing soccer, but has not been able to participate in the past two games due to his symptoms. He denies recent cough, chest pain, abdominal pain, nausea, or vomiting, but has had a diminished appetite. He complains of aching in his bilateral lower extremities. He denies any recent sick contacts.

Past Medical History

- None.

Medications

- None.

Allergies

- NKDA.

Physical Examination and Ancillary Studies

- *Vital signs*: T 100.8 °F, HR 134, BP 85/58, RR 26, O_2 sat 100% on room air.
- *General*: The patient is not in any acute distress and is cooperative.
- *HEENT*: PERRL. Mucous membranes moist. Tympanic membranes normal.
- *Neck*: Supple, with no lymphadenopathy and no JVD.
- *Cardiovascular*: His heart rate is tachycardic and regular. He has a grade 4/6 crescendo–decrescendo murmur best appreciated at the upper-right sternal border. There are no gallops or rubs. Peripheral pulses are palpable, but thready. Capillary refill > 3 seconds.
- *Lungs*: CTA bilaterally, with no W/R/R. No chest-wall tenderness.
- *Abdomen*: The patient's abdomen is soft, non-tender, and non-distended, without rebound or guarding. There are no palpable masses.
- *Extremities*: No deformity, no bruising, full range of motion.
- *Skin*: Pale and diaphoretic, without rashes or signs of trauma.
- *Neurologic*: Awake and interactive, but somewhat listless and fatigued.

Questions for Thought

- In what kind of shock is this child?
- How can this shock be differentiated from other forms of shock?
- What are some of the common causes of this kind of shock in children?
- How can cardiac output be improved in this kind of shock?
- What clues within a patient's history and physical examination help in the determination of the underlying cause of the patient's shock?

Diagnosis

- Cardiogenic shock secondary to endocarditis.

Discussion

- *Epidemiology*: Cardiac arrest in children is rarely caused by cardiac causes, but instead is more often secondary to respiratory failure and shock. In cases of shock, the most common cause in the pediatric population is hypovolemia. Cardiogenic shock is much less frequent in children; however, a multitude of both congenital and acquired conditions predispose a child to the development of cardiogenic shock, including congenital heart defects, arrhythmias, cardiomyopathies, myocarditis, endocarditis, toxin exposures, and ischemia.[1,2] About 12,000 children in the USA suffer from heart failure, the majority of which are the result of congenital heart diseases (usually presenting within the first year of life), followed by acquired dilated cardiomyopathy.[1-3]

- *Pathophysiology*: The pathophysiology of cardiogenic shock depends upon the underlying disease process. In infants with congenital heart defects dependent upon a patent ductus arteriosus, the closing of the ductus as the infant's circulation matures over the first days of life precipitates shock rapidly. Children with congenital defects causing volume- or pressure-overload may present in the first few months to years of life with slowly progressive heart failure. Additionally, children who have undergone repair of a congenital heart defect are at higher risk of arrhythmias or other complications from the repair which compromise pump function.

  Heart failure from acquired sources is most commonly infectious in origin. Myocarditis is usually of viral origin, but may also be caused by bacteria, fungi, rickettsia, spirochetes, autoimmune diseases, hypersensitivity reactions, and toxic exposures.[4] Endocarditis may involve the myocardium as well, or may cause valvular incompetency leading to cardiac pump failure.[5] Myocardial infarction is rare in children, but may occur as the result of Kawasaki disease, which typically presents in children under the age of 5.[3]

- *Presentation*: Infants with underlying congenital heart defects may initially have non-specific signs of congestive heart failure, such as feeding difficulties, failure to thrive, tachypnea, and agitation.[3] Children diagnosed with heart failure early in life tend to progress gradually in their illness despite medical interventions until inotropic support becomes necessary.

  In acquired cases of heart failure, such as myocarditis, the progression may be more sudden, with as many as 57 percent of myocarditis patients diagnosed on autopsy after sudden death.[3,4] Infective endocarditis often presents with a new or changing murmur, fever, malaise, as well as chest and abdominal complaints.[3,5] In patients with an underlying arrhythmia, episodes of syncope may precede their presentation.[3]

Regardless of cause, in the initial stages of cardiogenic shock, the patient often becomes tachycardic with prolonged capillary refill, cool/pale extremities, and weak peripheral pulses. At this point the body is able to compensate; however, as time progresses the patient's condition deteriorates with signs of decreased mental status, reduced urinary output, metabolic acidosis, tachypnea, hypotension, mottling of the skin, and weak central pulses with absent or weak peripheral pulses.

- *Diagnosis*: The diagnosis of cardiogenic shock is a clinical one, requiring emergent recognition and resuscitation with inotropes to improve cardiac output. A thorough history and physical examination should be performed after the initial resuscitation of the patient. A hallmark of cardiogenic shock that distinguishes it from hypovolemic or distributive shock is that cardiogenic shock is generally unresponsive to fluid resuscitation. Children will receive multiple boluses but will often have ongoing tachycardia and hypotension and may even develop worsening respiratory status from volume overload. Therefore, the clinician should suspect cardiogenic shock when fluid resuscitation fails to improve or worsens the child's clinical status.[3,4]

In terms of bedside and diagnostic testing, chest radiography may aid in the diagnosis of an abnormal size or shape to the heart, suggestive of cardiomyopathy or congenital defects. Blood pressure should be taken in all four extremities as a discrepancy may indicate obstruction along the aortic arch. An EKG should be performed to evaluate for ischemic changes and arrhythmias. An echocardiogram is useful in determining the ejection fraction of the heart, the extent of dilation or hypertrophy of the ventricles, the presence of pericardial effusion as well as the presence of lesions, stenosis, or regurgitation of heart valves. Biomarkers such as BNP and troponin may help in the determination of the cause of cardiogenic shock as BNP is often elevated in cases of heart failure and an elevation in troponin may be seen in cases of myocarditis, anthracycline toxicity, or cardiac ischemia.[4]

- *Treatment*: Prostaglandin may be considered in infants with cardiogenic shock and suspected ductal dependent lesions, to help maintain an open ductus arteriosus. These infants present precipitously in the first days to weeks of life. This therapy is not effective in older infants and children with cardiogenic shock. Arrhythmia management should be initiated in patients with shock from cardiac arrhythmia.

In suspected cases of endocarditis, blood cultures should be drawn and broad-spectrum antibiotics should be initiated. Emergency echocardiography may help define the extent of disease and need for operative repair.

In all cases of cardiogenic shock, including those with myocarditis, patients require resuscitation with respiratory support and inotropes such as dopamine.[6] These patients generally will not respond to fluid resuscitation as this form of shock is not caused by redistribution or loss of volume, but is instead due to the diminished contractility of the heart. At some centers, severe cases of refractory cardiogenic shock may be treated with ECMO and ventricular assist devices as a temporizing measure, prior to heart transplantation.[7] Therefore, when the diagnosis of cardiogenic shock is made in a child, consideration should be given to transferring the child to a center with these capabilities.

- *Disposition*: All children with cardiogenic shock require admission to a PICU, preferably at a facility with capacity for ECMO, pediatric cardiology, and pediatric cardiothoracic surgery capability.

Historical clues	Physical findings
• Fever	• Murmur on auscultation
• Fatigue	• Tachycardia
• Exercise intolerance	• Tachypnea
	• Diaphoresis
	• Delayed capillary refill
	• Hypotension
	• Weak peripheral pulses

Follow-Up

The patient was given two fluid boluses at 20 mL/kg, with no improvement in his tachycardia or hypotension. He was started on a dopamine drip, which improved his blood pressure. Broad-spectrum antibiotics were initiated for suspected endocarditis. An echocardiogram revealed a large vegetation on his aortic and mitral valves, with a diminished ejection fraction. He was admitted to the ICU where he received IV antibiotics. After a prolonged hospital stay, the patient had a full recovery and was discharged home.

References

1. Rossano J, Shaddy R. Heart failure in children: Etiology and treatment. *J Pediatr* 2014; 165: 228–33.

2. Hsu D, Pearson G. Heart failure in children part I: History, etiology and pathophysiology. *Circ Heart Fail* 2009; 2: 63–70.

3. Woods W, McCullock M. Cardiovascular emergencies in the pediatric patient. *Emerg Med Clin N Am* 2005; 23: 1233–49.

4. Canter C, Simpson K. Diagnosis and treatment of myocarditis in children in the current era. *Circulation* 2014; 129: 115–28.

5. Baltimore R, Gewitz M, Baddour L, et al. Infective endocarditis in childhood. 2015 Update: A scientific statement from the American Heart Association. *Circulation* 2015; 132: 1487–515.

6. Kleinman ME, Chameides L, Schexnayder S, et al. Part 14: Pediatric advanced life support – 2010 American Heart Association Guidelines for cardiopulmonary resuscitation and emergency cardiovascular care. *Circulation* 2010; 122 Suppl 3: S876–908.

7. Hetzer R, Potapov E, Alexi-Meskishvili V, et al. Single-center experience with treatment of cardiogenic shock in children by pediatric ventricular assist devices. *J Thorac Cardiovasc Surg* 2011; 141: 616–23.

Case 9

Contributing Author: Sean Zwiebel

History

The patient is a 15-month-old female brought in by her mother for difficulty breathing. The mother notes that the child has had 2 days of a moderate, non-productive cough and profuse anterior rhinorrhea. The patient was brought to the ED because her mother was concerned that the child's lips appeared blue and that she was breathing quickly. The mother states that the patient was otherwise in her usual health yesterday, with noted cough and runny nose, and that her respiratory symptoms have progressed rapidly over the last several hours. The mother adds that the patient has had decreased oral intake today. The child has no history of cardiopulmonary or infectious problems. Mom denies

fevers, ear tugging, change in bowels or bladder function, or rashes. No recent travel, sick contacts, or daycare.

Past Medical History

- Born at term with uncomplicated birth history.
- Immunizations are UTD.
- GERD.

Medications

- Ranitidine.

Allergies

- Sulfa-containing medications (rash).

Physical Examination and Ancillary Studies

- *Vital signs*: T 100.5 °F, HR 184, BP 82/58, RR 80, O_2 sat 78% on room air.
- *General*: She appears ill, drowsy, and fatigued, with marked increase in work of breathing.
- *Primary survey*:
  - *Airway*: Intact airway, no drooling or pooling of secretions, no stridor.
  - *Breathing*: Tachypneic, with intercostal, supraclavicular, and suprasternal retractions and decreased breath sounds.
  - *Circulation*: Tachycardic, with intact pulses and capillary refill 2 seconds.
  - *Disability*: Listless and lethargic, poor tone.
  - *Exposure*: The child is fully exposed. There are no signs of trauma.
- *Secondary survey*:
  - *HEENT*: Her head is atraumatic, PERRL, tympanic membranes clear, dry mucous membranes, her oropharyngeal structures are midline, without erythema or swelling.
  - *Neck*: Supple and non-tender, without adenopathy. Trachea is midline.
  - *Cardiovascular*: The patient's heart is tachycardic, without appreciable murmurs, rubs, or gallops. Her capillary refill is 2 seconds.
  - *Lungs*: Tachypneic, with increased work of breathing, decreased air movement. She has diffuse mild expiratory wheezing with scattered rhonchi.

- *Abdomen*: The patient's abdomen is soft, non-tender, non-distended, with bowel sounds throughout.
- *Skin and extremities*: The patient is diaphoretic, her lips and tongue are cyanotic, her skin is warm peripherally and centrally.
- *Neurologic*: The child moves all four extremities spontaneously. She has intact reflexes. Her mental status is depressed.

- *Pertinent ancillary studies*: WBC 12,000; CXR demonstrates diffuse patchy infiltrates throughout both lung fields.

Questions for Thought

- What steps would you take initially to stabilize this patient?
- When do you decide to establish a definitive airway in a patient like this?
- What are some therapeutic, procedural, and anatomic considerations to reflect upon before attempting to intubate a sick child or infant?
- After establishing a definitive airway, what type of settings will this patient require for mechanical ventilation?

Diagnosis

- Acute respiratory failure secondary to pneumonia.

Discussion

- *Epidemiology*: The epidemiology of pediatric respiratory distress and respiratory failure is difficult to define as it largely depends on the underlying cause. In general, two-thirds of all cases of respiratory failure occur in the first postnatal year, with one-half occurring in the neonatal period.[1] This is attributed primarily to anatomic and physiologic differences in young infants, who have developing airways and immature respiratory drive mechanisms.[1] However, respiratory failure is a broad category and is difficult to further define without discussing specific disease processes.
- *Pathophysiology*: Respiratory failure occurs when the rate of gas exchange between the atmosphere and the blood is unable to keep up with the body's metabolic demands. Respiratory failure can be subdivided into hypoxic (failure to oxygenate) or hypercarbic (failure to ventilate). Hypoxic respiratory failure is from inadequate delivery of oxygen from the alveoli to the pulmonary capillaries or from intrapulmonary shunting. This results in diminished oxygen dissolved in blood, or hypoxemia. Hypercarbic respiratory failure is from decreased minute ventilation and results in increased CO_2 dissolved in the blood, which causes acidemia and can suppress respiratory drive at higher levels. These two distinct processes coexist on a spectrum. For example, severe hypoxemia can cause increased work of breathing, which leads to fatigue and hypoventilation. This hypoventilation in turn results in hypercarbia, and as the $PaCO_2$ climbs, respiratory drive declines further, causing the PaO_2 to drop, and ultimately causing death. The underlying cause for these two entities is vast as further pathophysiology is dependent upon the underlying cause of respiratory distress and failure.
- *Presentation*: Respiratory distress and respiratory failure represent a broad spectrum of clinical presentations, depending on the underlying disease process. Children may be tachypneic or bradypneic, they may be hypoxic or have normal oxygen saturation, they may be alert or have altered mental status. Children may have abnormal lung sounds or essentially normal auscultation.

  Although the patient in the case above had a pneumonia causing respiratory distress, the differential should be broad and can be broken up into the following categories: central or upper-airway obstruction, peripheral or lower-airway obstruction, alveolar or interstitial airway disease, thoracic cage dysfunction, brainstem abnormality, spinal cord process, or neuromuscular disorder.
- *Diagnosis*: The diagnosis of respiratory distress and failure is primarily a clinical one. The clinician should focus on careful history and physical examination, with particular attention to work of breathing. The respiratory rate is the most misreported vital sign in a patient's chart and should be counted during physical examination with careful attention for tachypnea, nasal flaring, stridor, grunting, and retractions. Inspiratory stridor suggests an upper-airway obstruction while expiratory wheezes suggest lower-airway involvement. A decreased level of consciousness

or being poorly interactive can suggest hypercarbia and impending failure.

Although history and physical examination can provide clues to the underlying cause of respiratory distress and ancillary testing can confirm a diagnosis, recognizing respiratory distress is based on clinical impression and can be subtle. For example, it is easy to take a history from a parent as her 3-year-old sits on her lap with URI symptoms and the monitor reads 97% on room air and quickly listen to his lungs, which are clear but near silent. A careful clinician would note that same patient is breathing shallowly at 60 per minute, that removing the patient's shirt may reveal significant retractions and belly breathing, that the chest and back are diaphoretic, and that the lungs appear clear because the patient is so tachypneic he is not exchanging air. That same child cannot maintain that work of breathing for long without failure. It is important to identify those in distress and to act and intervene early to prevent failure. Although the diagnosis is primarily clinical, an ABG can help define impending failure, with an acute $PaO_2 < 60$ or $PaCO_2 > 50$ in the setting of new acidemia, and can also help guide therapy and aid in decision-making.

- *Treatment*: The patient in this case was in respiratory distress from pneumonia. The approach to all sick patients should include rapid IV access, oxygen administration, and cardiopulmonary monitoring. The child's airway, breathing, and circulation should be assessed almost simultaneously.

A patient's work of breathing and oxygenation may improve with simple nasal cannula and medical management aimed at the underlying cause. This may be escalated to high-flow nasal cannula, BiPAP, or CPAP. It is important to keep the child as calm as possible, as when children cry, not only do their metabolic demands increase, but the increased turbulence of airflow correlates to increased resistance to airflow. If these measures fail, the child should be intubated.

Indications to provide a definitive airway include failure to oxygenate, failure to ventilate, or anticipated clinical decline. The clinician should anticipate that children's airways differ from adults in that the child's head and occiput is disproportionately large compared to his/her neck and the rest of his/her body. This often requires special positioning, with a towel roll beneath the child's shoulders to align the oral, pharyngeal, and laryngeal axes. Regardless of child's age, the appropriate positioning places the child's earlobe at the level of the sternal notch, parallel to the floor. Children tend to have large tongues, with a large floppy epiglottis, often necessitating the use of a Miller blade for laryngoscopy, and their airways tend to be anterior. The narrowest portion of the airway is the cricoid ring, as opposed to the vocal cords in adults. Rapid sequence intubation may be safely employed using pediatric specific equipment and weight-based medication dosing. Pretreatment with atropine has shown no benefit and should not be used.[2]

During intubation, the clinician should anticipate that the child has a decreased safe apnea period as compared to an adult. This is because children consume more oxygen per kilogram than adults, and therefore desaturate faster.[2] Once intubated, the child should be placed on mechanical ventilation which is set to match the patient's minute ventilation, preferably on pressure control settings.

Circulation should be supported with fluids or pressors as needed. A Broselow tape or reliable pediatric dosing application should be utilized to reference airway and resuscitation medications for all sick pediatric patients. After stabilizing the patient, treatment is supportive and therapy should be aimed at the underlying cause. If the patient fails mechanical ventilation rescue, therapies include ECMO or bypass if available.

- *Disposition*: Children in respiratory failure, regardless of cause, should be admitted to an ICU setting.

Historical clues	Physical findings
• Lips turning blue	• Hypoxia
• Report of fast breathing	• Tachypnea/retractions
• Cough/runny nose	• Altered mental status

Follow-up

The patient was in severe respiratory distress, hypoxic, with clinical evidence to suggest hypercarbia and impending respiratory failure. A high-flow nasal cannula was used for pre-oxygenation to increase the working intubation time. Because the patient was severely hypoxic despite pre-oxygenation and she had a very high minute ventilation, ketamine was chosen without a paralytic drug to perform an awake intubation. The child was intubated with an uncuffed 4.5-mm ET tube, secured, and mechanically ventilated, matching her minute ventilation with pressure control settings. She was transferred to a PICU and remained intubated for 5 days. She was discharged from the hospital after 8 days with a diagnosis of rhinovirus pneumonia.

References

1. Nitue ME, Eigen H. Respiratory failure. *Pediatr Rev* 2009; 30: 470–7.

2. Walls RM, Murphy MF. *Manual of Emergency Airway Management*. Philadelphia (PA): Lippincott Williams & Wilkins, 2012.

Case 10

Contributing Author: Sean Zwiebel

History

The patient is a 5-year-old male presenting with parents for chief complaint of generalized weakness and fatigue. The parents note that the patient was recently diagnosed with acute lymphoblastic leukemia (ALL) and had his last dose of induction chemotherapy 8 days ago. He has mild persistent nausea with several episodes of non-bloody, non-bilious vomiting over the last week but has otherwise been doing well, without focal complaint. They went to wake him this morning, and found him poorly responsive. After rousing him, he complained of being fatigued and feeling generally unwell. The parents recorded an oral temperature of 102 °F and brought him to the ED for further evaluation. The patient is ill-appearing but interactive and states that he does not feel well and has ongoing nausea. The patient and parents otherwise deny headache, neck pain, URI symptoms, chest pain, cough, shortness of breath, abdominal pain, change in bowels/ bladder, rashes, or sick contacts. They do note there is increasing erythema around the port in his right chest.

Past Medical History

- Born at term with uncomplicated birth history.
- UTD on immunizations.

- Asthma, mild intermittent, well-controlled.
- ALL, diagnosed 6 weeks ago.
- Right internal jugular port, placed 4 weeks ago.

Medications

- Induction chemotherapy regimen via port, last dose 8 days ago.
- Dexamethasone.
- Ondansetron.
- Albuterol.

Allergies

- NKDA.

Physical Examination and Ancillary Studies

- *Vital signs*: T 101.7 °F, HR 145, BP 62/38, RR 22, O_2 sat 97% on room air.
- *General*: He appears ill, fatigued, but able to answer questions appropriately.
- *HEENT*: Head is atraumatic, PERRL, tympanic membranes clear, dry mucous membranes, oropharyngeal structures are midline without erythema or swelling.
- *Neck*: Supple and non-tender, without adenopathy. Trachea is midline. No nuchal rigidity or meningismus.
- *Cardiovascular*: Tachycardic, without appreciable murmurs, rubs, or gallops. Warm skin, capillary refill 5 seconds.
- *Lungs*: Clear and equal, with good breath sounds.
- *Abdomen*: Soft, non-tender, non-distended, with bowel sounds throughout.
- *Extremities and skin*: The skin is warm and dry. There is a 1 cm area of erythema with induration surrounding the port in the right chest, without fluctuance or purulence. The incision is well healed. There are no other rashes or other skin lesions noted, including the perirectal and perineal regions.
- *Neurologic*: The child is somewhat listless, but has normal mentation and a non-focal neurologic examination.
- *Pertinent ancillary studies:* WBC 600, polymorphonuclear cells 52%, bands 6%, absolute neutrophil count 348, Hb 10.1, Plt 22,000, BUN 32, Cr 2.2, INR 1.8, lactic acid 4.3, U/A negative, CXR negative.

Diagnosis

- Septic shock secondary to presumed line infection.

Discussion

- *Epidemiology*: Severe sepsis is a leading cause of death in infants and children with more than 44,000 cases annually in the USA.[1] Almost 50 percent of all pediatric sepsis involves infants less than 1 year of age, with 49–74 percent of children diagnosed with severe sepsis suffering from an underlying systemic disease process.[1,2] Mortality has improved significantly in recent decades in developed countries but the overall mortality is still estimated at 25 percent.[2] In the USA, mortality rate is still around 15–20 percent depending on the source cited with respiratory, bloodstream, and genitourinary infections accounting for the overwhelming majority of cases.[2,3] If the child survives to discharge, approximately 17 percent will have at least moderate disability.[2]

- *Pathophysiology*: Septic shock is truly a combination of distributive, hypovolemic, and cardiogenic shock.[4] The distributive component is from an inflammatory cascade or toxin-mediated decrease in systemic vascular resistance resulting in capillary leak and third-spacing, with intravascular losses and ensuing hypovolemia.[4,5] The cardiogenic component is from the myocardial-depressant effects from sepsis, the systemic inflammatory cascade, and acidosis. The resultant effect is hypoperfusion and end-organ dysfunction, which can be evident clinically or through laboratory values. Hypoperfusion and tissue hypoxia result in further cell damage, release of intracellular contents, lactic acidosis, and smooth muscle relaxation, which cause worsening vasodilation and release of further inflammatory mediators; this can result in multi-organ failure and fulminant cardiovascular collapse despite appropriate therapy and hemodynamic support.[4,5]

- *Presentation*: Sepsis and septic shock encompass a broad spectrum of disease, dependent largely on the type of infection and how far into the disease process the patient presents, ranging from well-appearing children with mildly deranged or normal vital signs to toxic-appearing children with multi-organ failure and cardiovascular collapse.[5] Well-appearing pediatric patients with early sepsis can progress very rapidly; the child can decompensate over the course of the provider's history and physical examination. Pediatric patients with severe sepsis and septic shock with clinical or laboratory evidence of end-organ dysfunction are well advanced into the clinical spectrum, and are at risk for increased morbidity and mortality.[2,5] The clinician must have a high index of suspicion for sepsis. A careful history and physical examination, taking note of subtle signs of organ dysfunction or shock, such as tachypnea, delayed capillary refill, or complaints of decreased wet diapers, are imperative.

- *Diagnosis*: For the emergency care provider, the diagnosis of severe sepsis and septic shock in a pediatric patient is primarily a clinical one. Traditionally, sepsis is defined as a presumed source of infection and the patient should meet SIRS criteria, with two or more of the following: a temperature less than 96.8 °F or greater than 100.4 °F, a HR greater than 90 BPM, a RR greater than 20 breaths per minute or $PaCO_2$ less than 32, or WBC less than 4,000 or greater than 12,000.[4,6] However, all children under 5 years of age could satisfy SIRS criteria using their normal age-appropriate vital signs. Furthermore, normal WBC also vary by age. For the pediatric population, a less stringent definition of sepsis includes a presumed source of infection with two or more of the following: temperature less than 96.8 °F or greater than 101.3 °F, age-specific tachycardia or bradycardia not from secondary causes (pain, fever), age-specific tachypnea, or an abnormal leukocyte count or greater than 10% bands.[2,5,7]

There is less consensus on the definition of severe sepsis and septic shock in pediatric patients, as children have excellent physiologic compensatory mechanisms. Age-specific hypotension is generally a late finding and should cause concern for impending cardiovascular collapse. Pediatric severe sepsis can be defined as sepsis with evidence of cardiovascular dysfunction, ARDS, or evidence of involvement of two or more organ systems.[2,5,7] This can include altered mental status, an acutely elevated Cr, INR, or liver enzymes, acute thrombocytopenia, or the need for increasing supplemental oxygen. Septic shock is sepsis with evidence of ongoing cardiovascular dysfunction despite adequate fluid resuscitation in the first hour. This is defined as hypotension less than 5th percentile for age or requiring pressors to support blood pressure, or at least two of the following: urine output less than 0.5 mL/kg per hour, capillary refill > 5 seconds, base deficit greater than 5 or lactic acid twice the upper limit of normal, or core to peripheral temperature gap of greater than 5.4 °F.[2,5,7]

Presumed sources of infection can include bacteria, viruses, fungi, and parasites. In the acute care setting, blood, urine, and viral cultures are not immediately available for clinical decision-making. Therefore, during the initial encounter with an ill pediatric patient, careful attention should be made to identify potential sources of infection, including meningitis, upper or lower respiratory infections, intra-abdominal sources, the skin (including perineal and peri-rectal areas), cardiac for new murmurs or stigmata of embolic phenomena, or risk factors for clinically significant viremia or fungemia. It is imperative to carefully take note of these patients' vital signs and perform a thorough history and physical examination to evaluate for evidence of end-organ dysfunction. Laboratory values may be of benefit in borderline-appearing or higher-risk children, but hypotension or lactic acidosis are often late findings and should not alone be relied upon to define severe sepsis or septic shock.

- *Treatment*: Treatment of severe sepsis and septic shock should focus on source control, if possible, and antibiotics directed towards presumed source of infection. The landmark study of early goal-directed therapy in 2001 demonstrated a significant improvement in mortality in adults with severe sepsis and septic shock by early antibiotic administration and aggressive hemodynamic support with invasive monitoring to meet predefined resuscitative endpoints.[4] This was the standard for over a decade until the ProCESS trial in 2014 refuted this and found that early identification of severe sepsis and septic shock along with early administration of antibiotics and aggressive fluid resuscitation was as effective in improving outcomes without the need for invasive monitoring. There is less robust information in the treatment and management in the pediatric population; however, early recognition is paramount and again the provider must maintain a high clinical suspicion to identify early sepsis.[5,7] Furthermore, antibiotics should be administered based on age, risk factors, and presumed source as soon as sepsis is identified. The patient should have an adequate IV/IO/CVC, and aggressive fluid resuscitation should be initiated in 20 mL/kg aliquots, with up to 60 mL/kg given in the first hour before pressors are initiated. Ongoing fluid resuscitation may be continued until the patient develops hepatomegaly, or respiratory distress with rales, and some children may require as much as 200 mL/kg intially. Although norepinephrine is recommended as a first-line pressor in adult septic shock, most sources cite dopamine as the first-line agent for blood pressure support if the pediatric patient has clinical signs of shock, which are not responsive to fluid boluses. Norepinephrine and epinephrine are recommended for hypotensive patients with *warm* or *cold* shock, respectively, or for shock refractory to dopamine. Consider hydrocortisone in patients with refractory hypotension on pressors or those with known adrenal insufficiency or prior steroid use.

  Careful monitoring of blood glucose and serum calcium is also crucial during resuscitation. Resuscitative endpoints in the acute care setting should include maintaining urine output > 1 mL/kg per hour, improving capillary refill to < 2 seconds, improving mentation, no difference between central and peripheral pulses, and the maintenance of an adequate blood pressure.

- *Disposition*: All pediatric patients with severe sepsis and septic shock have the potential for rapid decompensation, and should be evaluated for ICU-level admission, especially if pressors have been initiated.

Historical clues	Physical findings	Ancillary studies
• Underlying immunosuppression • Fatigue • Altered mental status • Indwelling line	• Fever • Tachycardia • Tachypnea • Hypotension • Skin changes at line site	• Leukopenia • Elevated Cr • Lactic acidosis • Elevated INR

Follow-Up

The patient was in septic shock, with evidence of cardiovascular dysfunction, end-organ failure, and lactic acidosis. He was persistently hypotensive despite three 20 mL/kg boluses of normal saline in the first hour. He was immediately started on weight-based cefepime, tobramycin, and vancomycin. Dopamine was initiated to support his blood pressure, in addition to aggressive fluid resuscitation, and the patient was transferred to a PICU with his oncologists consulting. His blood cultures grew out MSSA. His port was removed and a PICC line was placed. The patient's antibiotics were changed to cefazolin and he improved clinically, ultimately being discharged after 7 days in the hospital.

References

1. Watson RS, Carcillo JA. Scope and epidemiology of pediatric sepsis. *Pediatr Crit Care Med* 2005; 6 Suppl 3: S3–5.

2. Weiss SL, Fitzgerald JC, Pappachan J, et al. Global epidemiology of pediatric severe sepsis: The sepsis prevalence, outcomes, and therapies study. *Am J Respir Crit Care Med* 2015; 191: 1147–57.

3. Ruth A, McCracken CE, Fortenberry JD, et al. Pediatric severe sepsis: Current trends and outcomes from the Pediatric Health Information Systems database. *Pediatr Crit Care Med* 2014; 15: 828–38.

4. Rivers E, Nguyen B, Havstad S, et al. Early goal-directed therapy in the treatment of severe sepsis and septic shock. *N Engl J Med* 2001; 345: 1368–77.

5. Biban P, Gaffuri M, Spaggiari S, et al. Early recognition and management of septic shock in children. *Pediatr Rep* 2012; 4: e13.

6. Yearly DM, Kellum JA, Huang DT, et al. A randomized trial of protocol-based care for early septic shock. *N Engl J Med* 2014; 370: 1683–93.

7. Sepanski RJ, Godambe SA, Magnum CD, et al. Designing a pediatric severe sepsis screening tool. *Front Pediatr* 2014; 2: 56.

Case 11

Contributing Author: Ben Church

History

The patient is a 16-year-old male who initially presented to the local fire department with shortness of breath, which began approximately 20 minutes after being stung by a bee. He has a known anaphylactic bee allergy but did not have an epinephrine auto-injector with him. IM epinephrine and IV diphenhydramine and steroids were immediately given by paramedic staff, after which emergency transport was initiated. Associated symptoms include nausea, vomiting, extreme anxiety, and diaphoresis. The child arrives at the ED minimally responsive after decompensating in the ambulance bay.

Past Medical History

- Poorly controlled asthma.
- Immunizations are UTD.

Medications

- Albuterol.
- Fluticasone.

Allergies

- Bees and shellfish.
- No known drug allergies.

Physical Examination and Ancillary Studies

- *Vital signs*: T 98.8 °F, HR 116, BP 97/61, RR 34, O_2 sat 75% on room air per pre-hospital staff and 98% on 15 L O_2 non-rebreather in the ED.
- *General*: The patient has labored respirations and is responsive to painful stimuli only.
- *Primary survey*:
  - *Airway*: Child has drooling and some airway swelling, no stridor, gag intact. Vomitus is present on his cheek.
  - *Breathing*: Tachypneic, with severe intercostal and supraclavicular retractions. He has diffuse rhonchi and expiratory wheezing and little to no air movement.
  - *Circulation*: Tachycardic, with intact pulses and capillary refill 2 seconds.

- *Disability*: Responsive to painful stimuli only, no focal deficits appreciated.
- *Exposure*: The child is fully exposed. There are no signs of trauma. He has diffuse urticaria and is grossly diaphoretic, flushed, and warm.

Questions for Thought

- Are there interventions you should perform prior to continuing with your examination?
- How urgent is airway management in anaphylaxis?

- You intubate the child prior to continuing with your examination, because you recognize that, although the child does not have stridor and is breathing spontaneously, he is at high risk for losing his airway from ongoing edema or vomiting. You use ketamine as an induction agent because you know it is a bronchodilator, and you also use succinylcholine because you know that his airway may be difficult, and you want the best chance of success. You use a size 3 glidescope and a 7.5-mm cuffed tube, confirming airway positioning with end-tidal capnography. You also recognize the most likely diagnosis and start treatment.
- *Secondary survey*:
  - *HEENT*: PERRL, tympanic membranes clear, moist mucous membranes, increased secretions.
  - *Neck*: Supple, with midline trachea.
  - *Cardiovascular*: Tachycardic, regular rhythm, with no M/R/G. Radial and carotid pulses are present. He has erythematous skin, with brisk capillary refill.
  - *Lungs*: Tachypneic with rhonchi and wheezing, breath sounds are symmetric.
  - *Abdomen*: The patient's abdomen is soft and non-distended, with hyperactive bowel sounds. There is no guarding.
  - *Skin and extremities*: The patient is diaphoretic, and has diffuse erythroderma and urticaria.
  - *Neurologic*: The child moves all four extremities spontaneously. He responds to pain.
- *Pertinent ancillary studies*: WBC 19,100, ABG (pH 6.8, pCO_2 63, pO_2 241, bicarbonate 14), Na 141, K 3.9, Cl 101, serum bicarbonate 12, lactate 11.3.

Questions for Thought

- Should you have obtained laboratory tests prior to initiating therapy?
- How would you interpret this child's ABG?
- What are the treatment options for this disease entity?
- How would you monitor response to therapy in this patient?
- What anatomic differences unique to the pediatric airway must be considered?

Diagnosis

- Anaphylaxis secondary to insect envenomation.

Discussion

- *Epidemiology*: Insect envenomation leading to anaphylaxis can result from the sting of many different *Hymenoptera* species including Vespidae (wasps/hornets), Apidae (bees), and Formicidae (fire ants). Second only to antibiotic-related anaphylaxis, *Hymenoptera* anaphylaxis is the next most common etiology causing just under 100 deaths per year in the USA.[1,2] Food allergies affect 4–6 percent of children.[3] Surveys aimed at gauging anaphylactic reactions within the USA estimate that 1–3 percent of the general population will be affected in their lifetimes, with a mortality rate of 1 percent.[1,4] Limited data exist for the exact prevalence of insect stings within the USA. Those that spend more time outdoors and those living in rural areas are more prone to disease exposure. Poorly or uncontrolled reactive airway disease, namely asthma, is a major risk factor involved in increased morbidity and mortality of patients experiencing anaphylaxis.[4–6]
- *Pathophysiology*: Anaphylaxis develops via an immediate type I hypersensitivity reaction. Sensitization occurs when patients are initially exposed to an allergen triggering increased production of Immunoglobulin E antibodies. Early phase reaction then results from subsequent allergen exposure and massive degranulation of mast cells and basophils via receptor-mediated binding of antigen and preformed Immunoglobulin E complexes. Degranulation of histamine, leukotrienes, prostaglandins, and tumor necrosis factor-α are some of the many immunologic mediators implicated in the disease.

Late-phase reaction finally involves the continued production and release of additional inflammatory mediators. This all then leads to massive vasodilation and distributive shock.

- *Presentation*: Symptoms of anaphylaxis stem from the widespread vasodilatory effects of immune-cell degranulation and fall into a spectrum of mild to very severe disease. Presentation of symptoms can be categorized according to the organ system affected. For instance, patients may complain of pruritus and display diffuse urticaria with cutaneous involvement.[2,7,8] Respiratory-system signs and symptoms include dyspnea, rhinorrhea, stridor, and wheezing.[2,7,8] GI involvement includes nausea, vomiting, diarrhea, and abdominal pain.[2,7,8] Presyncope or syncope, tachycardia or bradycardia, hypotension, and altered mental status should all raise red flags of cardiovascular involvement and the possibility of impending cardiovascular collapse.[2,7,8] A complaint of "a lump in my throat" or of hoarseness may indicate impending and potentially lethal laryngeal edema. The vast majority of patients will experience symptom onset within 60 minutes of exposure, with those experiencing more rapid onset carrying a significantly higher rate of morbidity and mortality.[2,7,8] The overwhelming majority of patients will experience symptoms within 6 hours.[2,7,8]
- *Diagnosis*: There has been much controversy regarding the diagnosis of anaphylaxis as it is largely a clinical diagnosis. The most recent guidelines which outline a diagnosis of anaphylaxis come from the 2005 joint collaboration between the National Institute of Allergy and Infectious Disease and the Food Allergy and Anaphylaxis Network, and have been updated recently.[2,9] They describe three criteria for making the diagnosis. Fulfillment of one out of the three criteria is highly sensitive but not specific in recognizing the disease.[2,9]
  - Criteria 1 includes the rapid onset of symptoms (minutes to hours) involving skin, mucosa, or both *in addition to* respiratory compromise or hypotension.
  - Criteria 2 suggests the diagnosis if two of the following are present after exposure to a *likely* allergen: skin involvement, respiratory

compromise, hypotension or associated symptoms (presyncope/syncope), and/or persistent GI symptoms.
  - Criteria 3 suggests anaphylaxis if hypotension occurs in association with exposure to a *known* allergen. Laboratory testing in such a rapid and incredibly lethal disease is generally not helpful. Histamine levels, which are elevated for approximately 5–30 minutes post-reaction, begin to decline by the time patients present to the ED.

- *Treatment*: As with all emergencies, a focus on airway, breathing, and circulation is paramount. In anaphylaxis, IM epinephrine is the next most important treatment in life-saving therapy.[2,4] Epinephrine is the cornerstone of anaphylaxis treatment, with other therapies being complementary at best. Common pitfalls in anaphylaxis management include delayed or failed epinephrine administration, leading to significantly worsened outcomes. Preferred dosing is 0.01 mg/kg IM with an initial maximum dose of 0.3 mg of the 1:1,000 concentration in children.[2,4] IV epinephrine should be reserved for those with severe disease as the majority of adverse outcomes stem from IV administration. It is important to realize that compensated pediatric shock may initially present with tachycardia alone, as hypotension can occur quite late in the disease process.

Steroids, antihistamines, and inhaled bronchodilators comprise the list of adjunctive therapies only.[2] Steroids are used to dampen the continued production and release of inflammatory mediators, and adjunct therapy with a histamine blockade includes both H_1 and H_2 receptor blockers, such as diphenhydramine and famotidine, respectively.[2] None of these drugs act within a time frame to make them appropriate primary therapies for anaphylaxis.[2] Inhaled albuterol can be given to help correct bronchospasm, especially in light of the large proportion of these patients that have underlying bronchospastic disease/asthma.

- *Disposition*: The appropriate disposition of patients experiencing anaphylaxis can be difficult. Those with a rapid and severe onset of symptoms or those requiring airway interventions should be admitted to the hospital for further treatment and observation. Those with very mild disease can safely be discharged home. The difficulty arises as most patients fall somewhere in between these two extremes. Other aspects of the patient's presentation that may warrant admission include a history of severe or protracted anaphylaxis, a history of poorly controlled asthma, as well as various barriers to care or poor parental understanding of discharge instructions. There is no universally agreed-upon observation period in the ED but 6 hours is used as a general rule, to evaluate for any disease refractory to treatment or re-emergence of symptoms, known as the biphasic reaction.[2] A biphasic reaction has been reported to occur in approximately 11 percent of pediatric patients and can occur as far out as 72 hours. Those patients identified appropriate for outpatient treatment should receive an epinephrine auto-injector device, return precautions, education regarding allergen avoidance, indications for epinephrine administration, and outpatient follow-up instructions.[2] Traditionally, steroids and antihistamines have also been recommended.

Historical clues	Physical findings
• Known allergy to bees	• Hypoxia
• Vomiting	• Tachypnea/retractions
• Difficulty breathing	• Altered mental status

Follow-Up

The child was intubated. His ABG showed evidence of respiratory and metabolic acidosis, with elevated carbon dioxide as well as lactate. He was started on an epinephrine drip which was titrated to 0.3 µg/min per kg. This improved his symptoms. He was given in-line bronchodilators as well as IV antihistamines and steroids. He was admitted to the PICU where his epinephrine drip was weaned off over the course of 6 hours and he was extubated and ultimately discharged home in good condition. He was instructed to carry an epinephrine auto-injector with him at all times.

References

1. Centers for Disease Control and Prevention. Insects and scorpions. See www.cdc.gov/niosh/topics/insects/ (accessed February 2017).

2. Campbell RL, Li JTC, Nicklas RA. Emergency department diagnosis and treatment of anaphylaxis: A practice parameter. *Ann Allergy Asthma Immunol* 2014; 113: 599–608.

3. Centers for Disease Control and Prevention. Food allergies in schools. See www.cdc.gov/healthyschools/foodallergies/index.htm (accessed February 2017).

4. McLean-Tooke APC, Bethune CA, Fay AC, et al. Adrenaline in the treatment of anaphylaxis: What is the evidence? *BMJ* 2003; 327: 1332–5.

5. Bilò MB, Bonifazi F. The natural history and epidemiology of insect venom allergy: Clinical implications. *Clin Exp Allergy* 2009; 39: 1467–76.

6. Bock SA, Munoz-Furlong A, Sampson HA. Fatalities due to anaphylactic reactions to foods. *J Allergy Clin Immunol* 2001; 107: 191–3.

7. Lieberman P, Nicklas RA, Oppenheimer J, et al. The diagnosis and management of anaphylaxis practice parameter: 2010 update. *J Allergy Clin Immunol* 2010; 126: 477–80.

8. Golden DBK, Moffit J, Nicklas RA. Stinging insect hypersensitivity: A practice parameter update 2011. *J Allergy Clin Immunol* 2011; 127: e1–23.

9. Lieberman P, Nicklas RA, Randolph C, et al. Anaphylaxis: A practice parameter update 2015. *Ann Allergy Asthma Immunol* 2015; 115: 341–84.

Breathing Complaints

Chapter **3**

Case 1

Contributing Author: Lauren Snyder

History

The patient is a healthy 3-year-old male who presents to the ED after a choking episode just prior to arrival. The child's mother reports that they were at home getting ready for church when she felt the child tap the back of her leg. The mother turned around and found the child unable to breathe. She swept the child's mouth with her finger, but didn't feel anything so she began to implement the Heimlich maneuver. She delivered approximately five thrusts without dislodging anything from the child's airway. When she turned the child around, she noticed the child was blue in the face. She again placed her finger in the child's mouth and this time felt an object. She was unable to get a hold of the object in order to remove it, so instead she pushed the object downwards. The child began to breathe, mother called 911 for transport to the ED. Mother reports that the child has been acting normally since the event, without respiratory distress and without additional choking episodes.

Past Medical History

- No significant medical history, immunizations are UTD. He lives with both parents.

Medications

- None.

Allergies

- NKDA.

Physical Examination and Ancillary Studies

- *Vital signs*: T 97.4 °F, HR 92, RR 22, O_2 sat 98% on room air.

- *General*: The patient is alert, smiling, playful, and in no acute distress.
- *HEENT*: The patient's head is atraumatic and normocephalic. PERRL. No conjunctival injection or discharge. Tympanic membranes normal bilaterally. Nares are patent with small amount of clear rhinorrhea. Oral examination shows mucosa that is pink and moist, no tonsillar swelling or exudates, and no foreign body.
- *Neck*: Supple and non-tender, with no masses.
- *Cardiovascular*: Heart with regular rate and rhythm, no M/R/G. The patient has normal peripheral perfusion, with brisk capillary refill.
- *Lungs*: CTA, with non-labored breathing and equal breath sounds bilaterally. No W/R/R. No retractions with respiration.
- *Abdomen*: Soft and non-tender, with normal active bowel sounds and without distension.
- *Skin and extremities*: Warm, dry, and intact, with no signs of trauma and no rashes.
- *Neurologic*: No focal neurologic deficits.
- *Pertinent ancillary studies*: CXR and abdominal series both normal.

Questions for Thought

- What is the importance of a normal CXR in this case?
- What is the disposition of this child, now that he is in the ED with a normal examination and CXR?
- What services (if any) should be consulted?
- What is the definitive procedure to diagnose and treat this condition?

Diagnosis

- Foreign-body aspiration.

Discussion

- *Epidemiology*: Foreign-body aspiration is a common occurrence in children, especially in toddlers, due to increasing mobility and oral exploration. Foreign-body aspiration can occur at any age; however, peak incidence is between 1 and 2 years of age, with 80 percent of foreign-body aspiration occurring in children less than 3 years old.[1,2] Commonly aspirated objects include small toys and food items, such as peanuts and sunflower seeds.[2,3]

    Pathophysiology: Children have immature or incomplete dentition and an imature swallowing reflex, predisposing them to an aspirated foreign body.[2] Young children also have a smaller-diameter airway, which puts them at increased risk for partial or complete obstruction if a foreign body is aspirated. Depending on the object, the child may have an inflammatory reaction, particularly with lipophilic foreign bodies (for example, peanuts).[2] Organic material, such as popcorn or items with high starch content, may absorb water over time, converting a partial obstruction to a complete one.[2] Aspirated foreign bodies are most often located in the bronchial tree, with laryngeal and tracheal foreign bodies occurring less frequently. The location of a foreign body partially determines the patient's presentation.

- *Presentation*: The clinical signs of foreign-body aspiration are highly variable, and depend on the location of the object in the respiratory tract and whether the object is mildly or severely obstructing the airway.

    Severe obstruction includes complete or near-complete blockage of the airway. Children with severe airway obstruction by a foreign object will present in respiratory distress that may include the inability to speak or cough, cyanosis, and abnormal behavior, most commonly lethargy or listlessness from their inability to adequately oxygenate.

- More commonly, aspirated foreign bodies will not cause severe airway obstruction, and the child may have little or no acute distress. Children will have various respiratory symptoms, which may include cough, stridor, or wheezing.[2] Wheezing, if present, can be localized to a specific area or generalized throughout the lung fields. The classic triad of wheezing, cough, and diminished breath sounds is not always present. In patients with subacute or chronic foreign body, the child may develop infection (such as post-obstructive pneumonia) and may present with fever. Some children present with no symptoms at all, and a foreign body is only suspected based on history, or after an extensive work-up excluding other pathologies.

- *Diagnosis*: Historical clues that can help lead to a diagnosis of airway foreign body include a sudden onset of respiratory distress, cough, or wheezing. Parents or caretakers may also report a choking episode, defined as a sudden onset of any of the following symptoms in a previously healthy child: cough, dyspnea, and/or cyanosis. A witnessed choking episode is very sensitive for the diagnosis of foreign-body aspiration. In a child with respiratory symptoms and a history of choking, foreign-body aspiration should be assumed regardless of radiologic findings, and rigid bronchoscopy should be performed.[4]

    In some cases, the aspiration of a foreign object is unwitnessed, and the child is without severe respiratory symptoms, making the diagnosis difficult. For any pediatric patient with a respiratory complaint and no obvious etiology, the practitioner should consider foreign-body aspiration and inquire about choking or coughing episodes. For children with confirmed foreign-body aspirations, a history of choking is found in the majority of cases (80–90 percent).[2]

    Additionally, an unwitnessed aspiration with minimal symptoms may go unnoticed by caregivers, so that by the time the child presents for medical evaluation, the foreign body may have been in the airway for days or weeks, causing secondary infection or inflammation. These cases of unwitnessed aspiration may have additional symptoms of fever, sputum production, and other signs and symptoms of pneumonia, which often leads to misdiagnosis.[2] Therefore, it is imperative to consider foreign-body aspiration in a child with unusual respiratory symptoms (i.e. sudden onset coughing fits in the absence of nasal congestion and fever), failure of treatment for another diagnosis (i.e. asthma, pneumonia), or multiple healthcare visits (pediatrician office or ED) with little or no resolution of symptoms after treatment.[2]

Radiographs may be helpful in the evaluation of a child with a suspected airway foreign body, although this is dependent on whether the aspirated object is radiopaque and the degree of airway obstruction present.[2] Abnormalities, when they exist, are usually visualized foreign bodies or an area of hyperinflation, best seen in bilateral decubitus CXR. In most cases, CXR will be normal, without visualization of a foreign body. Therefore, the diagnosis of airway foreign body should come primarily from historical clues and physical examination findings.

- *Treatment:* For children presenting with severe airway obstruction and active respiratory distress, attempts to dislodge the object must be made immediately. As with any critical patient, the practitioner should follow the ABC method of primary assessment, evaluating the airway and breathing of the patient first. Look inside the mouth of the child to evaluate for a visible foreign body. If an object is visualized and appears easy to remove, an attempt should be made to retrieve the object.[5] The American Heart Association does not recommend sweeping the mouth blindly with a finger, as this could move a foreign object further into the airway or worsen obstruction.[5] Per American Heart Association recommendations for patients with foreign-body airway obstruction, infants less than 1 year of age should have five back slaps followed by five chest thrusts administered to attempt to dislodge the foreign body, repeating this pattern until the object is dislodged or the child becomes unresponsive.[5] For children over 1 year of age, the Heimlich maneuver (abdominal thrusts) should be done until the object is dislodged or the child becomes unresponsive.[5] Of note, these maneuvers (back slaps and chest compressions) should only be attempted in children that are unable to speak or cough. In children with mild airway obstruction, these maneuvers have the potential to convert a mild obstruction into a severe obstruction.

  If these maneuvers are unsuccessful in dislodging the foreign body, direct laryngoscopy should be performed, in an attempt to visualize the object. If an object is visualized, an attempt

can be made to remove the object with Magill forceps. If an object is not visualized or the removal is unsuccessful, intubation should be attempted, with dislodgement of the object distally, usually into the right mainstem bronchus. This will allow partial ventilation of the unobstructed lung while awaiting rigid bronchoscopy for definitive removal of the foreign body.

Foreign bodies in the lower airway are usually removed via rigid bronchoscopy. Therefore, a consult to pulmonology or surgical services proficient at bronchoscope should be placed. Rigid bronchoscopy under general anesthesia allows airway control, good visualization of the airway and any foreign objects, and allows for manipulation/removal of the object with a variety of forceps. The procedure is both diagnostic and therapeutic, as it can identify and remove foreign bodies from the airway successfully in 95 percent of cases.[4] In rare instances, thoracotomy is indicated for foreign-body removal, if bronchoscopy is unsuccessful.

- *Disposition:* Once an aspirated foreign body is suspected based on history or examination, consultation with pulmonology or surgical services that are proficient at bronchoscope should be obtained. Hospital admission might also be required for additional medical care related to complications such as pneumonia and continued respiratory distress.

Historical clues	Physical findings	Ancillary studies
• Sudden onset of difficulty in breathing • Visualized foreign body by mom • High-risk age group	• Normal examination	• Normal CXR

Follow-Up

The child underwent rigid bronchoscopy, and a piece of red crayon was removed from the child's right mainstem bronchus. The child was kept in the hospital for observation for 23 hours and discharged home with no sequelae.

References

1. Centers for Disease Control and Prevention. Non-fatal choking-related episodes among children – United States, 2001. *MMWR Morb Mortal Wkly Rep* 2002; 51: 945–8.

2. Salih AM, Alfaki M, Alam-Elhuda DM. Airway foreign bodies: A critical review for a common pediatric emergency. *World J Emerg Med* 2016; 7: 5–12.

3. Foltran F, Ballali S, Passali FM, et al. Foreign bodies in the airways: A meta-analysis of published papers. *Int J Pediatr Otorhinolaryngol* 2012; 76 Suppl 1: S12–19.

4. Martinot A, Closset M, Marquette CH, et al. Indications for flexible versus rigid bronchoscopy in children with suspected foreign-body aspiration. *Am J Respir Crit Care Med* 1997; 155: 1676–9.

5. Neumar RW, Shuster M, Callaway CW, et al. Part 1: Executive summary. 2015 American Heart Association Guidelines Update for Cardiopulmonary Resuscitation and Emergency Cardiovascular Care. *Circulation* 2015; 132 Suppl 2: S315–67.

Case 2

Contributing Author: Natalie Moore

History

The patient is an 11-day-old female born at 34 weeks via spontaneous vaginal delivery, who was brought into the ED because her mom was worried about "abnormal breathing spasms." Mom noted that while the infant was sleeping today, she had several episodes of breathing quickly followed by 4–5 seconds of apnea. The breathing spells have been intermittent but mostly while she is sleeping. Mom has otherwise not noted any changes in color, tone, or mental status. The baby has not had any fevers, cough, rhinorrhea, vomiting, or diarrhea. She has been breastfeeding well every three hours. Mom called her pediatrician after the fifth breathing spasm and was told that, given the child's prematurity, the child should be evaluated in the ED.

Past Medical History

- The patient was born prematurely via spontaneous vaginal delivery at 34 and 2/7 weeks to a group B streptococci-negative mother. There were no significant perinatal complications and the pregnancy was uncomplicated.

Medications

- None.

Allergies

- NKDA.

Physical Examination and Ancillary Studies

- *Vital signs*: T 98.9 °F, HR 168, RR 54, O_2 sat 99% on room air.
- *General*: Awake and alert.
- *Skin*: Warm, dry, and intact. She has milia on her nose.
- *HEENT*: Her head is normocephalic. Her anterior fontanelle is soft and flat. PERRL. Normal oropharynx, with moist mucous membranes.
- *Neck*: Normal.
- *Cardiovascular*: Regular rate and rhythm. Peripheral pulses normal throughout. < 2 second capillary refill.
- *Lungs*: The patient's lung sounds are CTA and respirations are non-labored. She has symmetric chest-wall expansion.
- *Abdomen*: Non-tender and non-distended.
- *Neurologic*: Moro, grasp, and suck reflexes normal and symmetric. Good tone.

> **Questions for Thought**
>
> - What is the differential diagnosis?
> - What is the definition of apnea?
> - What should the disposition be for the child?
> - What specific characteristics of these episodes support admission for observation?

Diagnosis

- Periodic breathing.

Discussion

- *Epidemiology*: Periodic breathing is defined as recurring cycles of regular respiration interrupted by short pauses in respiration, which typically last somewhere between 3 and 10 seconds and are followed by bursts of rapid shallow breaths.[1] Then breathing returns to normal. It is termed periodic breathing if these episodes occur at least three times within a minute. Periodic breathing is considered to be a normal respiratory pattern in both preterm and full-term infants although it is reported more frequently in preterm infants.[1,2] This breathing pattern is estimated to occur in almost all preterm infants and between 70 and 95 percent of full-term infants.[1,2] The episodes are observed more frequently when the infant is sleeping. This normal respiratory pattern must be distinguished from an ALTE or apnea, which is defined as the cessation of breaths for over 20 seconds at a time or if the infant has a skin color change (pale or blue), becomes bradycardic, has a drop in oxygen saturation, becomes limp, or requires stimulation for the episode to end.[3] These signs are not considered normal and do not happen in periodic breathing. If these are noted, further work-up should be pursued to assess for an underlying pathologic etiology, such as infection, CHD, metabolic derangements, airway obstruction, child abuse, or GI pathologies, among other causes.[4,5]

- *Pathophysiology*: Periodic breathing is thought to be a manifestation of immature ventilatory control and thus is common in preterm infants and occurs less frequently as the infant matures.[2] Periodic breathing typically begins around the first week of age, which corresponds to when the infant's peripheral chemoreceptors begin to mature. When the infant is born, the peripheral chemoreceptors are not sensitive, and as the chemoreceptors begin to mature, they become highly sensitive to changes in blood oxygen and carbon dioxide concentrations.[2] This leads to fluctuating breathing patterns of short periods of apnea followed by hyperventilation.

- *Presentation*: The classic presentation for periodic breathing is a preterm infant presenting with "abnormal breathing," or the chief complaint of "my infant stopped breathing." The caregiver describes a brief cessation of breathing, usually less than 10 seconds, followed by rapid, shallow breaths. This is normally observed while the infant is sleeping and occurs more often in rapid eye movement sleep and in a recurrent fashion.

  A patient with periodic breathing will have a completely normal physical examination. It is important to remember that this is a diagnosis of exclusion, and an assessment for other underlying pathology is required. A complete physical examination must include the following: assess vital signs for fever, bradycardia or tachycardia, and observe for an abnormal oxygen saturation; assess skin color and condition carefully for pallor or cyanosis; assess for nasal flaring, retractions, or any signs of increased respiratory difficulty; listen for murmurs and look for other signs of CHF and CHD; carefully assess the infant's tone and perform an abdominal examination; always assess for signs of non-accidental trauma.

- *Diagnosis*: Periodic breathing is a clinical diagnosis. Differential diagnosis includes apnea (and characteristics associated with an ALTE), respiratory disease (bronchiolitis, pneumonia), sepsis, CNS pathology, meningitis, seizures, increased intracranial pressure, metabolic derangements, CHD, upper-airway obstruction, aspiration, and GI pathology.[3-5] When the history is consistent with periodic breathing and the patient has a normal physical examination, the diagnosis can be made clinically. However, if any alternative diagnoses are considered, further diagnostic work-up should be performed. If the patient is having a significant amount of periodic breathing, the pediatrician may consider home-monitoring or polysomnography to assess the frequency of events and associated bradycardia or hypoxia, but these do not need to be performed in the ED.

- *Treatment*: None.

- *Disposition*: Patients with a normal physical examination and a clinical picture, consistent with periodic breathing, can be discharged home to follow up with their pediatrician. If any of the characteristics of apnea (cessation of breaths for over 20 seconds, skin color change, bradycardia, hypoxia, or change in tone) are present, or signs of underlying infection or other pathology are noted, further work-up should be pursued.

Historical clues	Physical findings
• Otherwise healthy preterm infant • Brief apnea with hyperventilation • Recurrent episodes	• Normal examination

Follow-Up

Mom was reassured and the child was discharged home. There were no sequelae at follow-up.

References

1. Glotzbach SF, Baldwin RB, Lederer NE, et al. Periodic breathing in preterm infants: Incidence and characteristics. *Pediatrics* 1989; 84: 785–92.

2. Mohr MA, Fairchild KD, Patel M, et al. Qualification of periodic breathing in premature infants. *Physiol Meas* 2015; 36: 1415–27.

3. American Academy of Pediatrics Policy Statement, Committee on Fetus and Newborn. Apnea, sudden infant death syndrome, and home monitoring. *Pediatrics* 2003; 111: 914–17.

4. Semmekrot BA, van Sleuwen BE, Engelberts AC, et al. Surveillance study of apparent life-threatening events (ALTE) in Netherlands. *Eur J Pediatr* 2010; 169: 229–36.

5. Tieder JS, Altman RL, Bonkowsky JL, et al. Management of apparent life threatening events in infants: A systematic review. *J Pediatr* 2013; 163: 94–9.

Case 3

Contributing Author: Dorka M. Jiménez Almonte

History

A 2-month-old baby girl presents with noisy breathing after feedings for the past 2 weeks, worsening over the last few days. The mother reports that the baby becomes fussy, sometimes appears breathless and sounds congested after feedings. She denies any fever, cough, nasal discharge, or cyanosis. The mother describes that the infant has had spit-ups with every feed since birth, but that more recently the amount she spits up has increased. She is very concerned that the baby appears to be in pain and has not been nursing as well in the last few days. The child latches to the breast and then unlatches before completing the feed and cries. The infant has also been arching her back during feedings. She has had no change in urination or stools. Mom specifically reports approximately eight wet diapers and two to three soft, yellowish, seedy bowel movements per day. The mother denies any skin rash or blood in the stool. There are no sick contacts at home.

Past Medical History

- The patient was born to a first-time mother via spontaneous vaginal delivery at 39 weeks' gestation, without complications. Mother had adequate prenatal care and denies any complications during pregnancy. The birth weight was 3.5 kg. The newborn screen was normal and the immunizations are current.

Medications

- Vitamin D drops.

Allergies

- NKDA.

Physical Examination and Ancillary Studies

- *Vital signs*: T 98.9 °F, HR 110, RR 35, O_2 sat on room air 100%, weight 5.4 kg.
- *General*: Awake, alert, and in no distress. She appears very comfortable in her mother's arms, turns toward mother's voice and smiles.
- *HEENT*: Anterior fontanelle is soft and flat. PERRL. Moist mucous membranes. There is no pharyngeal erythema, no whitish membranes, and no oral lesions. Tympanic membranes are clear. There is no nasal discharge. Mild audible upper-airway sounds, no stridor.
- *Cardiovascular*: Heart has regular rate and rhythm, with no M/R/G. Patient has equal femoral pulses. Capillary refill < 2 seconds.
- *Lungs*: Chest expansion symmetric. No retractions. CTA bilaterally, no W/R/R.
- *Abdomen*: The abdomen is not distended. The patient has normal bowel sounds. Her abdomen is soft and depressible. There is no tenderness to palpation and no masses or organomegaly.
- *Extremities and skin*: The patient has no rash or edema.
- *Neurologic*: Infant moves all four extremities well. Her tone is appropriate for her age. She has symmetric Moro reflex and has adequate head control for her age.

Questions for Thought

- What is the differential diagnosis for this patient's symptoms?
- What diagnostic modalities, if any, could you use to evaluate this patient?
- How would you describe this patient's airway?
- What interventions should be done in the ED?
- What is the prognosis for this condition?

Diagnosis

- GERD.

Discussion

- *Epidemiology*: Gastroesophageal reflux is the passage of stomach contents into the esophagus with or without regurgitation (spitting up) or vomiting. Gastroesophageal reflux is a normal physiologic process that occurs in more than two-thirds of healthy infants. The frequency of reflux episodes and the proportion of episodes that result in regurgitation peak at the age of 4 months and then resolves with age in most cases.[1,2] Physiologic spitting up affects only 5–10 percent of infants at 12 months of age and is very rare in children older than 18 months.[1-3] Gastroesophageal reflux disease (GERD) is significantly less common than gastroesophageal reflux and is characterized by troublesome symptoms or complications associated with the passage of stomach contents into the esophagus. Children with certain underlying conditions such as neurologic impairment, developmental delay, prematurity, anatomic abnormalities (esophageal atresia, hiatal hernia), and chronic respiratory disorders such as bronchopulmonary dysplasia, idiopathic interstitial fibrosis, and cystic fibrosis, are at high risk for developing severe chronic GERD.[1,2]

- *Pathophysiology*: The primary mechanism in reflux is transient lower esophageal sphincter relaxation, unaccompanied by swallowing. In addition, gastric distension due to large volume feeds in small stomachs, and delayed gastric emptying, increases the frequency of lower esophageal sphincter relaxation in infants. Also gravitational/positional factors (lying in a flat supine position) may predispose infants to gastroesophageal reflux. Alterations in protective mechanisms, such as the clearance of regurgitated gastric contents and gastric epithelium repair, enable physiologic reflux to develop into GERD.[1-3] Clustering of GERD symptoms in families suggests some heritability of the disease.

- *Presentation:* The most common presentation for gastroesophageal reflux is spitting up. Infants with physiologic reflux present with a history of regurgitation but have no signs of discomfort and no problems with weight gain.[1] These babies are typically described as "happy spitters" as they appear happy and undisturbed by spitting up although the caregivers often have significant concerns about it. Infants with GERD usually present with regurgitation or vomiting associated with irritability, feeding difficulties, poor weight-gain, arching of the back during feedings, or respiratory symptoms such as cough, gagging,

Table 3.1 Reflux differential diagnosis and associated red flags

Differential diagnosis	Red flags
• Pyloric stenosis	• Projectile vomiting
• Malrotation, volvulus	• Bilious vomiting, distension
• Cow milk protein intolerance	• Perianal rash, blood in the stool, diarrhea
• Gastroenteritis	• Fever, diarrhea
• UTI	• Fever
• Urinary obstruction	• Failure to thrive, recurrent UTIs
• Pneumonia, bronchiolitis	• Fever, cough, nasal discharge, wheezing, crackles, rhonchi, respiratory distress
• Meningitis	• Fever, altered mental status, petechial rash, bulging fontanelle, seizures
• Hydrocephalus	• Rapid increase in head circumference, downward deviation of eyes ("sun setting"), seizures, developmental delay
• Metabolic/genetic disorders	• Failure to thrive, developmental delay, seizures, hepatomegaly, macro/microcephaly

or wheezing. Rarely, infants may present with ALTEs and Sandifer syndrome (abnormal posturing or spells of generalized stiffening, occurring within 30 minutes following a feeding).

- *Diagnosis:* The diagnosis of physiologic gastroesophageal reflux in infants is a clinical diagnosis based on a thorough history and physical examination.[1-3] In older children, the clinical diagnosis of GERD is usually made when the characteristic symptoms of heartburn, regurgitation, and epigastric pain are present. A 2–4 week empiric treatment trial with acid suppressants is recommended for these children and a positive response to treatment is considered diagnostic.[1,2] No specific group of symptoms has been found to be reliable for the diagnosis of GERD in infants, however; it is still generally a clinical diagnosis. Laboratory studies are not necessary for the diagnosis of GERD but are utilized to investigate possible causes of failure to thrive in infants with a history of weight loss despite adequate caloric intake. Diagnostic evaluation is indicated only if there are the presence of red flags, concerns with complications related to GERD, or if the diagnosis is uncertain (Table 3.1).[1-3] Diagnostic methods most commonly used are barium upper GI series, esophageal and/or impedance pH monitoring, and upper endoscopy with biopsy.

- *Treatment*: Lifestyle modifications are emphasized as treatment of gastroesophageal reflux and GERD. In infants, feeding changes such as reducing the feeding volume, increasing the frequency of feedings, and positional changes such as keeping infants upright during feedings and for 30 minutes after feedings are recommended.[1-3] Semi-supine positioning (seating in a carrier or carseat) should be avoided as it may exacerbate reflux.[2] Prone position compared to supine position has been shown to decrease the number of episodes of gastroesophageal reflux in infants but infants should not sleep in the prone position because of the increased risk of sudden infant death syndrome (SIDS).[1,2] Current guidelines strongly recommend that infants should sleep in the supine position until the age of 12 months. For formula-fed infants, modifications including thickening the formula with rice cereal or changing to a commercially thickened formula may have some benefit.[1-3] First-line pharmacologic therapy for GERD consists of acid suppressants, specifically histamine 2-receptor antagonists and proton pump inhibitors.[1,2] Prokinetic agents and surface agents are also used in the treatment of GERD but are not as effective as acid suppressants. Finally, patients with severe symptoms or severe complications from GERD may benefit from surgical intervention (funduplication).

Historical clues	Physical findings
<ul><li>History of regurgitation</li><li>Presence of troublesome symptoms associated with regurgitation: irritability, discomfort with feedings, feeding refusal, respiratory symptoms in the absence of signs of infection</li><li>No red-flag historical items</li></ul>	<ul><li>Normal examination</li><li>Normal weight gain for age (1 kg per month in the first 3 months of life)</li></ul>

Follow-Up

The patient was observed during a feeding cycle and nursed well; however, she frequently unlatched from the breast. She was observed to occasionally arch her back when unlatching and did have a few non-bilious spit-ups. No signs of respiratory distress or significant changes in vital signs were noted and the physical examination was unchanged from previous. Lifestyle modifications (smaller, more frequent feedings and keeping the baby upright during and after feedings) were recommended. The patient was discharged with outpatient follow-up.

References

1. Vandenplas Y, Rudolh CD, DiLorenzo C, et al. Pediatric gastroesophageal reflux clinical practice guidelines: Joint recommendations of the North American Society for Pediatric Gastroenterology, Hepatology, and Nutrition (NASPGHAN) and the European Society for Pediatric Gastroenterology, Hepatology and Nutrition (ESPGHAN). *J Pediatr Gastroenterol Nutr* 2009; 49: 498–547.

2. Lightdale JR, Grense DA, Section on Gastroenterology, Hepatology and Nutrition. Gastroesophaegeal reflux: Management Guidance for the Pediatrician. *Pediatrics* 2013; 131: 1684–95.

3. Sullivan JS, Sundaram SS. Gastroesophageal reflux. *Pediatr Rev* 2012; 33: 243–53.

Case 4

Contributing Author: Amanda Shorette

History

The patient is a 5-week-old full-term infant female who presents by ambulance to a community hospital with difficulty in breathing. Her mother describes 2 days of fussiness followed by 1 day of cough, sneezing, watery eyes, and increased nasal and oral secretions. She has had two episodes of non-bloody, non-bilious emesis over the past couple days but otherwise has been breastfeeding and eliminating normally. Her mother denies fevers, cyanosis or color change, rash, or diarrhea. Per EMS, the child was noted to be tachypneic with grunting respirations and mild hypoxia (O_2 sat 91–92% on room air). They placed her on a non-rebreather mask with improvement in oxygen saturations to 99%.

Past Medical History

- The patient was born full-term via c-section for non-reassuring fetal heart rate tracings but had no significant perinatal complications. She has no chronic medical problems and lives at home with her parents.

Medications

- None.

Allergies

- NKDA.

Physical Examination and Ancillary Studies

- *Vital signs*: T 98.7 °F, HR 182, RR 62, BP 109/66. O_2 sat 82% on room air. She is placed on high-flow nasal cannula oxygen at 5 L/min and 30% oxygen, with improvement of her saturation to 96%.
- *General*: The patient is awake and alert but ill-appearing. She appears uncomfortable with labored respirations. She is pink in color and she has good tone.
- *HEENT*: Mucous membranes are moist with thick nasal secretions. There are no oropharyngeal lesions or exudates.
- *Cardiovascular*: The heart rate is tachycardic, with a regular rhythm. No M/R/G.
- *Lungs:* The child is grunting, tachypneic, and has intercostal retractions. Diffuse rhonchi are heard bilaterally as are transmitted upper-airway sounds.
- *Abdomen*: The abdomen is soft, non-tender, and non-distended, with normal bowel sounds.
- *Skin*: The skin is warm and well-perfused, without central or peripheral cyanosis. There is no rash visualized.
- *Neurologic*: Alert and interactive, with good tone, intact reflexes. Fussy.
- *Pertinent laboratory values*: WBC 6,400 with a differential of 77% lymphocytes. Hb 10.6. Plt 438,000. PCR positive for RSV.

Questions for Thought

- What are the typical presenting features of this diagnosis?
- Is ancillary testing helpful in the evaluation of this patient?
- When should more aggressive airway support be considered?
- Is there any benefit to beta-agonist therapy, hypertonic saline, or systemic glucocorticoids?
- When should inpatient admission for this condition be considered?

Diagnosis

- RSV bronchiolitis with impending respiratory failure.

Discussion

- *Epidemiology*: Bronchiolitis is an acute inflammatory disease caused by a viral, lower respiratory tract infection in infants. It is a clinical syndrome seen almost exclusively in children younger than 2 years of age and is the leading cause of hospitalization in infancy in the USA, accounting for about 3 percent of all hospitalizations in the first 12 months of life.[1,2] There are approximately 100,000 admissions for bronchiolitis in the USA annually, with an estimated cost of 1.73 billion dollars.[1] A CDC-sponsored study reported an average RSV hospitalization rate of 5.2 per 1,000 children under 24 months of age, with younger infants (30–60 days of age) and very preterm infants (born < 30 weeks' gestation) having the highest age-specific rate of RSV hospitalization.[1] Bronchiolitis has a seasonal pattern, with the highest rates of infection occurring between December and March in North America; however, regional variations do occur. RSV is the most common etiology of bronchiolitis, accounting for approximately 70 percent of all cases; however, other viruses can cause bronchiolitis. These include, but are not limited to, human rhinovirus, human metapneumovirus, influenza, adenovirus, coronavirus, and parainfluenza viruses. Infection with RSV does not confer permanent or long-term immunity so re-infections are common throughout life.
- *Pathophysiology*: Bronchiolitis is characterized by acute inflammation, edema, and necrosis of the epithelial cells which line small airways, with subsequent sloughing, accumulation of intraluminal debris, and increased mucous production.[1,2] Because non-ciliated cuboidal epithelial cells initially replace ciliated epithelial cells, there is inadequate mobilization of secretions and cellular debris, resulting in increased small airway obstruction and mucous plugging. This variable obstruction throughout the airways results in ventilation/perfusion mismatching, with resultant hypoxia and compensatory hyperventilation. In addition, air

trapping and atelectasis can occur distal to bronchiole obstruction. Hypercarbia may occur and is a very concerning finding, indicating that the obstructive process is severe and/or that the patient is experiencing respiratory fatigue. Functional regeneration of ciliated epithelium usually requires approximately 2 weeks, and children may continue coughing for over a month after infection.[2]

- *Presentation*: Regardless of the infectious etiologic agent, infants and children with bronchiolitis generally have a similar disease course, which typically begins as a viral upper respiratory tract prodrome followed by wheezing and increased respiratory effort. Symptoms include rhinorrhea, cough, low-grade fever, and anorexia in the first 1–2 days. As the lower airways become involved and obstruction occurs, this prodromal phase is then followed by tachypnea, wheezing, rales, and increased work of breathing, which can manifest as use of accessory muscles (intercostal retractions, substernal retractions, diaphragmatic breathing, tracheal tugging), grunting, head bobbing, and/or nasal flaring. Shallow respirations and a hyperinflated chest may be appreciated due to air trapping. Hypoxia is also a frequent finding. Children with bronchiolitis may be dehydrated due to a combination of limited oral intake from increased work of breathing and increased insensible losses from fever and tachypnea. Disease severity, however, can be quite variable, ranging from minimal cough to progressive respiratory distress, resulting in respiratory failure.

  Apnea is also associated with the disease process. Interestingly, apnea generally occurs very early on in the illness and often prior to the onset of other respiratory symptoms. Among patients infected with RSV, apnea occurs in about 1 percent of healthy term infants, with rates as high as 24 percent in those with risk factors such as very young age and prematurity.[3] The acute phase of bronchiolitis tends to be short-lived, with disease severity peaking around day 5–7 of illness; however, residual symptoms may persist for weeks.[2]

- *Diagnosis*: The diagnosis of bronchiolitis is a clinical one based on history and physical examination, specifically the history of viral URI prodromal symptoms followed by signs/symptoms of lower-airway-tract involvement in a child less than 2 years old. In addition, an assessment of disease severity should be made on a clinical basis. Specific variables have not been reliably correlated with outcomes but, in general, a child's respiratory rate, degree/persistence of hypoxia, work of breathing, mental status, and perfusion should be assessed. In addition, it is imperative that the clinician performs *serial examinations* in order to more accurately assess a child's respiratory status given the substantial temporal variability in physical findings in infants with bronchiolitis; at any given moment, a child's degree of agitation, mucous plugging, upper-airway obstruction, and even positioning can alter a respiratory examination.

  Ancillary tests, including laboratory studies, viral serology, and chest radiography, are generally not helpful in either the diagnosis or the assessment of disease severity and are therefore not routinely recommended per the AAP practice guidelines.[1-4] CXR in particular has not been demonstrated by current evidence to correlate with disease severity. CXR is likely to be abnormal in bronchiolitics, with findings including hyperinflation, peribronchial cuffing, and subsegmental atelectasis. Such findings may result in inappropriate antibiotics use, as suggested by one study cited by the AAP guidelines.[1] The AAP recommends CXR be reserved only for cases of severe respiratory distress, warranting ICU level of care, or where signs of airway complications (i.e. pneumothorax, foreign body) exist.

- *Treatment*: Therapy is supportive with analgesia, antipyretics, rehydration, and airway support.[1-4] The AAP does not recommend using beta-agonist therapy, antibiotics, systemic glucocorticoids, or chest physiotherapy in the treatment of bronchiolitis.[1-4] Hypertonic saline (3%) has been shown to have some benefit in the inpatient setting but has not been shown to reduce hospitalization rates in the ED setting.[1] Suctioning of the nasopharynx is a common practice, and may transiently improve nasal congestion and upper-airway obstruction; however, evidence is lacking to support routine use of this. Supplemental oxygen is indicated for SpO_2 persistently $< 90\%$ in previously healthy infants.[1-3] The AAP recommends discontinuing supplemental oxygen for $SpO_2 > 90\%$.[1]

Increasing evidence suggests that continuous pulse oximetry monitoring is not required, especially in stable and overall well-appearing bronchiolitics. This may lead to unnecessary hospital stays and prolonged length of stay given that normal, healthy infants often have transient desaturations into the low 80s. If indicated, there are multiple methods of oxygen delivery including nasal cannula, non-rebreather, and high-flow nasal cannula. There are retrospective studies showing that a high-flow nasal cannula reduces the work of breathing through generation of CPAP, with a decline in the need for intubation; however, given the lack of data, the AAP cannot make specific recommendations regarding its use.[1] There are no absolute criteria for endotracheal intubation and mechanical ventilation; however, the following indicators should prompt consideration for more aggressive airway management: hypercarbia greater than 60–65 mmHg, poor respiratory effort or fatigue, depressed mental status, recurrent apneic spells, and persistent hypoxia despite oxygen therapy.[1-4]

- *Disposition*: The clinician should assess both disease severity and risk for apnea. Full-term infants < 1 month of age, preterm infants < 2 months of age, children with underlying neuromuscular disorders, those with chronic lung disease or congenital heart disease, and children with a history of previous apneic events are at a higher risk for apnea and warrant admission and monitoring.[1,2] Other indications for admission include recurrent apneic episodes, persistent tachypnea greater than 70, severe work of breathing, alterations in mental status, inability to tolerate feeds as a result of work of breathing, and poor hydration status.[1-3] In addition, it is important to assess the ability of the family to care for the child and their ability to return for further evaluation if needed. Children with unreliable follow-up may need to be observed in the hospital.

Historical clues	Physical findings	Ancillary studies
• Viral prodromal symptoms • Progressive respiratory distress • High-risk age group	• Tachypnea • Increased work of breathing • Retractions • Hypoxia • Diffuse rhonchi and wheezing	• PCR positive for RSV

Follow-Up

This patient was stabilized in the ED after brief suctioning of copious thick, yellow secretions and placement on high-flow nasal cannula. Despite supportive therapy and titration of her high-flow settings on the floor, her work of breathing progressively worsened. Approximately 12 hours after admission, the patient went into hypercarbic respiratory failure due to fatigue and severe mucous plugging, ultimately requiring intubation and transfer to the PICU. She was weaned from the ventilator 1 week later and quickly transitioned to room air. She was discharged in good health from the hospital without need for further respiratory support after a 2-week hospital stay.

Further reading

1. Ralston SL, Lieberthal AS, Meissner HC, et al. Clinical practice guideline: The diagnosis, management, and prevention of bronchiolitis. *Pediatrics* 2014; 134: 1474–89.

2. Joseph M, Witt M, Sharieff GG. Evidence-based assessment and management of acute bronchiolitis in the emergency department. *Emerg Med Pract* 2011; 8: 1–20.

3. Ravaglia C, Poletti V. Recent advances in the management of acute bronchiolitis. *F1000Prime Rep* 2014; 6: 103.

4. Johnson LW, Robles J, Hudgins A, et al. Management of bronchiolitis in the emergency department: Impact of evidence-based guidelines? *Pediatrics* 2013; 131 Suppl 1: S103–9.

Case 5

Contributing Author: M. Bryan Dalla Betta

History

A 6-year-old male presents to the ED with shortness of breath and wheezing for the last day. His mother states that he began having nasal congestion, cough, and rhinorrhea 3 days ago. She notes that he has had similar difficulty in breathing in the past that has sometimes been associated with changes in temperatures or "colds." Symptoms became worse overnight and the patient had difficulty sleeping due to increasing cough. There has been no fever, nausea, vomiting, rash, or complaints of abdominal discomfort. The mother says the child has been less active over the last day but has been eating and drinking normally. The cough is non-productive and there are no known family sick contacts, although she notes some of the child's class-mates have had similar symptoms recently. The child has been using an albuterol inhaler over the last day every four hours, which provides only temporary relief of his symptoms.

Past Medical History

- The patient has a history of both asthma and eczema. Immunizations are UTD.

Medications

- Intermittent albuterol.

Allergies

- NKDA.

Physical Examination and Ancillary Studies

- *Vital signs*: T 99 °F, HR 115, RR 28, BP 122/78, O_2 sat 91% on room air.
- *General*: Awake and alert, looking around the room. He is well-nourished but tired-appearing, sitting forward slightly and appearing mildly anxious. He has a normal body habitus for his age.
- *HEENT*: Posterior pharyngeal erythema but no exudate. There is slight cobble-stoning to the posterior pharynx. There is clear rhinorrhea about the nares.
- *Neck*: Supple, with no JVD or subcutaneous air. Trachea is midline.
- *Cardiovascular*: The heart rate is increased but the rhythm is regular. No M/R/G.
- *Lungs*: The respiratory rate is increased and there are intercostal retractions bilaterally, with some suprasternal retractions. There is bilateral inspiratory and expiratory wheezing on auscultation, without rhonchi.
- *Abdomen*: Abdomen is soft, non-tender, and non-distended, without masses or scars.
- *Skin and extremities*: No rashes or pallor. No peripheral edema, swelling, or deformity.
- *Neurologic*: PERRL. Cranial nerves intact. No focal deficit. Normal alertness.
- *Pertinent laboratory values*: WBC 13,300, Hb 13.9, Plt 234,000, bicarbonate 21, all others normal.
- *Pertinent radiologic studies:* CXR with hyperinflation, no pneumothorax, no infiltrate.

Questions for Thought

- What about this patient's physical examination is concerning?
- What therapies are indicated immediately?
- How would you treat this patient if he worsens or does not respond to initial treatment?
- Does a CXR need to be done in all children with these symptoms?

Diagnosis

- Acute asthma exacerbation.

Discussion

- *Epidemiology*: Asthma affected 25 million people in the USA in 2010, including 7 million children under 18 years of age.[1] Asthma prevalence in the USA increased from 5.5 percent in 1996 to 8.4 percent in 2010.[1] In pediatrics, asthma prevalence is highest in males of 5–14 years of age, and is more prevalent in African Americans than any other race.[1] Geographically, the Northeast and Midwest have the highest prevalence of asthma in the USA.
- *Pathophysiology*: Much remains to be learned about the exact mechanism of airflow obstruction in asthma. Asthma is an obstructive process that often begins when a stimulus or "trigger" precipitates inflammatory change in the peripheral airways. Triggers can range from exercise to viral respiratory infection, exposure to pharmacologic agents, or contact with allergens.[2,3] These triggering molecules activate mast cells, eosinophils, and other cells of the immune system that cause the release of histamine, cytokines, and other inflammatory mediators into the lung vasculature.
- Build-up of inflammatory mediators causes mucous hypersecretion, increased bronchial blood flow, and increased vascular permeability. As the tissues around the bronchioles swell and smooth muscles around the airways contract, mucous plugs form in the bronchioles.[2–4] Air-trapping in the distal airways causes impaired exhalation and eventually dyspnea, as less and less air is able to enter the alveoli.
- *Presentation*: Acute asthma exacerbations can present with great variability. Some patients will have only dry cough, variable wheezing, and

subjective difficulty breathing or chest tightness with normal vital signs.[2,3] Others present in extremis, with tachycardia, decreased oxygen saturation, increased respiratory rate, and accessory muscle use.[2,3] Patients with severe exacerbations typically have poor air movement on auscultation and appear anxious. Wheezing can be variable and does not necessarily correlate with the severity of airway compromise.

Typically, children will present with a history of dry, non-productive cough, chest tightness, and worsening shortness of breath. Symptoms are frequently worse at night and wheezing is common, but not always present. In patients with an established diagnosis of asthma, it can be helpful to ask about exacerbating factors or triggers. Symptom onset after respiratory infections, exercise, allergen or smoke exposure, or a history of seasonal allergy symptoms can aid in diagnosis when the presentation is atypical.

- *Diagnosis*: Asthma should be suspected based on the presence of typical symptoms and suggestive physical examination findings such as retractions or wheezing.[2-4] Elements of history supporting the diagnosis consist of non-productive cough that can be nocturnal or seasonal, with chest tightness and dyspnea. Many patients will have symptom onset after precipitating factors or "triggers." Examples include respiratory infections, smoke, allergens (dust, pollen), exercise, or changes in weather and temperature. Characteristically, cough is accompanied by wheezing – a high-pitched musical sound – that can be heard on auscultation. Patients with more severe symptoms will have retractions.

When asthma is suspected, spirometry is commonly used to confirm the diagnosis.[2-4] Spirometry measurements of interest include the forced expiratory volume in 1 second (FEV1), and the forced vital capacity (FVC).[2-4] It is important to note that spirometry plays virtually no role in the ED management of a child with suspected asthma exacerbation, and should be done outpatient, after the acute exacerbation has been managed.

In patients with suspected or known prior asthma and typical symptoms, CXR is not necessary. When patients fail to improve with appropriate therapy, CXR is reasonable to rule out comorbid processes, such as pneumonia or foreign body, and to assess for complications of asthma such as pneumothorax. Most of the time, CXR during an acute asthma exacerbation will be normal or demonstrate hyperinflation.

- *Treatment*: There are multiple treatment options for children presenting to the ED with asthma exacerbation, with the mainstays being inhaled beta-agonists and systemic glucocorticoids.[5-8] Inhaled beta-agonists are the most effective means for rapidly improving symptoms, and they should be started as soon as possible in the child presenting with respiratory difficulty due to asthma exacerbation.[4-7] Administration via metered-dose inhaler, intermittent nebulizer, and continuous nebulizer are all acceptable, but continuous nebulization is usually reserved for children with symptoms refractory to initial treatment with a metered-dose inhaler or intermittent nebulized albuterol.

Glucocorticoids should also be started as soon as possible in the child with asthma exacerbation.[9,10] Prednisone and dexamethasone are both reasonable choices and have been shown to be similarly effective as treatment options.[9,10] Dosing is weight-based and duration of treatment is typically 3–5 days for prednisone. There does not seem to be added benefit of IV administration over oral administration if the child is capable of tolerating oral steroids.

Another treatment option for asthma exacerbations includes inhaled ipratropium, an anticholinergic agent that can be given with albuterol. This drug facilitates relaxation of smooth muscles and decreases bronchospasm. When co-administered with albuterol it can improve lung function and decrease admission rates in children with moderate to severe exacerbations.[8]

Additional treatment options exist for more serious exacerbations, or if initial interventions fail to significantly improve symptoms. One such agent is IV magnesium sulfate. It is thought to aid smooth muscle relaxation and bronchodilation, and may decrease the need for hospital admission.[11] When inhaled beta-agonists fail, IV or IM beta-agonists like epinephrine or terbutaline can be used.[6,7] Both can be given as an IM injection to patients presenting with severe symptoms who may be anxious, uncooperative, or have poor inspiratory flow, preventing effective inhaled beta-agonist treatment. Patients with rapid deterioration or persistent worsening of symptoms may require intubation and sedation for continued treatment or respiratory support.

- *Disposition*: Several factors are involved when deciding to discharge a patient home or admit to the hospital following an asthma exacerbation. Chief among these is the amount of clinical improvement the patient has made, and the amount of therapy required in the ED. Patients requiring high doses of inhaled beta-agonists, IM or IV beta-agonists, or those who have had minimal or transient improvement should be admitted for further therapy. However, use of second-tier therapies like magnesium sulfate do not always mandate admission. Clinicians should use clinical judgment when determining the disposition of these patients.

Conversely, patients presenting with mild to moderate symptoms that respond well to inhaled beta-agonists and glucocorticoids should be considered for discharge home if they appear clinically improved. Social factors, such as the ability to return for worsening symptoms, the reliability of parents to notice worsening symptoms, and the means to obtain and reliably follow an outpatient treatment plan, should also be assessed when attempting to determine disposition. Also important is the ability for discharged patients to be seen in follow-up for reassessment and continued treatment by their clinician.

Historical clues	Physical findings	Ancillary studies
• Recent URI • Exposure to known trigger • Non-productive cough • Cough worse at night	• Dry cough • Wheezes • Retractions/accessory muscle use • Tachypnea • Relative hypoxia	• Hyperinflated CXR • Respiratory alkalosis

Follow-Up

The patient in this case received oral steroids and two treatments of 7.5 mg nebulized albuterol as well as ipratropium in the ED. After interventions he was still found to be wheezing diffusely and slightly tachypnic, with no improvement in oral intake or activity. He was admitted to the pediatric ward for further treatment of his asthma exacerbation and was discharged the

following day after significant improvement in respiratory status.

References

1. Centers for Disease Control and Prevention. Most recent asthma data. http://www.cdc.gov/asthma/most_recent_data.htm (accessed February 2016).
2. Wood PR, Hill VL. Practical management of asthma. *Pediatr Rev* 2009; 30: 375–85.
3. Bush A, Fleming L. Diagnosis and management of asthma in children. *BMJ* 2015; 350: h996.
4. National Heart, Blood, and Lung Institute. National Asthma Education and Prevention Program. Expert Panel Report 3: Guidelines for the Diagnosis and Management of Asthma. Bethesda, MD: National Institutes of Health, 2007.
5. Scarfone RJ, Friedlaender EY. β2-Agonists in acute asthma: The evolving state of the art. *Pediatr Emerg Care* 2002; 18: 442–7.
6. Sellers WF. Inhaled and intravenous treatment in acute severe and life-threatening asthma. *Br J Anaesth* 2013; 110: 183–90.
7. Suau SJ, DeBlieux PM. Management of acute exacerbation of asthma and chronic obstructive pulmonary disease in the emergency department. *Med Clin North Am* 2016; 34: 15–37.
8. Griffiths B, Ducharme FM. Combined inhaled anticholinergics and short-acting beta 2-agonists for initial treatment of acute asthma in children. *Cochrane Database Syst Rev* 2013; 8: CD000060.
9. Rowe BH, Spooner C, Ducharme F, et al. Early emergency department treatment of acute asthma with systemic corticosteroids. *Cochrane Database Syst Rev* 2001; 1: CD002178.
10. Keeney GE, Gray MP, Morrison AK, et al. Dexamethasone for acute asthma exacerbations in children: A meta-analysis. *Pediatrics* 2014; 133: 493–9.
11. Rowe BH, Bretzlaff JA, Bourdon C, et al. Intravenous magnesium sulfate treatment for acute asthma in the emergency department: A systematic review of the literature. *Ann Emerg Med* 2000; 36: 181–90.

Case 6

Contributing Authors: Daniel K. Pauzé and Denis R. Pauzé

History

The patient is a 25-day-old girl who presents after having an episode where she stopped breathing and changed color. This child was born 4 weeks early by spontaneous vaginal delivery. She has been completely well until today, when the father noticed that the child had an episode where she stopped breathing, turned blue, and went limp. This lasted for about 30 seconds and then the baby returned back to normal. This has never occurred before. The episode occurred about an hour after her noon feed. The dad notes she has no fever, irritability, lethargy, vomiting, diarrhea, or cough. She has been eating normally and has had good urine output. She has no history of trauma, no previous ED visits, and no family history of similar events.

Past Medical History

- The patient was born at 36 weeks and has no significant past medical history. The mother has no significant perinatal history.

Medications

- The patient takes no medications.

Allergies

- NKDA.

Physical Examination and Ancillary Studies

- *Vital signs*: T 97.9 °F, HR 148, RR 40, BP 80/40, O_2 sat 99% on room air.
- *General*: The patient is a well-developed female, in no apparent distress.
- *HEENT*: No facial bruising or scalp hematoma. The anterior fontanelle is soft and flat. Mucous membranes are moist and tympanic membranes are clear. The oropharynx is without erythema exudate, or ulcers. PERRL. No conjunctival injection or scleral icterus.
- *Neck*: Supple and with no cervical adenopathy.
- *Cardiovascular*: The heart is regular, with no M/R/G. Brisk capillary refill and equal pulses.
- *Lungs*: CTA bilaterally, with no W/R/R. No retractions.
- *Abdomen*: Soft, non-distended, with no masses or organomegaly. Normal bowel sounds.
- *Skin and extremities*: Normal range of motion, no joint swelling or redness, well-perfused without rashes. No contusions, ecchymoses, or abrasions.
- *Neurologic*: Facial muscles activate symmetrically. Extraocular movements are intact with midline tongue. Spontaneously moves all four extremities with no obvious focal weakness. Normal Moro

and grasp reflex. The patient has normal tone and suck.

Questions for Thought

- What are the possible etiologies of this condition?
- What are some components of history that could help narrow the diagnosis?
- What are some considerations to guide the use of diagnostic modalities?
- What is the appropriate disposition of this child?

Diagnosis

- Brief resolved unexplained event (BRUE), formerly known as apparent life-threatening event (ALTE).

Discussion

- *Epidemiology*: In 2016, the AAP offered a clinical practice guideline for infants with an ALTE.[1] They decided to replace the ALTE term with BRUE. The new AAP specific BRUE guideline offers an approach to patient evaluation and recommendations for management.

  Under the prior definition of ALTE, the incidence of children with similar events varied between 0.05 and 1 percent.[2] The incidence under the new definition of BRUE is unknown. A BRUE typically occurs in the first 2 months of life and most often occurs between 8 am and 8 pm.[1] Risk factors for occurrence include apnea history, feeding difficulties, and younger age (< 10 weeks).[1-5] Prematurity may also contribute to risk.[1-5]

- *Pathophysiology*: There is not one single unifying pathophysiology for a BRUE as the cause depends upon the underlying disease process. In extrapolating causality from the prior definition of ALTE, BRUEs may commonly be caused by gastroesophageal reflux, clinically non-apparent respiratory tract infections, and seizures.[1,4-10] Other less-common but serious causes of BRUEs include bacterial infections, congenital cardiac abnormalities, poisoning, and inborn errors of metabolism.[1,11] Non-accidental trauma, especially abusive head trauma, should always be considered in these patients.[1,7,12]

- *Presentation*: An ALTE was initially defined by a consensus panel of experts at the National

Institutes of Health in 1986 as "an episode that is frightening to the observer and that is characterized by some combination of apnea (central or occasionally obstructive), color change (usually cyanotic or pallid but occasionally erythematous or plethoric), marked change in muscle tone (usually marked limpness), choking or gagging."[13] Such a definition provides a large umbrella for potential presentations. Today, this term has been replaced by BRUE - a brief resolved unexplained event. The AAP defines a BRUE as "an event occurring in an infant younger than 1 year when the observer reports a sudden, brief, and now resolved episode of ≥1 of the following: (1) cyanosis or pallor; (2) absent, decreased, or irregular breathing; (3) marked change in tone (hyper- or hypotonia); and (4) altered level of responsiveness."[1] The AAP goes on to say that a BRUE may only be diagnosed after a history and physical examination do not yield an explanation.

- *Diagnosis*: Patients presenting with BRUEs are a significant diagnostic challenge to the practitioner as symptoms are brief and have resolved by the time the child arrives at the ED. New diagnostic criteria mandate that a BRUE is only diagnosed after a complete and reassuring history and physical examination. Children who are unwell or present with systemic findings do not qualify for the definition of a BRUE.[1] Therefore, obtaining a careful history and examination is imperative and may either elicit a diagnosis without unnecessary testing or drive further investigation. If the infant's complete history and physical examination do not identify causality, infants are then evaluated to be classified as "low risk" or "high risk."

  Low-risk patients are those who have a reassuring history and a normal physical examination, are greater than 60 days old, have a gestational age of greater than 35 weeks, and did not have CPR performed by a medical provider.[1,14] The event must be brief (less than 60 seconds) and must be a first-time event for the infant.[1]

  Higher-risk patients are those less than 2 months old, premature babies with a gestational age of less than 32 weeks, and those with multiple events.[1] CPR by medical providers also places an infant into the high-risk category.

- *Treatment*: While most episodes of BRUE have good outcomes, serious adverse events can occur

in this population. In one study of children admitted for an ALTE, 13.6 percent had a subsequent extreme cardiorespiratory event.[4] Other prospective studies where all children with an ALTE were admitted showed that up to 12 percent of children had recurrent episodes as well as 9 percent needing stimulation and 3 percent requiring resuscitation.[15] Risk factors for subsequent and serious events include prematurity, prior history of an ALTE, and suspected child abuse.[1,3] Additional concerning findings included prolonged unresponsiveness and/or cyanosis during the episode or a history of resuscitation by the caregiver.[3]

Therefore, for low-risk infants, the guidelines recommend monitoring, observation, and potentially EKG and pertussis testing.[1,6,9] Patients may be observed and, when appropriate, monitored with pulse oximetry. Laboratory work, LPs, chest radiographs, echocardiograms, and hospital admission are not recommended for these low-risk patients.[1] Additionally, parents and/or caregivers can be offered resources for CPR training. The child should receive a repeat assessment by their physician within 24 hours to evaluate for developing illness.[1] High-risk infants should have the same evaluation as their low-risk counterparts, but should be admitted to the hospital for monitoring because of their higher risk for adverse events.[1]

Infants with a non-reassuring history or an abnormal physical examination no longer represent the BRUE population, and are high-risk infants who should be cared for based upon historical and physical examination findings. Potential etiologies of BRUE are multifold. Infections, including those from a respiratory etiology, are common and may be not clinically evident, especially in the younger and premature child.[1] Pertussis may be present without respiratory symptoms or other findings on examination. If available, testing may be done to confirm this etiology. Gastroesophageal reflux may be suggested by episodes occurring during or after feeding.[1] Seizures may be associated with tonic-clonic type activity, as well as unresponsiveness and poor muscle tone.[1] Congenital arrhythmias, such as neonatal supraventricular tachycardia, ventricular tachycardia, and abnormal conduction pathways such as Wolff–Parkinson–White syndrome are also possible causes in this population.[1] Family history of similar events, sudden death, long QT syndrome, or Wolff–Parkinson–White syndrome, should be obtained. EKG and cardiac monitoring may be considered.

Non-accidental trauma must always be on the differential diagnosis, and may be manifested as abusive head trauma, suffocation, or even poisoning. Previous studies have found up to 10 percent of ALTEs may be caused by some form of abuse.[1] A high index of suspicion and careful dissection of the presenting story is required in these patients as physical findings are not always evident. Was there a previous event or 911 call? Is the story consistent with the developmental abilities of the infant? Does the story change? Is there a prior injury? A thorough physical examination should evaluate for bruising, as bruises in non-ambulatory infants are a red flag for potential abuse. The examination should further look for bulging fontanelles, irritability, blood from the nose/mouth, or extremity swelling. Funduscopic examination can also detect retinal hemorrhages. Additionally, poisoning is possible in a child who has altered sensorium. Over-the-counter medicines or ethanol may be the offending culprits. One study found over 18 percent of children with ALTE had a positive toxicology screen, many of these from over-the-counter preparations such as ephedrine, pseudoephedrine, and diphenhydramine.[11] Appropriate toxicologic testing is indicated in these situations.

- *Disposition*: Low-risk infants with BRUE may be discharged after EKG and pertussis swab with close follow-up precautions, shared decision-making with the caregivers, and a recheck at 24 hours.[1] Additionally, resources and information for learning CPR should be made available to the parents or caregiver. High-risk infants should be admitted for monitoring because of their higher risk of events.

Historical clues	Physical findings
- Apnea	- Entirely normal examination
- Color change (cyanosis)	
- Limp tone	
- Less than a year old	

Follow-Up

This 25-day-old girl did not meet low-risk criteria due to the child's age being less than 60 days. She had laboratory evaluation, EKG, and pertussis swab. Because she appeared well and was afebrile, a spinal tap was not performed. She was admitted to the hospital, where all diagnostic testing was negative.

References

1. Tieder JS, Bonkowsky JL, Etzel RA, et al. Clinical practice guideline: Brief resolved unexplained events (formerly apparent life-threatening events) and evaluation of lower-risk infants. *Pediatrics* 2016; 137: e20161487.

2. Kiechl-Kohlendorfer U, Hof D, Pupp Peglow U, et al. Epidemiology of apparent life threatening events. *Arch Dis Child* 2004; 90: 297–300.

3. Tieder JS, Altman RL, Bonkowsky JL, et al. Management of apparent life-threatening events in infants: A systematic review. *J Pediatr* 2013; 163: 94–9.

4. Al-Kindy HA, Gelinas JF, Hatzakis G, et al. Risk factors for extreme events in infants hospitalized for apparent life-threating events. *J Pediatr* 2009; 154: 332–7.

5. Monti MC, Borrelli P, Nosetti L, et al. Incidence of apparent life-threatening events and post-neonatal risk factors. *Acta Paediatr* 2017; 106: 204–10. doi: 10.1111/apa.13391. Epub 2016 Apr 22.

6. Santiago-Burruchaga M, Sanchez-Etxaniz J, Benito-Fernandez J, et al. Assessment and management of infants with apparent life-threatening events in the paediatric emergency department. *Eur J Emerg Med* 2008; 15: 203–8.

7. Guenther E, Powers A, Srivastava R, et al. Abusive head trauma in children presenting with an apparent life-threatening event. *J Pediatr* 2010; 157: 821–5.

8. Esani N, Hodgman JE, Ehsani N, et al. Apparent life-threatening events and sudden infant death syndrome: Comparison of risk factors. *J Pediatr* 2008; 152: 365–70.

9. De Piero AD, Teach SJ, Chamberlain JM. ED evaluation of infants after an apparent life-threatening event. *Am J Emerg Med* 2004; 22: 83–6.

10. Doshi A, Bernard-Stover L, Kuelbs C, et al. Apparent life-threatening event admissions and gastroesophageal reflux disease: The value of hospitalization. *Pediatr Emerg Care* 2012; 28: 17–21.

11. Pitteti RD, Whitman E, Zaylor A. Accidental and non-accidental poisonings as a cause of apparent life-threatening events in infants. *Pediatrics* 2008; 122: e359-62.

12. McGovern MC, Smith MB. Causes of apparent life threatening events in infants: A systematic review. *Arch Dis Child* 2004; 89: 1043–8.

13. Little GA, Ballard RA, Borooks JG, et al. National Institutes of Health consensus development conference on infantile apnea and home monitoring, Sept 29 to Oct 1, 1986. *Pediatrics* 1987; 79: 292–9

14. Claudius I, Keens T. Do all infants with apparent life threatening events need to be admitted? *Pediatrics* 2007; 119: 679–83.

15. Mittal MK, Sun G, Baren JM. A clinical decision rule to identify infants with apparent life-threatening event who can be safely discharged from the emergency department. *Pediatr Emerg Care* 2012; 28: 599–605.

Case 7

Contributing Authors: Ben Church and Rebecca Jeanmonod

History

A 4-week-old boy is brought into the ED by his mother because of "breathing really fast." Mom reports that the child has had fussiness for the last day and "seems to be working hard when he breathes." She reports that he felt cold at home, especially in his hands and feet, which prompted her visit. Mom denies decreased feeding or change in urine output. There have been no fevers, vomiting, or rash. He has been stooling normally. He has had some difficulties with weight gain since birth, and is on high-calorie formula for this. He is not in daycare and is an only child.

Past Medical History

- The patient's mother has a history of depression and lupus. There were no complications with the patient's birth, and prenatal vitamins were taken throughout the entire pregnancy. The patient was born full-term at 39 weeks via c-section.

Medications

- None.

Allergies

- NKDA.

Physical Examination and Ancillary Studies

- *Vital signs*: T 91.6 °F, HR 154, RR 40, BP 96/56, O_2 sat 100% on 0.5 L nasal cannula.
- *General*: Mild respiratory distress, weak cry.

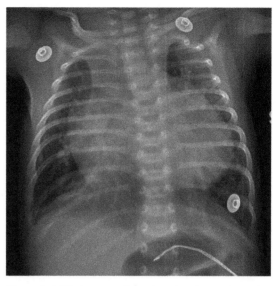

Figure 3.1 CXR demonstrating enlarged cardiac-mediastinal silhouette. The lungs are clear with no evidence of effusion, infiltrate, or pneumothorax.

- *HEENT*: Anterior fontanelle soft and flat. No signs of trauma. Mucous membranes moist. Oropharynx clear.
- *Neck*: Supple, with midline trachea.
- *Cardiovascular*: The heart has a regular rate and rhythm, without murmurs, rubs, or gallops. Pulses are intact. Capillary refill > 3 seconds.
- *Lungs*: The lungs are CTA but the patient is tachypneic, with mild supraclavicular retractions.
- *Abdomen*: Soft and non-tender. Normal bowel sounds.
- *Skin and extremities*: No bony deformity. Skin is cool, pale, and intact.
- *Neurologic*: Intact reflexes. Poor overall tone. Weak suck.
- *Pertinent ancillary studies*: CXR and EKG shown in Figures 3.1 and 3.2, respectively.

Questions for Thought

- How does this patient's EKG help you determine pathology? How does the EKG help you in general when considering congenital heart disease (CHD)?
- What are the diagnostic modalities you need to make a diagnosis of CHD?
- What treatment would you initiate on this patient?

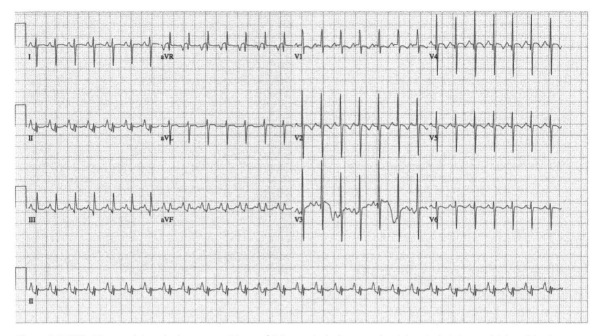

Figure 3.2 EKG with normal sinus rhythm, some evidence of right ventricular hypertrophy, right-axis deviation, and right atrial enlargement. There are ST elevations in the inferolateral leads and inverted T waves in the lateral leads.

- How would you monitor response to therapy in this patient?
- What is the definitive treatment for this condition?

Diagnosis

- Congestive heart failure (CHF) secondary to large septal defect and volume overload.

Discussion

- *Epidemiology*: CHD, including both cyanotic and acyanotic lesions, is the most common congenital disease in newborns, occurring in an estimated 6 to 13 per every 1,000 live births.[1,2] Although there have been major advances in the management of the disease, CHD remains the leading cause of perinatal and infant death. The most common malformation is a ventricular septal defect with Tetralogy of Fallot being the most commonly occurring cause of cyanotic CHD. There are many risk factors involved with the development of CHD, including prematurity, first-degree relative with CHD, maternal comorbidities such as hypertension and diabetes, maternal alcohol/tobacco/drug use, certain in utero infections including rubella, medications like ACE inhibitors and lithium, as well as various genetic syndromes.[1]

- *Pathophysiology*: CHD can be roughly divided into cyanotic ("blue") and acyanotic ("pink") lesions. Blue CHD typically involves one of the following: right-sided *obstructive* processes with *shunting* (for example, Tetralogy of Fallot, in which subpulmonic stenosis obstructs right ventricular outflow, and there is some degree of right-to-left shunting through either a ventricular septal defect or a patent ductus arteriosus) or *mixing* of oxygenated and deoxygenated blood (for example, in truncus arteriosus, where a single outflow tract provides both right- and left-sided circulation).

    Pink CHD most commonly involves anatomic derangements that result in either *pressure overload* (such as in coarctation of the aorta, where the left ventricle must pump against the obstruction posed by the narrowed aorta) or *volume overload* with left-to-right shunting (as in the case of this patient, where a large septal defect results in increased volume delivery to the right heart).

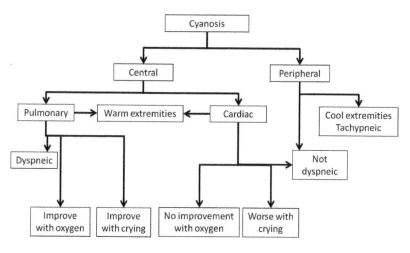

Figure 3.3 Differentiating features of cyanosis.

CHF, defined as inability of the heart to meet the blood supply demands of the body, can occur with any kind of CHD. CHF can also result from arrhythmia or from acquired cardiomyopathy, as can occur from viral or bacterial etiologies. In children who do not have evidence of cardiovascular compromise at birth and who are discharged home with undiagnosed or asymptomatic CHD, the typical presenting age for CHF is 4–6 weeks. This is because there is persistently high pulmonary resistance immediately following birth (reducing the pressure gradient for left-to-right flow), which slowly decreases over time, reaching its nadir at about 6 weeks. At this point, the decrease in pulmonary pressure may hit a tipping point, with high left-sided pressures causing pulmonary overcirculation through septal defects. Our patient suffered from CHF due to increases in preload from left-to-right shunting secondary to an atrial septal defect and ventricular septal defect causing ventricular hypertrophy and eventual heart failure.

- *Presentation*: Patients with CHD with CHF often display lethargy and poor or prolonged feeding.[3–6] There may also be increased cyanosis and sweating with feeding.[5,6] The extremities can be cool and mottled, with delayed capillary refill.[5] Tachypnea from metabolic acidosis is common and tachycardia is frequently profound.[5,6] Other common findings include murmurs, failure to thrive, and hepatomegaly.[5,6] These patients may appear septic but will only worsen with IV fluid resuscitation. Do not rely on peripheral and generalized edema as infants usually do not display these physical examination findings like adult patients.

- *Diagnosis*: In cases of cyanotic infants, the provider should first determine if the cyanosis is central or peripheral. A cool or dehydrated infant may have peripheral cyanosis with neither cardiac nor pulmonary abnormality. Central cyanosis is typically cardiac or pulmonary in etiology. Some distinguishing factors are that cardiac cyanosis does not typically improve with administration of oxygen (because of shunt physiology), and typically worsens with crying (which increases cardiac work), while pulmonary cyanosis often improves with crying (because of increased recruitment of alveoli) and improves with oxygen (Figure 3.3). Once cyanosis is suspected to be of cardiac origin, the provider should perform a CXR and an EKG to support or refute the diagnosis and to potentially narrow down the diagnosis to specific pathologic entities (Figure 3.4).

Pink babies with CHD may present in more subtle fashion. Cardiac disease should be considered in any neonate or child presenting with poor feeding, diaphoresis, respiratory distress, or hepatomegaly.[5] All these children should undergo CXR and EKG, as well. In addition to assisting in diagnosis of specific cardiac lesions, these tests can help rule out other diagnostic possibilities, such as pneumonia or arrhythmia (Figure 3.5). Although laboratory testing is non-specific, it may reveal hyponatremia, renal dysfunction, or elevated LFTs secondary to hepatic congestion.

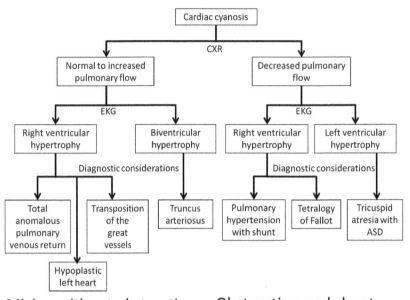

Figure 3.4 Differential of cardiac cyanosis based on CXR and EKG findings.

Echocardiography is the modality used to make a definitive diagnosis of CHD by providing information regarding both cardiac anatomy and function.[3–5]

- *Treatment*: The EM provider does not need to know the specific cardiac lesion in order to begin treating the child with symptomatic CHD. Generally, in any ill-appearing child, the provider will begin with the ABC algorithm and address respiratory and circulatory issues. If the diagnosis is uncertain, the provider should consider the entire differential diagnosis for the unwell infant, *THE MISFITS* (*T*rauma, *H*ypovolemia/heart, *E*ndocrine, *M*etabolic, *I*ntestinal disasters, *S*eizures, *F*ormula misadventures, *I*nborn errors of metabolism, *T*oxicologic, and *S*epsis), and simultaneously treat for sepsis during evaluation. Definitive treatment for patients with CHD is emergent consultation with a pediatric cardiologist and eventual operative repair of the underlying defect, but this can clearly not be accomplished in every ED. Emergency

Figure 3.5 Differential of acyanotic cardiac lesions based on CXR and EKG findings.

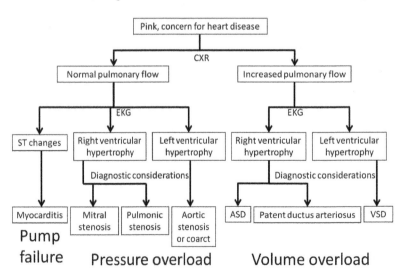

therapeutic modalities important to pediatric CHF management include airway control, diuretics, and vasopressor support.[6,7] Oxygen administration for the most part is helpful in the majority of cyanotic babies but keep in mind that oxygen is a potent vasodilator and can actually lead to increased pulmonary vascular flow leading to "steal" from the systemic circulation in those patent ductus ateriosus-dependent patients.[6,7]

Patients with evidence of shock or heart failure should initially be thought to be septic and treated with weight-based IV fluid administration, as well as antibiotics, as sepsis is by far much more common than CHD. Those with CHF will likely worsen clinically with IV fluid administration, and this may be the clue to the provider that he or she is dealing with CHD. In patients in shock who are unresponsive to other therapies, a trial of IV prostaglandin E_1 therapy should be initiated.[6–8] These refractory infants, who most commonly present in the first month of life, typically have either a cyanotic or an acyanotic lesion that is so severe that they require blood shunting through the ductus arteriosus in order to sustain life. The lesions are varied – Tetralogy of Fallot, left ventricular hypoplasia, transposition, and many other lesions may be ductal dependent, if severe enough. The key is that, when every other modality has failed to improve the clinical picture of a neonate in shock, prostaglandin should be tried. A well-known serious side effect of prostaglandin is apnea, which may require intubation.[8] If prostaglandin seems to be improving the child's clinical status, the child's supplemental oxygen should be decreased, as a high arterial oxygen tension promotes ductus closure. An oxygen saturation in the 80s is acceptable in these children. Diuresis with furosemide can be given to help improve oxygenation.[6,7] Cardiac output can be improved with a number of inotropes.[6,7]

- *Disposition*: Patients with new-onset CHD will need admission for hemodynamic monitoring and treatment, depending primarily on the type of lesion and severity of symptoms. Transfer of patients to a tertiary facility with more expertise is also appropriate, depending on the hospital's capabilities. Disposition decisions are usually made in consultation with a pediatric cardiologist. In patients on prostaglandin therapy, prophylactic endotracheal intubation should be considered before transport.[8]

Historical clues	Physical findings	Ancillary studies
• Failure to thrive • Dyspnea	• Poor perfusion • Tachypnea • Hypothermia • Ill-appearing	• EKG with right ventricular hypertrophy and right atrial hypertrophy • CXR with cardiomegaly

Follow-Up

The child's echocardiogram demonstrated moderate to severely depressed left ventricular function, with a moderately dilated left ventricle. There was a moderate muscular ventricular septal defect and a moderate-sized secundum atrial septal defect, both with left-to-right flow, and bilateral dilated atria. There was moderate tricuspid insufficiency with elevated right-sided ventricular pressures. There was no patent ductus arteriosus. The child was treated for sepsis and also underwent pediatric cardiology consultation. He was transferred to a tertiary care center with pediatric cardiac surgery capabilities. The child's septic work-up was ultimately negative, and he underwent surgical correction of his heart defects and had an uneventful postoperative course.

References

1. van der Linde D, Konings EE, Slager MA, et al. Birth prevalence of congenital heart disease worldwide: A systematic review and meta-analysis. *J Am Coll Cardiol* 2011; 58: 2241–7.

2. Peterson C, Ailes E, Riehle-Colarusso T, et al. Late detection of critical congenital heart disease among US infants: Estimation of the potential impact of proposed universal screening using pulse oximetry. *JAMA Pediatr* 2014; 168: 361–70.

3. Kuehl KS, Loffredo CA, Ferencz C. Failure to diagnose congenital heart disease in infancy. *Pediatrics* 1999; 103: 743–7.

4. Eckersley L, Sadler L, Parry E, et al. Timing of diagnosis affects mortality in critical congenital heart disease. *Arch Dis Child* 2016; 101: 516–20.

5. Ross RD, Bollinger RO, Pinsky WW. Grading the severity of congestive heart failure in infants. *Pediatr Cardiol* 1992; 13: 72–5.

6. Rosenthal D, Chrisant MR, Edens E, et al. International Society for Heart and Lung Transplantation: Practice guidelines for management

of heart failure in children. *J Heart Lung Transplant* 2004; 23: 1313–33.

7. Brooks PA, Penny DJ. Management of the sick neonate with suspected heart disease. *Early Hum Dev* 2008; 84: 155–9.

8. Meckler GD, Lowe C. To intubate or not to intubate? Transporting infants on prostaglandin E_1. *Pediatrics* 2009; 123: e25–30.

Case 8

Contributing Authors: Natalie Moore and Rebecca Jeanmonod

History

The patient is a previously healthy 17-month-old male who presents to the ED because his mother notes that he has been breathing increasingly hard over the past week. The labored breathing was particularly noted when playing with his sister. Mom also notes general fatigue over the past week and some swelling around his eyes. Over the past 3 days, he began to have swelling in his legs as well. On further questioning, mom states that he had been sick with a viral URI about 10 days ago. He also had four to five episodes of non-bloody, non-bilious vomiting and six to seven episodes of diarrhea about 1–2 weeks before these symptoms started. He otherwise has had no recent travel, is not prone to bruising or frequent infections, and has not experienced any recent visual blood loss from stool, gums, or nose. The mother notes that he is a picky eater and has a limited solid food intake and drinks over 40 ounces of cow's milk daily.

Past Medical History

- No significant past medical or family history. Vaccinations are UTD.

Medications

- None.

Allergies

- NKDA.

Physical Examination and Ancillary Studies

- *Vital signs*: T 98.7 °F, HR 170, RR 38, BP 139/100, O_2 sat 98% on room air.
- *General*: Awake and alert in his mother's arms. He appears pale and in mild respiratory distress.
- *HEENT*: Bilateral eyelid swelling. No scleral icterus. PERRL. Mouth and oropharynx without lesions.
- *Neck*: Supple, with no adenopathy.
- *Cardiovascular*: The patient is tachycardic, with no M/R/G.
- *Lungs*: Tachypneic, with increased work of breathing and mild intercostal retractions. Lungs are CTA, with no W/R/R.
- *Abdomen and genitourinary*: Distended but not tender to palpation. No hepatosplenomegaly or masses. The child has mild scrotal edema.
- *Extremities and skin*: The patient has 1+ pitting edema of both upper and lower extremities. His skin is warm, dry, and intact, with no petichiae, jaundice, or bruising.
- *Neurologic*: He has a non-focal neurologic examination.
- *Pertinent laboratory values*: WBC 11,500, Hb 7.5, HCT 24.6, MCV 70, MCHC 30, Plt 499,000, Cr 0.2, BUN 15, ALT 13, AST 36, total bilirubin 0.1, lipase 47, albumin 1.3, LDH 169, iron level 7, TIBC 159, iron saturation 4%, ferritin level 4. His stool is positive for occult blood. The urine dip is negative for protein, WBC, RBC, nitrites, or leukocyte esterase.
- *Pertinent radiographs*: CXR with bilateral small pleural effusions. Otherwise, clear lungs, without consolidation or interstitial edema.

Questions for Thought

- Once you have found that a patient has decreased hemoglobin, what other diagnostic tests should be sent to assess for the etiology of anemia?
- In what category of anemia would you place this child given his Hb, MCV, MCHC, and iron studies?
- What other types of anemia cause microcytic red blood cells?
- What are other causes of anemia?

Diagnosis

- Iron-deficiency anemia caused by inappropriate diet with excessive intake of cow's milk. Also contributing to his anemia was enteropathic protein loss from destruction of the epithelial lining of his gut from his recent viral illness.

Discussion

- *Epidemiology*: Anemia is a common condition that affects approximately 20 percent of children in the USA at some point during their childhoods.[1] Globally, anemia affects approximately 50 percent of children.[2] Anemia is defined as a reduction in hemoglobin concentration two standard deviations below the mean hemoglobin for age and gender.[3]

  Iron deficiency is the most common nutritional deficiency in children, and iron-deficiency anemia is particularly high in African American and Hispanic populations as well as children who live in poverty.[1–4] It affects approximately 4 percent of patients between 6 and 12 months, 12 percent over 12 months, and 7–9 percent of toddlers.[1–4]

- *Pathophysiology*: Anemia has numerous causes, and any of them may present with shortness of breath. Oxygen delivery to tissues requires intact lungs, a working pump, and blood for delivery. Therefore, a breakdown in any step of this process can result in dyspnea, weakness, or syncope. Ultimately, it is this failure in oxygen delivery that causes dyspnea.

  Iron-deficiency anemia is a specific subset of anemia. Iron is absorbed in the intestines, primarily in the duodenum and upper jejunum. After absorption by the mucosal cells, iron binds to transferrin, which delivers the iron to the liver, where it is primarily stored in a form called ferritin.[5] When erythropoietin is released from the kidney, iron is released to make red blood cells in the bone marrow. A normal red blood cell circulates for approximately 120 days; it is then reabsorbed by the spleen and the iron is recycled.

  Iron-deficiency anemia is caused by either insufficient dietary intake of iron, inadequate iron absorption, or increased intestinal blood loss. Infants have enough iron stores for the first 6 months of life and then they require iron in their diet. Per AAP guidelines, infants who are breastfed should be given daily iron supplementation until iron-rich foods can be introduced into their diet.[3] They also recommend screening for anemia at 9–12 months of age.[3] Inadequate dietary intake is common in children between 6 months and 24 months of age, especially in children who are picky eaters and those who drink excessive amounts of non-modified cow's milk. Cow's milk should not be introduced into the diet prior to 12 months of age secondary to the decreased concentration of iron in the milk and because protein present in cow's milk may cause a colitis, leading to occult intestinal blood loss.[3] Inadequate iron absorption occurs when there is malabsorption in the intestine secondary to chronic disease such as celiac disease, inflammatory bowel diseases, or iatrogenic causes from bowel resection. Inadequate absorption can also occur acutely from GI illness causing inflammation and destruction of the lining of mucosal cells. Finally, iron-deficiency anemia can also be caused by increased blood loss.

- *Presentation*: The most common presentation of anemia is an asymptomatic patient. However, other symptoms of iron-deficiency anemia are fatigue, irritability, shortness of breath, not being able to keep up with the other children, decreased performance or attention in school, and cold intolerance.[2] Another presenting symptom is pica, which is when the patient eats non-food substances such as sand, clay, dirt, or paper, and craves ice. Physical examination findings include lethargy, tachypnea, tachycardia, flow murmur, pallor (which is best seen on the palms, nail beds, and conjunctiva), glossitis (swelling and redness of the tongue and disappearance of the papillae), angular stomatitis (fissures in the corner of the mouth), splenomegaly, koilonychias (concave/spoon-shaped nails), and impaired growth.

- *Diagnosis*: Diagnosis of anemia requires laboratory measurement of Hb and HCT. The differential diagnosis for anemia is broad, and can be roughly divided into anemia from *losing* red blood cells, anemia from *destroying* red blood cells, and anemia from *failing to make* red blood cells. Although a complete discussion of all subsets of anemia is beyond the scope of this book, there are laboratory tests that can help determine the category into which a given patient's anemia falls.

  Patients with anemia from *losing* red blood cells will, by definition, have a low Hb and HCT. They should also have an elevated reticulocyte count, which is evidence of the patient's bone marrow increasing red blood cell production in response to the losses. Since the body relies on recycling of iron from "expired" red blood cells by the spleen, when blood is lost externally over time, the patient will eventually additionally develop iron-deficiency anemia. They will then drop their reticulocyte counts as well, because of an inability to produce cells. Occult blood loss most commonly occurs from the GI tract or from menorrhagia in adolescent girls.[2] In anemic patients, therefore, a stool guaiac and menstrual history should be obtained. Acute blood-loss anemia tends to be normocytic.

Patients with anemia from red blood cell *destruction* may have an intrinsic process, such as an inherited problem with making red blood cell walls (for instance, spherocytosis) or problems that interfere with glycolysis (such as G6PD deficiency), both of which will cause a shortened red blood cell lifespan.[2] They may also have an extrinsic process, such as autoimmune hemolytic anemia or hemolytic uremic syndrome.[2] In addition to anemia, these patients will have an elevated reticulocyte count as well as elevated levels of the products of hemolysis, including indirect bilirubin, increased lactate dehydrogenase, and decreased haptoglobin.[2] These anemias tend to be normocytic.

Patients with anemia from *failure to make* red blood cells are the largest group of pediatric anemic patients. These patients have an inappropriately low reticulocyte count for their anemia. Their bone marrow cannot respond to the low HCT with increased red blood cell production. This can occur from primary bone-marrow failure or malignancy, from viral infections (such as parvovirus B19 or hepatitis), or, most commonly, from iron-deficiency anemia. These anemias tend to be macrocytic or microcytic.

In diagnosis of iron-deficiency anemia, a CBC will reveal decreased Hb and HCT. These patients also tend to have an elevation in platelet count from increased erythropoietin release, which cross reacts with thrombopoietin receptors leading to an elevation in platelet count.[6] When evaluating red blood cell indices, a patient with iron-deficiency anemia will have a low MCV, which is a measure of average volume of red blood cells in a specimen. They will also have a decreased MCHC, which is the measure of the concentration of hemoglobin in a given red blood cell. The reticulocyte count will be low because the bone marrow is lacking one of the building blocks for the production of red blood cells, iron. In patients with microcytic anemia, iron studies should also be obtained, as this is the most common cause of microcytic anemia. Patients with iron-deficiency anemia will have low serum iron, low ferritin level, increased total iron binding capacity, and low transferrin saturation.[6]

- *Treatment*: Treatment for iron-deficiency anemia depends on the cause and severity. If it is caused by inadequate intake of iron, treatment is to increase dietary iron and take an iron supplement. Iron-rich foods include meat (especially beef and liver), eggs, lentils, dark-green leafy vegetables, and iron-fortified cereals. Ferrous sulfate supplement is recommended. Enteral iron side effects include GI symptoms such as abdominal pain, nausea, diarrhea, constipation, and black stool. Parenteral iron may also be a good option for iron-deficiency anemia in children who cannot absorb iron or have undergone surgery which has limited their ability to absorb iron. There are no guidelines for an absolute hemoglobin threshold for transfusion of packed red blood cells for patients with iron-deficiency anemia, thus the decision to transfuse would be dependent on the child's clinical picture.

- *Disposition*: Most children with iron-deficiency anemia can be discharged home, with follow-up with their pediatricians for a recheck of hemoglobin or potentially for further testing and referral to hematology. Children with severe symptomatic anemia should be transfused and admitted to the hospital.

Historical clues	Physical findings	Ancillary studies
• Recent viral illness, which likely caused destruction of the intestinal mucosal lining • Excessive cow's milk intake • Increased fatigue • Increased work of breathing	• Pallor • Tachycardia • Tachypnea • Fatigue	• Decreased Hb and HCT • Low MCV and MCHC • Low serum iron and serum ferritin • Elevated total iron binding capacity • Low transferrin saturation

Follow-Up

Due to his abnormal vital signs and anasarca, the child was admitted to the PICU for his symptoms. While inpatient, he began having desaturations to 92 percent and was placed on oxygen. He was also treated with furosemide and albumin, and was transfused for his anemia. His clinical picture eventually improved, and he was discharged home 6 days later, with parental counseling regarding excessive milk intake.

References

1. Centers for Disease Control and Prevention. Iron Deficiency – United States, 1999–2000. See www.cdc .gov/mmwr/preview/mmwrhtml/mm5140a1.htm.

2. Recht M. Thrombocytopenia and anemia in infants and children. *Emerg Med Clin N Am* 2009; 27: 505–23.

3. Baker RD, Greer FR, and the Committee on Nutrition. Clinical report: Diagnosis and prevention of iron-deficiency anemia in infants and young children (0–3 years of age). *Pediatrics* 2010; 126: 1040–50.

4. Short MW, Domagalski JE. Iron deficiency anemia: Evaluation and management. *Am Fam Phys* 2013; 87: 98–104.

5. Waldvogel-Abramowski S, Waeber G, Gassner C, et al. Physiology of iron metabolism. *Transfus Med Hemother* 2014; 41: 213–21.

6. Walters MC, Abelson HT. Interpretation of the complete blood count. *Pediatr Clin North Am* 1996; 43: 599–622.

Chapter 4

Fever

Case 1

Contributing Author: Rebecca Jeanmonod

History

A 14-month-old girl is brought into the ED by her grandmother for fever and abnormal movement. The child has had a runny nose, dry cough, and low-grade fever for the last 2 days. Grandma has been giving her acetaminophen intermittently and suctioning her nose before bed. The child has continued to be active and playful, and Grandma reports that the child has been making a usual number of wet and dirty diapers, although she has a slightly decreased oral intake, particularly for solids. She has not been vomiting or had any diarrhea. This afternoon, the child became pale and listless. Grandma took her temperature rectally and noted that it was 103.7 °F. The child started to have twitching in her left face, which progressed to involve the whole left side of her body. The child did not respond to Grandma during the episode, which lasted for about 3–4 minutes. Grandma lives two blocks from the hospital, and ran with the child down the street to the ED, thinking the child was dying, and not willing to wait for an ambulance. Grandma reports that the child has been somnolent and irritable since the event, but has been breathing the whole time. Grandma reports that nothing like this has ever happened to the child before.

Past Medical History

- Term neonate, mom with narcotic addiction. Child underwent inpatient detoxification after birth and has been in Grandma's custody since then, although she has regular contact with mom. She is UTD on immunizations and developmentally normal, just beginning to walk.

Medications

- Acetaminophen.

Allergies

- Penicillin – gets rash.

Physical Examination and Ancillary Studies

- *Vital signs*: T 103.5 °F, HR 170, RR 38, BP 93/62, O_2 sat 99% on room air.
- *General*: The child is somnolent but rouseable. She is irritable.
- *HEENT*: There are no signs of head trauma. PERRL. The child has moderate nasal discharge. She has mild bilateral tonsillar hypertrophy and erythema, without exudate. Her tympanic membranes are normal.
- *Neck*: Supple, with bilateral shotty adenopathy.
- *Cardiovascular*: Regular tachycardia, with no M/R/G. Normal capillary refill.
- *Lungs*: CTA bilaterally, with good air movement. She has an intermittent dry cough.
- *Abdomen and genitourinary*: Soft and non-tender/non-distended, with no masses or organomegaly. Normal genitalia.
- *Skin and extremities*: Hot to touch. No rashes or vesicles. No signs of trauma.
- *Neurologic*: The child is fussy and sleepy. She moves all four extremities spontaneously and is purposeful. She has normal reflexes. She responds to her grandmother's voice.
- *Pertinent laboratory values*: Fingerstick glucose 87.

Questions for Thought

- In this clinical scenario, when does the child require extensive testing to determine the source of fever?
- Do children with this diagnosis require LP?
- When is it necessary to perform neuroimaging of children with this diagnosis?
- What counseling can you provide the caregivers regarding prevention of further episodes?

Diagnosis

- Complex febrile seizure.

Discussion

- *Epidemiology*: Seizure disorders are common in children. 0.05–1 percent of children will have a seizure from a metabolic or neurologic process, 0.1 percent will develop repetitive seizure episodes, and 2–4 percent will have at least one febrile seizure.[1,2] Febrile seizures are defined as a seizure that occurs in the setting of fever in the absence of intracranial infection, metabolic cause, or prior afebrile seizure history.[3] First febrile seizure typically occurs between age 6 months and 5 years, with peak onset at 18 months of age.[3] About 30 percent of children have a family history of febrile seizures, suggesting a genetic component to its etiology.[3] Children with developmental delay are most susceptible.[4]
- *Pathophysiology*: All seizures are a result of an abnormal discharge of electrical activity in the brain. Febrile seizures are thought to be related to the increased excitability of neurons in the developing brain.[5] Hyperthermia generates seizures in animal models, as well.[5] This may occur secondary to disrupted function of temperature-sensitive ion channels or due to inflammatory mediators from underlying infection, combined with a genetic predisposition.[5] About two-thirds of febrile seizures are defined as simple, meaning that they meet all of the following criteria: duration less than 15 minutes, generalized seizure, single episode in 24 hours, in children age 6–60 months.[4,6] All others are characterized as complex. Although the majority of febrile seizures are generalized, they may present with focal

symptoms, abnormalities in behavior, staring spells, syncope, thought disturbances, visual symptoms, or prominent autonomic symptoms. Simple febrile seizures marginally increase the risk of adult epilepsy (2 percent, compared to background risk of 1 percent in the general population), while complex seizures increase risk to 4–6 percent.[4]

- *Presentation*: Most children will present after their seizure is over. Seizures in general typically last about 3 minutes, so most patients will have stopped seizing in the time it takes to travel to the ED. Most children will present in a post-ictal state, which should resolve within the hour. Some children may have a prolonged post-ictal period, or Todd's paralysis, but this is atypical. Since children who are post-ictal are usually somnolent or irritable, it can be difficult to determine which children with seizure are "sick" versus "not sick." In the child with febrile seizure who is no longer post-ictal, presentation is largely dependent upon the underlying process that is causing the fever. Most febrile seizures have URI as the underlying source of fever, and human herpes virus 6 has an association with febrile seizure,[3,4] but the clinician should consider the possibility of other serious bacterial infection (UTI, meningitis, bacteremia, soft-tissue infection) as well as toxins and environmental sources of fever.
- *Diagnosis*: The diagnosis of febrile seizure is clinical. In well-appearing children with an uncomplicated febrile seizure, there is no role for routine laboratory work or neuroimaging.[4,6] The AAP does not advocate for routine LP in cases of simple febrile seizure.[6] They do state that LP is an option in the child with febrile seizure between the ages of 6 and 12 months whose vaccination status is incomplete or unknown, and in those who are taking antibiotics, which might mask meningitis symptoms.[4,6] Likewise, in children with complex febrile seizure, there is no evidence that CT should be performed,[7] nor has it been demonstrated that these children benefit from routine LP.[4] Performing an EEG has also been shown to be unhelpful in the febrile seizure population.[4] Instead, the clinician should focus on the child's overall status. An ill-appearing child or a child with altered mental status requires a full evaluation, including LP. A young child with a fever of no apparent source also requires some

evaluation, in keeping with standard guidelines, most commonly CBC, blood culture, and urine culture. The ED provider should perform a thorough history, including family history, feeding/formula history, and a complete examination in all these children, and order ancillary studies as indicated by the history and physical examination. In any child with altered sensorium and abnormal vital signs, the provider should consider the dangerous differential diagnosis, *THE MISFITS* (*T*rauma, *H*ypovolemia/heart, *E*ndocrine, *M*etabolic, *I*ntestinal disasters, *S*eizures, *F*ormula misadventures, *I*nborn errors of metabolism, *T*oxicologic, and *S*epsis). In this case, the child remains post-ictal with altered mental status, and it is appropriate to initiate neuroimaging (especially given the focality of the seizure), blood work, cultures, and metabolic studies. The provider for the child in this particular case should consider traumatic injury, CNS infection or masses, hypoglycemia, or toxins as possible seizure causes. The child should only be diagnosed with a complex febrile seizure after these other possibilities are eliminated. On the other hand, if the child returns to her normal functioning and is well-appearing in the ED, with a benign examination and reassuring history, no further studies are necessary, as the child has a source for her fever.

- *Treatment*: Treatment of ongoing seizure activity in the ED is usually accomplished with benzodiazepines as a first-line agent, and any patient in status epilepticus should receive benzodiazepines. Status epilepticus is rare in febrile seizures, and most children require only supportive care. Acetaminophen or other antipyretics may be given for the child's comfort, but these do not reduce recurrence or incidence of febrile seizure.[8] Although some providers prescribe intermittent benzodiazepines or phenobarbital to children with recurrent febrile seizures, there are no data that this has any clinical benefits to the child.[8]

- *Disposition*: The majority of children with febrile seizures have a benign course, and most are discharged home with reassurance and instructions to family regarding safe positioning of the child during seizure, and other supportive measures. Parents should know that febrile

seizures can recur in 30 percent of children, and that there are no preventative measures that have been identified.

Historical clues	Physical findings	Ancillary studies
• History of febrile illness • Focal seizure witnessed by caregiver • Altered mental status	• Post-ictal state • Examination consistent with URI • Fever	• Normal glucose

Follow-Up

The provider ordered CT scanning, blood work, and urine studies and planned to perform LP. The child was given rectal acetaminophen for her fever. While the child was waiting for her CT, she rapidly returned to her normal self, awake, and interacting with Grandma. On reassessment, she had an entirely non-focal examination, with the exception of her runny nose and dry cough. All diagnostic studies were cancelled, and the child was discharged home with her grandmother to follow up with her pediatrician in the next 24–48 hours.

References

1. Panayiotopoulos CP. Benign childhood epilepsy with occipital paroxysms: A 15-year prospective study. *Ann Neurol* 1989; 26: 51–6.

2. Hauser WA. The prevalence and incidence of convulsive disorders in children. *Epilepsia* 1994; 35 Suppl 2: S1–6.

3. Sharawat IK, Singh J, Dawman L, et al. Evaluation of risk factors associated with first episode febrile seizure. *J Clin Diagn Res* 2016; 10: SC10–13.

4. Graves RC, Oehler K, Tingle LE. Febrile seizures: risks, evaluation, and prognosis. *Am Fam Phys* 2012; 85: 149–53.

5. Dube CM, Brewster AL, Baram TZ. Febrile seizures: Mechanisms and relationship to epilepsy. *Brain Dev* 2009; 31: 366–71.

6. Subcommittee on febrile seizures. Febrile seizures: Guideline for the neurodiagnostic evaluation of the child with a simple febrile seizure. *Pediatrics* 2011; 127: 389–94.

7. DiMario FJ. Children presenting with complex febrile seizures do not routinely need computed tomography scanning in the emergency department. *Pediatrics* 2006; 117: 528–30.

8. Offringa M, Newton R. Prophylactic drug management for febrile seizures in children (review). *Evid Based Child Health* 2013; 8: 1376–485.

Case 2

Contributing Author: Shellie Asher

History

The patient is a 3-week-old female brought to the ED by her mother after the patient's rectal temperature was found to be 100.8 °F. The patient's mother states that she took the baby's temperature because she seemed more fussy than usual, but was consolable. There has been no vomiting or diarrhea, no rashes, and no cough or other symptoms of URI. She has been breastfeeding well with normal urinary and stool output. She is an only child and there are no known sick contacts. The patient's mother reports that the infant was born via spontaneous vaginal delivery at 39 weeks' gestation, and that she had a normal, healthy pregnancy. Mother had normal prenatal care without any concerns for maternal infection.

Past Medical History

- None.

Medications

- None.

Allergies

- NKDA.

Physical Examination and Ancillary Studies

- *Vital signs*: T 101 °F, HR 167, RR 32, O_2 sat 99% on room air.
- *General*: Resting comfortably in mom's arms, no acute distress.
- *HEENT*: Anterior fontanelle is open and flat. Neck is supple. Oropharynx is moist and pink, no evidence of thrush.
- *Cardiovascular*: Regular rhythm, with no M/R/G. Capillary refill < 2 seconds
- *Lungs*: Equal expansion, without retractions. Equal breath sounds, without crackles or wheezing.
- *Abdomen and urogenital*: Soft, non-distended, normoactive bowel sounds. No masses or organomegaly. Normal genitalia with no rash.
- *Skin and extremities*: Skin warm to touch. No rashes appreciated.
- *Neurologic*: Moves all extremities. Fussy but consolable. Normal neonatal reflexes.
- *Pertinent laboratory values*:
  · U/A: 2+ leukocytes, moderate bacteria;
  · CBC: WBC 15,000, remainder within normal limits;
  · Electrolytes, renal function, and glucose: normal;
  · Blood culture: pending;
  · CSF: 0 WBC, 1 RBC per high-powered field. Gram's stain negative.
- *Pertinent radiologic studies*: CXR with no cardiomegaly, effusions, consolidations, or infiltrates.

Questions for Thought

- What are the primary sources of infection to be concerned about in this patient?
- What maternal factors should be considered in the evaluation of a neonate with a fever?
- What type of laboratory testing/imaging should be performed in this type of patient?
- How is a definitive diagnosis made in the ED, and what treatment is necessary?

Diagnosis

- Neonatal fever secondary to UTI.

Discussion

- *Epidemiology*: The evaluation and management of neonates (age < 28 days) and young infants (age 28–60 days) with fever (defined in this age group as a temperature > 100.4 °F) is focused on serious bacterial infections. Up to 3 percent of neonates presenting with fever have a serious bacterial infection, including UTI, meningitis, pneumonia, and bacteremia.[1] Infections in the first 7 days of life are typically associated with vertical transmission, or infection that is transmitted from the mother to the infant.[1] After the first 7 days of life, infections are typically acquired from sick contacts in the home, community, or hospital environment. The rate of serious bacterial infection in infants 28–60 days of age may be as high as 6–10 percent, with the most common etiology being UTI.[1]

- *Pathophysiology*: Bacterial and viral infections in the neonatal and young infant period may result from vertical (maternal to fetal) transmission or community exposure (household, child care, hospital, etc.). While the prenatal environment is ideally sterile, infection may be introduced through amniotic membrane disturbance prior to labor, resulting in clinical presentations that range from occult infection to chorioamnionitis. Risk factors for early-onset neonatal sepsis include preterm birth, group B streptococci positivity in mother, prolonged rupture of membranes, and maternal fever and tachycardia.[1] Immature immune systems and a less-developed blood–brain barrier in the neonate and infant result in increased susceptibility to bacterial infections. Serious etiologies of bacterial infection include meningitis, pneumonia, UTI, and bacteremia. Significant viral infections may also occur, with serious sequelae.

- *Presentation*: Although there are no historical factors that rule out serious infection in neonates and young infants, there are several that increase the likelihood that fever is associated with a serious bacterial infection, including cough, poor feeding, irritability, lethargy, diarrhea, and seizures.[1] That said, many children present with isolated fever.

- *Diagnosis*: The critical evaluation of the neonate or young infant with fever starts with a careful history and physical examination. This evaluation may be challenging due to lack of clinical signs or symptoms of focal infection in this age group. Historical elements should include thorough prenatal and maternal history, birth history, presence of underlying diseases or conditions, medications used (including herbal or over-the-counter), presence of sick contacts, diet (breast- or bottle-fed and how feedings are prepared), signs or symptoms of focal bacterial infection as described above, previously diagnosed infections, and antibiotic use, presently or in the recent past.

  Pertinent physical examination elements include vital signs with rectal temperature; general appearance, including activity level, tone, presence of cyanosis or jaundice, and irritability or lethargy; signs of focal infection including skin, HEENT including fontanelles, lungs, abdomen including the umbilical stump, and GU, noting circumcision status if pertinent.

  All neonates with a documented rectal temperature greater than 100.4 °F should have a full sepsis evaluation including CXR, peripheral WBC, blood cultures, U/A, urine culture, and CSF studies including cell count, Gram's stain, glucose, protein, enterovirus/herpes PCR, and culture. Stool culture is indicated if there are any changes to the infant's usual stooling habits or if there is blood or mucous in the stool.

  In the 29–60 day age group, there is more of a role for clinical evaluation in the decision-making process regarding fever evaluation. The ill-appearing child (lethargic, irritable, poor perfusion, or clinical impression) should have a full sepsis work-up as previously described. The well-appearing child without clinical evidence of acute viral bronchiolitis (tachypnea, hypoxia, wheezing in the setting of fever) should have laboratory tests, including CBC and blood cultures drawn, as well as U/A and urine culture.[1,2] CXR and stool studies may be performed per clinical indications. "Low-risk" infants (previously healthy, full-term, well-appearing, WBC 5,000–15,000 without bandemia, negative urine and no clinical signs of focal infection) may have LP and CSF studies performed depending on the clinician's assessment.[1,2]

- *Treatment*: Management of the neonate and young infant with a fever depends on the patient's age group, risk factors, and clinical presentation. Any diagnosed focal infection such as pneumonia or UTI should be treated according to clinical guidelines, with patterns of local bacterial antibiotic resistance taken into account. All neonates with a documented rectal temperature greater than 100.4 °F should be admitted to the hospital and empiric antibiotic/antiviral treatment should be started while sepsis work-up results are pending. Empiric antibiotic treatment in neonates includes coverage for group B streptococci, *Escherichia coli*, *Haemophilus influenzae*, *Moraxella catarrhalis*, *Neisseria meningitidis*, *Staphylococcus aureus*, and *Listeria monocytogenes* with ampicillin and an aminoglycoside such as gentamycin, or ampicillin and cefotaxime.[1,2] In addition, empiric treatment with acyclovir should be administered for possible HSV infection, especially if there is any positive history of maternal herpes, prolonged vaginal delivery, or vesicular rash in the infant.[1,2]

Older infants (age 29–60 days) who are well-appearing may be treated empirically with ceftriaxone while cultures are pending.[1,2] If sepsis is suspected in this age group, empiric therapy for the organisms listed above includes ampicillin, cefotaxime, and vancomycin.

- *Disposition*: All neonates with fever should be admitted to the hospital for empiric therapy as described while cultures are pending. Infants 28 days and greater, who look well and are classified as low risk for bacterial infection, may be admitted to the hospital or discharged home depending on clinical evaluation, social factors, including ability to return to the hospital, and the established local standard of care for these patients.

Historical clues	Physical findings	Ancillary studies
• Neonate < 28 days old • T > 100.4 °F • Fussy	• Fever • Otherwise normal examination	• U/A positive for WBC and bacteria • Other studies unremarkable for infectious source

Follow-Up

Clinical evaluation of the infant did not reveal any evidence of focal bacterial infection, and U/A was positive for leukocytes. The patient was admitted to the hospital and started empirically on ampicillin and gentamicin. Urine culture grew out *E. coli*. Blood and CSF cultures were negative. The patient completed her course of antibiotics and was discharged home after an uneventful hospital course.

References

1. Hamilton J, John S. Evaluation of fever in infants and young children. *Am Fam Phys* 2013; 87: 254–60.
2. Polin R. Management of neonates with suspected or proven early-onset bacterial sepsis. *Pediatrics* 2012; 129: 1006–15.

Case 3

Contributing Authors: David H. Long and Janet Young

History

The patient is a 7-year-old female brought to the ED by her mother after the patient's oral temperature was found to be 101.8 °F. Her fever was preceded by four bouts of vomiting that started earlier in the day while she was at school. The patient was diagnosed with ALL 9 months ago; otherwise she had been a healthy child prior to her leukemia diagnosis. She is on chemotherapy managed by her oncologist, and her last maintenance dose was 6 days ago. Prior to today the patient had been in good spirits, eating and drinking well, and tolerating her chemotherapy regimen with minimal side effects. The mother states that the oncologist provided strict precautions to go immediately to the ED for evaluation if the patient ever develops a fever. The patient has had one episode of non-bloody, non-bilious vomiting upon arrival to the ED, but otherwise has had no associated symptoms.

Past Medical History

- ALL, diagnosed 9 months ago.

Medications

- Methotrexate.
- 6-Mercaptopurine.
- Prednisone.
- Ondansetron (as needed for nausea).

Allergies

- NKDA.

Physical Examination and Ancillary Studies

- *Vital signs*: T 102.1 °F, HR 167, BP 90/50, RR 24, O$_2$ sat 97% on room air.
- *General*: Female child lying supine, tearful. She withdraws to her mother several times during examination as she appears fearful and states she wants to go home.
- *HEENT*: Normocephalic, atraumatic. PERRL. No conjunctival pallor. Tympanic membranes clear, nares clear. No pharyngeal erythema or oral lesions.
- *Neck*: Supple, with no adenopathy.

- *Cardiovascular*: Tachycardic, otherwise regular rhythm, with no M/R/G. < 2 second capillary refill.
- *Lungs*: Mild expiratory coarse breath sounds bilateral upper and lower lung fields; otherwise good air movement.
- *Abdomen and genitourinary*: Soft, non-distended, normoactive bowel sounds. No rectal or vaginal bleeding, no fissures or abscesses.
- *Skin and extremities*: Skin warm to touch. Well-appearing nail beds upper and lower extremities. Tunneled IV port upper-left chest wall with no tenderness to palpation, well-healed surgical scar. No erythema, induration, or purulence around port site.
- *Neurologic*: Oriented to time, person, and place. Cranial nerves II–XII grossly intact. Cerebellum testing normal (rapid alternating movements, heel to shin, finger to nose), negative pronator drift and Romberg. Reflexes +2 upper and lower extremities. Normal gait.
- *Pertinent laboratory values*: ANC of 234 cells/μL.
- *Pertinent radiologic studies*: CXR with no cardiomegaly, effusions, consolidation, or infiltrates. Tunneled IV catheter tip visualized in superior vena cava–atrial junction.

Questions for Thought

- Why is this type of patient at high risk in regards to infection?
- Are there any "typical" signs and symptoms for this patient's diagnosis?
- What type of laboratory testing/imaging should be performed in this type of patient?
- How is a definitive diagnosis made in the ED, and what treatment is necessary?

Diagnosis

- Neutropenic fever in pediatric patient with cancer (chemotherapy-induced neutropenia).

Discussion

- *Epidemiology*: Neutropenic fever in cancer patients is considered a medical emergency. Infections left untreated can lead to life-threatening complications and death. The rate of documented infections in the neutropenic febrile patient is approximately 10–40 percent.[1] Gram-positive and Gram-negative organisms account for 85–90 percent of documented infections.[1,2] Common sites of infection include the respiratory tract, urinary tract, skin, GI/GU tract, and oral cavity.[1-3] Bacteremia is the most common infection. Viral infections must also be considered in the neutropenic patient, with Varicella zoster virus and HSV being the most common viral etiologies.[1] Patients are also susceptible to fungal infections. These are less common but more likely to occur in the setting of prolonged neutropenia (> 10 days), prolonged antibiotic use, steroid use, or after bone marrow transplant in the setting of chronic immunosuppression therapy.
- *Pathophysiology*: Chemotherapy treatment places a burden on both the patient's innate and adaptive immune system. The innate immune system provides protection through *non-specific* recognition of pathogens. Common components include mucosal barriers, natural killer cells, phagocytic cells, macrophages, and monocytes. The adaptive immune system mounts an immune response by producing *specific* antibodies and lymphocytes to target invading pathogens. Chemotherapy treatment causes bone marrow suppression, which in turn causes the immune system to become weakened due to the decrease in immune cells available to fight infection. Another side effect of chemotherapy is its non-specific destruction of rapidly dividing cells, such as mucosal and epithelial cells. Breakdown of oral and intestinal mucosa, as well as skin, allows invasion of pathogens. Many patients also are on steroid treatment, which also suppresses the immune system. All of these factors place the patient at increased risk of bacterial, viral, and fungal infections.
- *Presentation*: Neutropenic patients have a depressed immune system, so it is important to remember the patient may not mount a response to an infection. Therefore, finding a source of infection may be challenging. In fact, fever may be the only sign of infection in a neutropenic patient. Due diligence in obtaining a detailed history, full set of vitals, complete review of systems, and a thorough physical can all lead to finding a primary source of infection. The nadir for absolute neutrophil count (ANC) is typically

5–10 days after the last chemotherapy treatment, although neutropenic fever can occur at any time.

- *Diagnosis*: The critical evaluation of a child with febrile neutropenia is a careful history and physical examination. Neutropenia in a febrile pediatric cancer patient is defined as an ANC of < 500 cells/μL, or an ANC expected to drop < 500 cells/μL in the next 48 hours. The lower the ANC and the greater duration of neutropenia (> 7 days), the greater the risk of infection.[1–3] Fever is defined as a single temperature of 101 °F in neutropenic patients, or a temperature > 100.4 °F for longer than 1 hour, or a temperature > 100.4 °F recorded at least two times within a 24-hour period.[1] Temperatures should be taken orally or in the axilla. Rectal temperatures are contraindicated as they can increase the risk of mucosal damage leading to bacteremia. As already discussed, fever is often the only sign of infection in a neutropenic patient. On the other hand, patients may not mount a fever (due to poor immune function and immunosuppressive medications), and their only sign of infection may be an abnormal vital sign. Tachypnea, tachycardia, hypothermia, or hypotension should always be considered critical findings. Regardless of temperature, the risk of infection in a neutropenic pediatric patient should be considered if the patient has unstable vitals or has signs of clinical deterioration. A thorough history should include a list of chemotherapy agents, the last treatment date, a list of all other medications prescribed to the patient, the duration and intensity of the fever, as well as any exposure to sick contacts at home or school. A complete head-to-toe examination should be performed to search for possible sources of infection. Symptoms or physical findings such as headache, cough, congestion, sore throat, ear pain, difficulty breathing, chest pain, abdominal pain, dysuria, rectal pain, and skin lesions can lead to a primary source of infection. Pay careful attention to indwelling catheter sites, oral lesions, and nailbed lesions due to the risk of skin and mucosal breakdown in these patients. Indicated laboratory studies include a complete blood count with differential and platelet count, complete metabolic profile (electrolytes, Cr, BUN, liver transaminases, total bilirubin), and blood cultures from all CVC ports. Urine cultures can also be ordered if a clean-catch sample can be collected. Other laboratory studies, including peripheral blood cultures, skin swabs, throat cultures, and LP are not routinely useful and should be ordered based on clinical indications. Imaging should also be ordered as clinically warranted.

- *Treatment*: Current evidence recommends providing prompt administration of antibiotic therapy within 1 hour of presentation for the febrile, neutropenic pediatric patient.[1–3] Administration of antibiotics greater than 60 minutes after presentation has been associated with increased morbidity and mortality. Antibiotic selection will be based on regional resistance patterns and hospital protocols. Recommended initial therapy for febrile neutropenia includes monotherapy with a broad-spectrum third- or fourth-generation antipseudomonal cephalosporin (ceftazidime or cefepime), an antipseudomonal penicillin (piperacillin/tazobactam), or a carbapenem (meropenem or imipenem–cilastin).[1–3] Randomized controlled studies have shown monotherapy to be as efficacious as combination therapy, with fewer side effects. However, additional therapies should be added based on clinical presentation. For example, overt infection at indwelling catheter sites or skin breakdown warrants adding vancomycin to the antibiotic regimen. If an intra-abdominal infection is suspected or diagnosed, metronidazole should be administered. Lastly, if the patient is clinically unstable with no source of infection, a second Gram-negative antibiotic (aminoglycoside) should be started. Antivirals are not considered first-line treatments, but should be administered if clinically warranted. Lastly, fungal therapy is also not considered first-line treatment, but should be administered for persistent fever more than 4 days after the initial antibiotic therapy.[1–3]

- *Disposition*: Increasing evidence has shown that febrile neutropenic patients can be treated based on categorization into high- and low-risk categories using clinical decision rules.[1–3] Placing patients into these groups can assist in deciding if a patient is a candidate for either inpatient or outpatient therapy, and IV versus oral antibiotics. Unfortunately, current clinical decision rules are only validated for adults. Although there are at least 16 clinical decision rules proposed for children, none of them have met the rigorous requirements for validation.[1-3] The patient's oncologist should *always* be consulted for further recommendations, modification of therapy, and determination as to whether the patient is suitable for inpatient or outpatient therapy. Developing a final disposition will be dictated by the patient's clinical presentation, the patient's oncologist, and local hospital protocols that are put in place for pediatric patients with febrile neutropenia.

Historical clues	Physical findings	Ancillary studies
• History of ALL • Last chemotherapy 6 days ago • Vomiting	• Fever • Tachycardia	• ANC < 500/μL

Follow-Up

Due to her temperature and absolute neutrophil count, the patient was started on broad-spectrum antibiotic monotherapy with cefepime after blood cultures were drawn. After consulting her oncologist, it was decided to admit the patient for IV antibiotic treatment and observation.

Two days later her blood cultures came back positive for Gram-negative rods. She was kept in the hospital until culture sensitivities were reported. On day three cultures grew *Pseudomonas aeruginosa* susceptible to cefepime. She was discharged by her oncologist with daily IV antibiotic administration through a home health provider. Antibiotics were continued for a total of 14 days. Blood cultures were redrawn after finishing her antibiotic regimen, and the results came back negative.

References

1. Villafuerte-Gutierrez P, Villalon L, Losa JE, et al. Treatment of febrile neutropenia and prophylaxis in hematologic malignancies: A critical review and update. *Adv Hematol* 2014; 2014: 986938. doi: 10.1155/2014/986938.

2. Dubos F, Delebarre M, Martinot A. Predicting the risk of severe infection in children with chemotherapy-induced febrile neutropenia. *Curr Opin Hematol* 2012; 19: 39–43.

3. Lehrnbecher T, Phillips R, Alexander S, et al. Guideline for the management of fever and neutropenia in children with cancer and/or

undergoing hematopoietic stem-cell transplantation. *J Clin Oncol* 2012; 30: 4427–38.

Case 4

Contributing Author: Shellie Asher

History

The patient is a 17-year-old male with autism spectrum disorder who presents to the ED with fever, irritability, and muscle stiffness. The patient's parents state that he was in his usual state of health until about 2 days ago when he developed low-grade fever, muscle aches, and repetitive right arm movements. Today his symptoms worsened, he became irritable, had difficulty walking, and his temperature increased to 103 °F. They deny any other recent illnesses, nausea/vomiting, diarrhea, rash, respiratory symptoms, or any other concerns.

Past Medical History

- Autism spectrum disorder.

Medications

- Aripiprazole (Abilify®).
- Melatonin as needed for sleep.

Allergies

- NKDA.

Physical Examination and Ancillary Studies

- *Vital signs*: T 104.5 °F, HR 122, RR 28, O_2 sat 99% on room air.
- *General*: Agitated, restless.
- *HEENT*: Drooling, slurred speech. Tympanic membranes normal, pharyngeal structures midline. PERRL.
- *Neck*: No adenopathy. Patient resists ranging, but does not seem tender.
- *Cardiovascular*: Tachycardic, regular, with no M/R/G. < 2 second capillary refill.
- *Lungs*: Equal expansion, without retractions. Equal breath sounds, without W/R/R.
- *Abdomen*: Firm, no apparent tenderness.
- *Skin and extremities*: Skin warm to touch and diaphoretic.
- *Neurologic*: Confused and agitated. Unable to assess orientation. Increased muscle tone throughout. Unable to assess sensory examination or gait. Diminished reflexes.

- *Pertinent laboratory values*:
  - WBC 16,000;
  - CPK 898 U/L (normal range 22–198);
  - AST 92 U/L, ALT 85 U/L;
  - LDH 440 U/L.

Questions for Thought

- What is the differential diagnosis for this patient's presentation?
- What type of laboratory tests/imaging should be performed in this type of patient?
- How is a definitive diagnosis made in the ED, and what are the priorities in management?

Diagnosis

- Neuroleptic malignant syndrome (NMS).

Discussion

- *Epidemiology*: NMS may develop in 0.07–2.2 percent of patients taking neuroleptic medications.[1,2] Mean onset is 10 days after initiation of therapy, but may occur much later, even years, into treatment.[1,2] NMS is more common in males, with a male:female ratio of 2:1, and may occur at any age with the mean age being 40 years.[1] In pediatric cases, 9 percent result in death, with 20 percent of survivors going on to have significant sequelae.[1,2]
- *Pathophysiology*: The generally accepted mechanism for NMS is dopamine receptor antagonism in the hypothalamus, nigrostriatal pathways, and spinal cord.[2] This blockade results in extrapyramidal symptoms such as muscle rigidity and tremor. Dopamine receptor blockade also results in a dysfunction of temperature autoregulation and a blockade of cooling mechanisms such as vasodilation and sweating.[2] Increased calcium release from the sarcoplasmic reticulum may result in increased contractility, hyperthermia, rigidity, and muscle cell breakdown.[2] "Traditional" neuroleptic drugs, such as haloperidol, act directly through the inhibition of dopamine receptors, while "atypical" agents, such as olanzapine, risperidone, and in this case aripiprazole, primarily cause a blockade of serotonin receptors but may have secondary dopaminergic effects. Risk factors for NMS include use of high-potency agents, high doses, a rapid increase in dose, long-acting depot agents, prior episodes of NMS, and a recent history of catatonia. Illness, dehydration, concurrent medication use (especially lithium), and genetic factors may also play a role in the development of NMS.[2]

- *Presentation*: NMS occurs in the setting of neuroleptic medication use and is characterized by hyperpyrexia (temperature > 100.4 °F), muscle rigidity, altered mental status, and autonomic dysfunction (sialorrhea, diaphoresis, incontinence, tachycardia, labile blood pressure).[2] Children with NMS tend to present with dystonia, as opposed to the prominent tremor typically seen in adults.[2] Symptoms tend to develop over approximately 24–72 hours.[2] Signs and symptoms of a dopaminergic blockade include muscle rigidity, dysphagia, shuffling gait, tremor, dystonia, and dyskinesia.[2] Psychomotor agitation is evidenced by excessive or purposeless motor activity and/or tremor. Mental status alteration may progress from agitation to delirium to coma.[2]

- *Diagnosis*: The diagnosis of NMS depends on a careful and accurate history (particularly medication history) and physical examination. Diagnostic criteria include recent treatment with neuroleptics, hyperthermia > 100.4 °F, and muscle rigidity in addition to at least five of the following: altered mental status, tachycardia, hyper- or hypotension, diaphoresis or sialorrhea, tremor, incontinence, increased CPK or urinary myoglobin, leukocytosis, metabolic acidosis, or other evidence of autonomic instability. In addition, alternate diagnoses must be excluded. Differential diagnoses to consider include, but are not limited to, withdrawal of dopaminergic medications (such as those used for Parkinson disease), acute dystonia, acute akathisia, tardive dyskinesia, Parkinsonism, pseudoparkinsonism, catatonia, serotonin syndrome, CNS infections, status epilepticus, tetanus, thyroid storm, heat stroke, sepsis, and toxic exposures.[2–4]

  The distinction between serotonin syndrome and NMS can be difficult, especially in patients taking both serotonergic and neuroleptic medications. Some helpful differentiating features include:

- Serotonin syndrome is characterized by altered mental status, autonomic nervous system disturbances, neurologic dysfunction, *clonus*, and hyperthermia in the setting of serotonergic medication use.[3,4]
- NMS is characterized by *muscle rigidity*, hyperpyrexia, altered mental status, and autonomic instability in the setting of neuroleptic medication use.[3,4]
- In patients taking both serotonergic and neuroleptic medications, laboratory findings of elevated CPK, abnormal liver function tests, low serum iron and leukocytosis favor a diagnosis of NMS over serotonin syndrome.[3,4]
- *Treatment*: Neuroleptic medications must be stopped immediately as soon as the diagnosis of NMS is considered.[2-4] Most patients with NMS respond well to supportive management including IV fluid resuscitation, benzodiazepines for rigidity and agitation, cooling measures, and respiratory support as needed.[3,4] Rarely, paralysis and intubation as well as dantrolene may be used in refractory cases.[3,4]
- *Disposition*: Patients with NMS should be admitted to an intensive care setting for close respiratory and cardiovascular monitoring. Most patients with NMS will be able to tolerate a different antipsychotic medication after a washout period of at least 2 weeks.

Historical clues	Physical findings	Ancillary studies
• History of autism • Atypical antipsychotic use	• Fever • Agitation • Muscle rigidity	• Elevated CPK • No infectious source

Follow-Up

The patient's aripiprazole was stopped immediately. He was actively cooled with a cooling blanket. Benzodiazepines were administered for agitation and muscle rigidity, and fluid resuscitation was started. The patient was admitted to the ICU and improved over 48 hours. He was discharged home to follow up with his outpatient provider.

References

1. Silva RR, Munoz DM, Alpert M, et al. Neuroleptic malignant syndrome in children and adolescents. *J Am Acad Child Adolesc Psychiatry* 1999; 38: 187–94.
2. Neuhut R, Lindenmayer J-P, Silva R. Neuroleptic malignant syndrome in children and adolescents on atypical antipsychotic medication: A review. *J Child Adolesc Psychopharmacol* 2009; 19: 415–22.
3. Katus LE, Frucht SJ. Management of serotonin syndrome and neuroleptic malignant syndrome. *Curr Treat Options Neurol* 2016; 18: 39.
4. Perry PJ, Wilborn CA. Serotonin syndrome vs neuroleptic malignant syndrome: A contrast of causes, diagnoses, and management. *Ann Clin Psychiatry* 2012; 24: 155–62.

Case 5

Contributing Authors: Kristine Marie J. Casal and Melanie K. Prusakowski

History

The patient is a 15-month-old African American male with a history of wheezing in the past who presents with increased work of breathing, rhinorrhea, cough, and wheezing for one day. Mother gave albuterol at home; however, the patient did not appear to respond to treatments. The patient was seen by his primary physician where he had tachypnea of 56 breaths per minute, O_2 sat 96% on room air and HR 194. He received oral steroids, an albuterol nebulizer treatment, and supplemental oxygen, with only mild improvement. Due to the severity of his illness he was referred to the ED where he was found to have a fever of 101.2 °F.

Past Medical History

- Sickle cell disease, type SC.
- Mild intermittent asthma.

Medications

- Penicillin daily.
- Albuterol nebulized as needed.

Allergies

- NKDA.

Physical Examination and Ancillary Studies

- *Vital signs*: T 101.2 °F, HR 178, RR 44, BP 129/69, O_2 sat 96% on room air.

- *General*: Very playful, well-developed, and non-toxic toddler, who appears to be in mild respiratory distress.
- *HEENT*: Moist mucous membranes, normal tympanic membranes, PERRL, no mucosal lesions.
- *Neck*: Supple, with no tenderness or adenopathy.
- *Cardiovascular*: Tachycardia, normal S1, S2, no audible M/R/G.
- *Lungs*: Tachypnea, with fair air entry on lung fields bilaterally, prolonged expiratory phase with wheezing and mild subcostal retractions. No nasal flaring or supraclavicular retractions.
- *Abdomen*: Normal scaphoid appearance, soft, non-tender, without hepatomegaly.
- *Skin and extremities*: No rashes, jaundice, or pallor. No signs of trauma. No joint pain.
- *Neurologic*: Awake, interactive, and appropriate, with normal tone and reflexes.
- *Pertinent laboratory values*: WBC 8,500, Hb 10.4.
- *Pertinent radiographs*: CXR with no infiltrates, effusions, or consolidations.

Questions for Thought

- What other laboratory tests are necessary at this time?
- What complications are associated with this condition?
- What treatments need to be initiated in the ED?
- What is the management of this condition?

Diagnosis

- Fever in a patient with sickle cell disease.

Discussion

- *Epidemiology*: Sickle cell disease is an autosomal recessive disorder that affects about 250,000 children worldwide and occurs in approximately one out of every 500 black or African American births.[1] One in 12 blacks or African Americans carries sickle cell trait. It affects up to 2,000 US born infants annually and it is the most common disease detected by routine newborn screening.[1]
- *Pathophysiology*: Sickle cell disease is an autosomal recessive genetic disorder where the amino acid valine is substituted for glutamic acid, causing a mutation in the beta-globulin structure of hemoglobin. This defect causes hemoglobin to have reduced plasticity and to polymerize and sickle when deoxygenated.[1] This abnormal shape results in more rapid filtering and destruction in the spleen, leading to anemia. The shape of sickled hemoglobin causes it to adhere to the endothelium, leading to chronic inflammation and reperfusion injury. When this damage occurs in the spleen, it results in autoinfarction of the small vessels, decreased splenic function, and an increased risk of infections due to encapsulated bacterial organisms.[1]
- *Presentation*: Acute illness in children with sickle cell disease may have a similar presentation to typical childhood ailments, such as fever, common cold, and pneumonia. However, bacterial infections can rapidly progress to fulminant sepsis; thus, timely recognition and management of these children is important.[2-5] Fever may be the first sign of sepsis.

  Other presentations of illness in sickle cell disease can vary from generalized fatigue and pallor during episodes of acute anemia or splenic sequestration to severe pain. Pain crises can occur in the digits (dactyitis), skeleton, chest, and abdomen. Children often have a typical site of pain for their crises, but pain crisis should be considered in pain of any location in a child with sickle cell disease, especially in the absence of a known injury. Fever can be the presenting symptom of each of these serious sequelae of sickle cell disease in the absence of infection, as well.

  Infants with sickle cell disease may also present with jaundice, splenomegaly, and increased irritability. In some patients who have not been diagnosed with sickle cell disease on newborn screening, first presentation may be with disseminated encapsulated infection (such as pneumococcus) or sepsis.
- *Diagnosis*: Fever may be the initial presentation for acute chest syndrome or sepsis. Patients older than 2 months with a known history of sickle cell disease, who present with a temperature of $> 101.3 \,°F$ (38.5 °C), should be promptly evaluated by performing a history and physical examination, and laboratory studies including a CBC with differential, reticulocyte count, and

blood culture should be performed.[6] Urine culture should be strongly considered in patients with past history of UTI, current symptoms of dysuria, or young age at risk for pyelonephritis.[6] Fever in infants less than 2 months requires a full sepsis work-up and empiric antibiotics.[6]

Children with sickle cell disease who have fever and dyspnea, tachypnea, cough, or rales require CXR immediately to evaluate for acute chest syndrome.[6] Similarly, bone pain in an atypical location or pain associated with local swelling or erythema may indicate osteomyelitis. In these cases, radiographs may determine the etiology of the pain, although bony changes on plain film in osteomyelitis tend to be a late finding. With a high index of suspicion, consideration should be given to MRI.

- *Treatment*: Fever in a patient with sickle cell disease is an emergency because these children are at an increased risk for severe bacterial infection due to reduced splenic function.[1-5] Empiric antibiotics with appropriate coverage for *Streptococcus pneumoniae* and Gram-negative enteric organisms (ceftriaxone or cefotaxime, for example) should be utilized while cultures are pending.[3-7] Parenteral antibiotics are recommended even if the presenting illness appears to have a focal source (for example, viral URI). Supplemental oxygen should be provided to patients who present with hypoxia. If acute chest syndrome is suspected, CXR and pulse oximetry should be obtained for further evaluation. Immediate IV fluid resuscitation should be initiated in cases of hypovolemia or hypotension. Pain control in patients with sickle cell disease is important in treating an acute vaso-occlusive crisis. Mild to moderate pain may be controlled with NSAIDs such as parenteral ketorolac, while opioids may be added for severe pain.

- *Disposition*: Patients with a history of sickle cell disease who present with fevers should be promptly evaluated for sepsis, started on IV antibiotics, and admitted for further management. In addition, other acute complications of sickle cell disease including acute chest syndrome, splenic sequestration, and aplastic crisis should be considered during febrile illnesses. Infection is the major cause of death in children with sickle cell disease. With the introduction of *Haemophilus influenzae* type B and pneumococcal vaccinations,

the risk for developing sepsis has dramatically decreased; however, patients with sickle cell disease are immunocompromised, and maintaining a high index of suspicion for sepsis is an important step in preventing morbidity and mortality.

Historical clues	Physical findings	Ancillary studies
• Fever • History of sickle cell disease • Cough and respiratory difficulty	• Fever • Tachycardia • Tachypnea • Abnormal lung examination	• Negative CXR

Follow-Up

The patient was admitted to the hospital and started on empiric antibiotics even though his CXR and symptoms suggested a viral source. Blood cultures drawn prior to antibiotic administration were negative, and a respiratory swab was positive for human metapneumovirus. The patient recovered well with appropriate treatment for bronchospasm, which was likely due to his viral infection, and was discharged home on hospital day 4.

References

1. Centers for Disease Control and Prevention. Sickle cell disease: Data and statistics. See https://www.cdc.gov/ncbddd/sicklecell/data.html (accessed December 2016).

2. Bansil NH et al. Incidence of serious bacterial infections in febrile children with sickle cell disease. *Clin Pediatr* 2013; 52: 661–6.

3. Morrissey BJ et al. Incidence and predictors of bacterial infection in febrile children with sickle cell disease. *Hemoglobin* 2015; 39: 316–19.

4. Narang S et al. Bacteremia in children with sickle hemoglobinopathies. *J Pediatr Hematol Oncol* 2012; 34: 13–16.

5. Savlov D et al. Predictors of bacteremia among children with sickle cell disease presenting with fever. *J Pediatr Hematol Oncol* 2014; 36: 384–8.

6. Schultz CL et al. Adherence to prompt fever evaluation in children with sickle cell disease and the health belief model. *Pediatr Blood Cancer* 2015; 62: 1968–73.

7. Shihabuddin BS, Scarfi CA. Fever in children with sickle cell disease: Are all fevers equal? *J Emerg Med* 2014; 47: 395–400.

Case 6

Contributing Author: Taylor R. Spencer

History

The patient is a 12-year-old female with a history of a renal transplant, who presents for fever. Her family reports that she has had increased fatigue over the past 2 days. She has had fever measured orally to 101.8 °F at home. This is associated with weight loss, myalgias, fatigue, and nausea without vomiting. She notes a mild diffuse abdominal discomfort without exacerbating or alleviating factors. There have been multiple episodes of non-bloody diarrhea. She has no head or neck pain. She has no congestion, cough, sore throat, or chest pain. She has no dysuria or pelvic pain, and reports no rash. The patient denies prior similar episodes. She has no sick contacts or recent travel. After calling her transplant team, the family was instructed to go to the ED for further evaluation.

Past Medical History

- Renal transplant 2 years previous, without complications. Transplant was the result of focal segmental glomerulosclerosis leading to chronic renal failure.

Medications

- Mycophenolate mofetil.
- Tacrolimus.
- Prednisone.

Allergies

- Penicillin, which causes a rash.

Physical Examination and Ancillary Studies

- *Vital signs*: T 100.5 °F, HR 108, RR 14, BP 138/82.
- *General*: Awake and alert, in no acute distress.
- *HEENT*: No tympanic membrane erythema, no sinus tenderness, no rhinorrhea, and no pharyngeal injection or exudates.
- *Neck*: Moderate shotty cervical lymphadenopathy is seen.
- *Cardiovascular*: Regular, with no M/R/G.
- *Lungs*: Normal work of breathing, lungs clear and equal, with no W/R/R.
- *Abdomen*: Vague diffuse discomfort on palpation, without Murphy's sign, Rovsing's sign, or McBurney's point tenderness. Soft without organomegaly. No tenderness overlying the kidney transplant site.
- *Skin and extremities*: Somewhat warm to the touch but dry without rashes. No cellulitic changes. A well-healed surgical scar is noted on the abdomen, without any acute findings.
- *Neurologic*: Cranial nerves intact, no focal neurologic deficits, normal alertness.
- *Pertinent laboratory values*:
  - WBC 14,300, including absolute neutrophil count of 3,400;
  - Cr 1.3, consistent with baseline laboratory values;
  - U/A with trace protein, but no evidence of leukocytes, nitrites, or bacteria;
  - Lactate is within normal limits;
  - Stool has no fecal leukocytes, and negative for *Clostridium difficile* and for ova and parasites;
  - Cytomegalovirus (CMV) serology is positive.
- *Pertinent radiographs*: CXR with no infiltrates or other acute pathology. Non-contrasted CT of the abdomen and pelvis with non-specific small bowel wall thickening.

Questions for Thought

- What sources of fever are unique to patients with transplant?
- What non-infectious causes of fever must be considered after transplant?
- How do anti-rejection drugs influence the presentation of infectious processes?
- What findings on history or examination are suggestive of CMV infection?
- When may it be appropriate to decrease immunosuppressant therapy in transplant patients with fever?

Diagnosis

- Transplant-associated CMV infection.

Discussion

- *Epidemiology*: In the USA, nearly 30,000 organ transplantations are performed annually. Renal transplants are most common, followed by liver, heart, and lung. While only a small proportion of these are pediatric cases, fever is not an uncommon complication in the pediatric transplant population.

Infection is the most common cause of fever after pediatric transplant.[1-3] Epidemiologically, these may be divided into patient-derived infections, host-derived infections, healthcare-acquired infections, and community-acquired infections. Certain patient characteristics are associated with increased risk for infection, including black or Hispanic race, the nature of the transplant and pre-transplant health status, and age.[1,2] For example, RSV and influenza may present with more severe infection in younger transplant recipients compared with older children. However, younger patients are also less likely to have acquired pathogens that induce lifelong latent infection.[2]

The time since transplantation also influences infectious risk.[1-3] In the first month, bacterial post-operative infections are most likely. Opportunistic infections and latent pathogens from the recipient or donor are more prevalent in the next 6 months. After 6 months, community-acquired infections and those associated with chronic graft dysfunction predominate.

Of significant concern is the subset of infections particularly associated with transplantation and immunosuppression. CMV is one of the most common and important viral pathogens. Infection can be asymptomatic or symptomatic. It can be due to primary infection, reactivation, or superinfection.[2] CMV is one of the most common infectious diarrheas in this population, although *Clostridium difficile* must also be considered. EBV is also important to consider in transplant recipients. Presentations range from a non-specific viral illness to post-transplant lymphoproliferative disease (PTLD), including lymphoma.[2] BK viral infection is an important cause of nephropathy and renal dysfunction in pediatric renal transplant with a 5 percent incidence.[4]

- *Pneumocystis jirovecii* (formerly *Pneumocystis carinii* or PCP) is a fungal pneumonia with an incidence of roughly 5–15 percent after transplantation. Like the aforementioned viral infections, this is of particular concern in patients who are immunosuppressed, and fungal infections show increased prevalence in this group.[4]

Consideration must be given for common community-acquired infections in the pediatric transplant patient with fever. Pneumonia may be community- or healthcare-acquired, and accounts for a large portion of infections seen. The incidence varies based upon the type of transplant. For example, UTI is the most common bacterial infection in kidney transplant recipients.[1-3] Antimicrobial resistance must be considered due to the possibility for prior antibiotic exposures and recurrent infections in this group. Other community bacterial or viral infectious may also be seen in patients who are immunosuppressed due to transplantation and anti-rejection medications. Vaccine-preventable infections are in the differential diagnosis, particularly with an incomplete vaccination record or without previously developed immunity.

Non-infectious etiologies may cause fever in the pediatric transplant recipient, with estimates ranging from one in four to one in eight of transplant patients presenting with fever.[1,2] Rejection, malignancy, adrenal insufficiency, and drug fever are common non-infectious causes.[1-3] Rejection accounts for around 4 percent of episodes.[1] Especially of concern among malignancy is PTLD as a complication of EBV in transplant patients, and 80 percent of these cases initially present with fever.[1,2]

All of the relevant exposures and risk factors must be considered in the evaluation of fever in the pediatric transplant recipient.

- *Pathophysiology*: The pathophysiology of fever is influenced by a variety of factors, including aspects related to host, donor, infection, and the type of transplantation.

Many infections in transplant recipients may be a reactivation of a latent infection to which the patient has been previously exposed. CMV and EBV are associated with such reactivation. This occurs in the transplant patient because anti-rejection medications blunt the immune response that would normally keep such infections dormant. Therapeutic immunosuppression can also decrease the immunogenicity of vaccines, increasing susceptibility to these infections. Neutropenia may be seen in transplant recipients and can directly increase the risk for infection in patients with organ transplantation. Management of febrile neutropenia is discussed in this chapter, Case 3.

Alternatively, the transplanted organ may contribute to fever in the pediatric transplant population. Donor infections have a high risk of transmission to the recipient.[1-4] Organ mismatch can be another source for fever, mostly as human leukocyte antigen mismatch can precipitate organ rejection.[1] Rejection can be acute or chronic, and mediated by cellular, antibody, and humoral mechanisms. Fevers result from the immunologic and inflammatory response in these cases.

The nature of the transplantation itself can also contribute to pathophysiologic processes in some cases. Pediatric transplant recipients often receive organs from adult donors, with a resultant discrepancy in organ size, which can lead to an increased risk for anastomotic complications such as leakage, thrombosis, or necrosis.[1]

- *Presentation:* In transplant recipients, fever is defined as a temperature of at least 101 °F at least twice in a 24-hour period.[4] However, the antimetabolite immunosuppressive drugs mycophenolate mofetil and azathioprine are associated with lower maximum temperatures and leukocyte counts. One of the great challenges with fever in the transplant patient is the broad array of potential etiologies and degrees of severity, which leads to a wide range of associated presentations. The clinician must be vigilant to subtle and atypical presentations, particularly given the potential for immunosuppression to blunt the infectious and inflammatory response.

Clinical presentation can suggest the underlying source of infection, yet the severity of these symptoms is hard to predict. For example, most pediatric organ recipients experience typical childhood respiratory and GI illnesses without significant issues.[3] In contrast, some viral infections, such as RSV, influenza virus, or parainfluenza, can cause severe disease, especially if they occur soon after transplant and during maximal immunosuppression.

Malignancy such as PTLD, thromboembolic disease including pulmonary embolism, drug fever, and acute allograft rejection must also be considered in the setting of transplant-associated fever.[1] The classic presentation of acute rejection with fever and graft tenderness is observed less commonly with current immunosuppressive

regimens. With newer regimens, acute rejection episodes may only be detected by laboratory testing.

- *Diagnosis:* Physical examination is crucial in identifying subtle sources for infection. In the absence of localizing findings, consideration should be given for the following:
  - CBC with differential, particularly for identification of neutropenia;
  - U/A and urine culture, including pyuria that may suggest renal rejection;
  - CXR;
  - Blood cultures;
  - CMV PCR;
  - Purified protein derivative or QuantiFERON testing;
  - Antigen detection tests available for adenovirus, influenza A, RSV, and rotavirus; PCR may also be available.
  - U/S or CT imaging may help to diagnose rejection or deep-tissue infection.

While all of these tests need not be pursued in all patients, they should be considered as a means to identify common triggers and causes of subtle presentations following pediatric transplants.

While a broad evaluation can be considered for fever in the child with a transplantation, work-ups should focus on likely sources of infection. When pulmonary symptoms predominate, this could include sputum cultures, *Legionella* antigen, sputum acid-fast bacillus testing, or direct fluorescent antibody for *P. jirovecii*.[2,4] In contrast, LP and CSF analysis can evaluate fever with neurologic symptoms.[4] Up to 20 percent of these patients will also require an MRI for abscesses, non-focal lesion, and other pathology. Diarrhea can suggest initial evaluation with fecal leukocytes and cultures, *C. difficile* testing, and ova and parasites.[4] Endoscopy may ultimately be needed, with mucosal biopsy and immunohistochemical stains for CMV. In the interim, blood tests for CMV PCR can help to diagnose. When lymphadenopathy is noted in the febrile transplant patient, serum EBV and CMV are particularly warranted. Serologic evaluation for EBV antibodies is unreliable in the transplant patient, and PCR testing of viremia may be preferred when a clinical concern exists. In addition, *Bartonella* (catscratch disease) and

Toxoplasmosis gondii may be assessed. Lymph-node biopsy is often diagnostic for EBV and PTLD, augmented by using the Epstein–Barr encoded RNA probe. CT scanning of the neck, chest, abdomen, and pelvis in these patients can characterize the extent of nodal involvement.

- *Treatment*: With regard to management of fever after a transplant, properly targeting the source is crucial. However, the etiology is often unknown in the early stages and empiric therapy may be necessary. For example, unless another source of fever is apparent, a febrile kidney transplant patient who demonstrates acute renal injury should be treated with empiric antibiotics, including Gram-negative coverage, particularly *Pseudomonas*. When prescribing such empiric antibiotics, the provider should consider the most likely site of infection, the possibility of antimicrobial resistance, and prior antibiotic use. If broad-spectrum antibiotics are used, the spectrum should be narrowed as soon as is feasible, to target the specific identified organism.

A low threshold for antiviral therapy is appropriate in the transplant patient. Initial treatment of CMV includes IV ganciclovir with concomitant reduction of immunosuppression (unless there is evidence of rejection).[1-4] The use of effective antiviral therapy has improved outcomes in this population. For EBV, a stepwise approach to therapy is recommended, starting with reduced immunosuppression. Similarly, the consensus supports reducing immunosuppression to treat polyomavirus-associated nephropathy due to BK viral infection.

Empiric antifungal treatment can be considered, particularly if the immune suppression is associated with neutropenia.[2,4] When diagnosed, fungal pneumonia from *P. jirovecii* can be managed with trimethoprim–sulfamethoxazole.[2,4]

With the potential for non-infectious causes, treatment should address these alternative etiologies if they are identified (for example, treating acute rejection or a pulmonary embolism).

Antipyretics can be considered but are not necessarily routinely recommended due to potential for masking of symptoms and drug interactions.

- *Disposition*: Most patients with fever and immunocompromise related to transplantation require hospitalization. In some cases, children with a low-risk fever may be considered for initial or step-down outpatient care, with oral antibiotics as needed. This determination should be based on a clinical risk stratification strategy. Given the complexity of pediatric transplantation, close collaboration with the patient's primary care and specialist providers is essential for all management and disposition planning.

Historical clues	Physical findings	Ancillary studies
• Immunosuppression due to anti-rejection medications • Fever with abdominal pain and diarrhea	• Fever • Non-specific physical examination findings	• Renal function with no findings of acute kidney injury • No neutropenia • CMV serology positive

Follow-Up

In the hospital, the patient's transplant surgeon and nephrologist were consulted. Infectious disease was consulted, too. The patient was initially placed on broad-spectrum antibiotics with meropenem and admitted for further care. Blood cultures and stool cultures ultimately returned negative. Antibiotics were discontinued based upon this further evaluation. Due to the positive CMV serology, IV ganciclovir was administered with concomitant reduction of immunosuppression. Her renal function remained unaffected, and her symptoms resolved with treatment. She was discharged following the course of IV antiviral therapy.

References

1. Bouza E, Loeches B, Muñoz P. Fever of unknown origin in solid organ transplant recipients. *Infect Dis Clin North Am* 2007; 21: 1033–54, ix-x.

2. Green M, Michaels MG. Infections in pediatric solid organ transplant recipients. *J Pediatric Infect Dis Soc* 2012; 1: 144–51.

3. Lau KK, Giglia L, Chan H, et al. Management of children after renal transplantation: Highlights for general pediatricians. *Transl Pediatr* 2012; 1: 35–46.

4. Muñoz P, Singh N, Bouza E. Fever in organ transplant recipients. *Antimicrobe: Infect Dis Antimicrob Agents.* Available online at http://www.antimicrobe.org/e54.asp (accessed December 2016).

Case 7

Contributing Author: Sarah Hudgins

History

A 20-month-old female presents to the ED with her mother for an evaluation of fever. The mother states that the child is not acting normally and has had several episodes of vomiting as well as difficulty breathing (she described this as "breathing fast as if she cannot catch her breath"). The mother first noticed these symptoms after waking the child for daycare this morning. The mother states the child is healthy at baseline and had no symptoms when she went to bed last night. The child has had no cough or cold symptoms, wheezing or stridor, diarrhea, blood in her vomit or stool, dysuria, or rash. She has had no known sick contacts at school or home, has a PCP, and is UTD on vaccinations. She lives with her mother and father. She is the middle child of three children with the youngest sibling being less than a month old.

Upon further questioning, mom conveys that the child was found yesterday rifling through one of the medicine cabinets. The mother states that although her child was trying to drink from a small bottle in the cabinet she was stopped just as she was placing it to her lips so "she couldn't have drank very much." The child's father has left work to go home in order to determine the name of the liquid to which the child was exposed. The child has had no resolution of dyspnea using her older sibling's albuterol nebulizer prior to arrival.

Past Medical History

- None. Vaccinations are UTD.

Medications

- No routine medications.

Allergies

- NKDA.

Physical Examination and Ancillary Studies

- *Vital signs*: T 103.8 °F, HR 156, RR 60, BP 100/60, O_2 sat 100% on room air.
- *General*: The child appears to be in moderate to severe distress, she is tachypneic and lethargic, she will open her eyes on occasion but is not tracking or following commands.
- *HEENT*: Her head is normocephalic and atraumatic. PERRL. No nasal congestion or rhinorrhea. Tympanic membranes normal. Tacky mucous membranes, no pharyngeal erythema, no tonsillar edema/exudates.
- *Neck*: Supple, with no lymphadenopathy.
- *Cardiovascular*: Heart rate is tachycardic, with a regular rhythm, no audible M/R/G. Peripheral pulses are thready. Capillary refill > 3 seconds.
- *Lungs*: Tachypneic, with equal but diminished breath sounds bilaterally. Scattered rales, no wheezing or rhonchi.
- *Abdomen*: Soft, non-distended, diffusely tender abdomen, with decreased bowel sounds. No hepatosplenomegaly. No palpable masses. One episode of hematemesis shortly after arrival.
- *Skin and extremities*: Skin is intact and dry, no signs of trauma. No edema.
- *Neurologic*: Child moves all four extremities symmetrically, but does not follow commands. She is lethargic.

Questions for Thought

- Based on this child's history and physical examination, what tests should be considered?
- Knowing the potential time of ingestion, would lavage be indicated? How about activated charcoal?
- What other toxins can present in this way? What non-toxicologic etiologies are there?
- What tests would help you exclude non-toxicologic causes for this presentation?

Diagnosis

- Acute salicylate toxicity secondary to methyl salicylate overdose.

Discussion

- *Epidemiology*: The unintentional ingestion of pharmaceutical agents is a leading cause of morbidity and mortality in children. Children less than 3 years old account for greater than 35 percent of toxic ingestions, with almost half of all unintentional ingestions occurring in children less than 6 years of age.[1] Annually, approximately 20,000 of those unintentional ingestions are from salicylate products.[1] Fatal poisonings from salicylates have been reported in ~5 percent of ingestions secondary to pulmonary and cerebral edema, renal failure, and severe acid–base imbalances.[2,3] Delay in diagnosis is a large contributing factor in fatal outcomes.

- The number of salicylate-related fatalities has decreased since the 1980s as a result of aspirin no longer being a prevalent treatment for children due to its association with Reye's syndrome, more child-resistant packaging methods, and manufacturing limits on the quantities per bottle distributed.[3] Aspirin and its derivatives are found in many formulations and are also a component of several well-known over-the-counter products such as Excedrin, Percodan, Bengay creams, and Pepto-Bismol. Methyl salicylate (oil of wintergreen) remains the most potent form of salicylate available. As little as 5 mL equates to 7,000 mg of aspirin, over 85 baby aspirin tablets. Lethal doses have been reported in young children with exposure to as little as one teaspoon of methyl salicylate.

- *Pathophysiology*: Once consumed, aspirin products are quickly converted to salicylic acid, where they are primarily absorbed in the small intestine. Salicylic acid is metabolized by the liver and excreted in small quantities in the urine, but in large doses, the liver cannot adequately metabolize the drug load, and urinary excretion becomes increasingly important.[3]

  Salicylates typically cause a respiratory alkalosis followed by an anion gap metabolic acidosis.[2,3] The first phase of salicylate toxicity is the direct stimulation of the respiratory center of the brain that causes tachypnea, hyperventilation, and respiratory alkalosis.[2,3] Salicylic acid then causes a metabolic acidosis through the uncoupling of oxidative phosphorylation in mitochondria and the inhibition of the Krebs cycle. This increase in metabolic demand combines with the inability to utilize aerobic metabolism to shift the cells to anaerobic and lipid metabolism, producing large quantities of lactic acid and ketone bodies.[2,3]

  As only non-ionized salicylic acid is able to cross cell membranes, serum and urine pH are major contributors of salicylic acid distribution and elimination. As non-ionized salicylic acid more readily crosses the blood–brain barrier, worsening metabolic acidosis can cause a greater degree of neurotoxicity.[2,3] The non-ionized salicylic acid decreases renal excretion, resulting

in a downward spiral of complications, in which acidosis leads to excretion issues, which again leads to worsening acidosis.[2,3]

Acid–base imbalances are not the only concerning outcomes of salicylate toxicity. GI toxicity can result from either the direct interaction of salicylate with the gastric mucosa or secondarily from neurotoxic effects.[2,3] Dehydration is a common complication of salicylate toxicity. Up to 10 percent of total body water can be lost as a result of vomiting, hyperpnea, and fever.[2,3]

- *Presentation*: Patient presentation varies greatly based on the quantity and timing of toxic ingestion. The classic triad of salicylism is tinnitus, hyperventilation, and GI irritation.[3,4] Early manifestations are a combination of potentially reversible respiratory, GI, and neurologic complications.[3,5] Symptoms early in the overdose include: nausea and vomiting, tinnitus and/or vertigo, and anorexia. On presentation, patients can appear well although they will often appear ill. Patients can be diaphoretic and tachycardic, with hyperventilation that can appear as respiratory distress. Later symptoms of salicylism are the result of severe acid–base abnormalities as well as pulmonary and cerebral edema.[3,5] These symptoms can include: fever, lethargy, altered mental status, agitation, seizures, hallucinations, and renal and respiratory failure. A high index of suspicion should be maintained in children and adolescents presenting with these features as a toxic ingestion history is not always easily divulged and delayed treatment can cause significant morbidity or even mortality.

- *Diagnosis*: Although the patient history often leads the clinician to consider a toxic ingestion, the diagnosis of salicylate toxicity is obtained with serum salicylate levels. Based solely on reported ingestion, a mild toxicity is defined as consuming between 150 and 300 mg/kg of salicylate.[5] A moderate to severe toxicity will range from 300 to 500 mg/kg and a severe toxicity can be found with any ingestion greater than 500 mg/kg.[5] For serum salicylate levels, a toxic ingestion is any level greater than 30 mg/dL.[5] Lethal toxicity can occur with an acute ingestion level of greater than 100 mg/dL or a chronic ingestion level of 60 mg/dL.

  Additional laboratory studies that should be obtained with salicylate toxicity include: ABG, electrolytes, glucose, BUN/Cr, LFTs, coagulation studies, CBC, serum calcium, U/A, and urine pH. These laboratory studies guide treatment by determining the extent of acid–base disorders, severity of dehydration, metabolic abnormalities, and underlying organ damage.[3]

EKG, CXR, and abdominal X-ray are the standard diagnostic studies used to evaluate for complications of overdose. Additional tests are often used to exclude other diagnoses when the history does not definitively lead to salicylate overdose. Differential diagnoses that can mimic salicylate poisoning include diabetic ketoacidosis, sepsis, and other ingestions such as iron or toxic alcohols.

- *Treatment*: Treatment for salicylate toxicity will depend on the time elapsed between the patient's ingestion and presentation to the hospital as well as the salicylate level and symptom manifestations.[3,5] Patients with known or suspected salicylate ingestion should be immediately stabilized.[3] Patients with toxic salicylate levels (greater than 30 mg/dL) should be treated quickly and monitored closely for acute changes. If the patient has presented within 1 hour of ingestion, gastric lavage is a reasonable decontamination strategy.[5] Activated charcoal should be given at a 1–2 g/kg dose, and repeated every 3 hours during management while repeating salicylate levels to determine the peak.[3,5] The provider should gain IV access, pursue aggressive fluid resuscitation, and correct any metabolic derangements.[3,5] Patients with salicylate toxicity can be severely dehydrated upon presentation, often losing several liters of fluid prior to arrival. Bicarbonate drips should be adjusted to maximize urine output and urine pH (goal of at least 7.5).[3,5] Patients will require repeat laboratory tests (ABG, electrolytes, and salicylate levels) every 1–2 hours as well as close monitoring of blood glucose levels.[3]

Hemodialysis will be necessary for patients who have salicylate toxicity levels greater than 100 mg/dL, critical symptoms (defined as signs of either pulmonary or cerebral edema or a severe acid–base imbalance), or those patients not responding to conservative treatment.[3,5] Exchange transfusions can be considered for young infants when there is significant hemodynamic instability. Once a method of dialysis or filtration system is initiated, it should be continued until serum salicylate levels are less than 20 mg/dL.[3]

Intubation may be required for patients who present with severe toxicity, signs of cerebral/pulmonary edema or refractory shock. The underlying severe metabolic acidosis in combination with the increased metabolic demand of salicylate overdose raises specific intubation concerns.[3] Ventilator settings such as PEEP and respiratory rate will have to be secondarily adjusted based on ABG analyses, and it is challenging to meet the patient's ventilatory requirements to allow adequate compensation for metabolic acidosis.[3] Patients will often require an additional bicarbonate bolus as a buffer for the transition, and providers should be prepared to provide emergent hemodialysis upon intubation as ventilator settings are incapable of adequately compensating for the effects of salicylate poisoning.[3]

- *Disposition*: If the provider is sure of the dose, the dose is less than 125 mg/kg, and the patient is asymptomatic, he or she may be discharged home.[5] The remainder should be observed with repeat aspirin levels, as levels may not peak for 12 hours.[5] Obviously, any symptomatic patient or any patient requiring intubation or dialysis should be admitted to an ICU.

Historical clues	Physical findings
• History of witnessed accidental ingestion	• Fever
	• Tachypnea
• Altered mental status	• Signs of cerebral edema (lethargy)
• Vomiting	• Signs of GI toxicity (hematemesis)
• Tachypnea by report	• Signs of pulmonary edema (rales)

Follow-Up

Father called the hospital 20 minutes later stating that he found a partially empty bottle of wintergreen oil in the medicine cabinet. He was asked to measure the remaining liquid from the 100 mL bottle which revealed 12 mL, a little over two teaspoons, was missing.

After arriving to the hospital, the child rapidly deteriorated and required intubation. Her salicylate levels returned at 110 mg/dL. The child was treated with IV fluids as well as bicarbonate infusions and immediately transitioned to hemodialysis. She was sent to the PICU where she continued to have hourly laboratory tests (ABG, electrolytes, salicylate levels). Despite the provider's exhaustion of all available treatment options, the child continued to clinically deteriorate, progressed to a coma, and died later that afternoon. Based on the missing amount of liquid from the bottle of wintergreen oil, the maximum amount the child could have consumed would have been the equivalent of 16,000 mg of aspirin – over twice the lethal dose for her age.

References

1. Poison Control: National Capital Poison Center. Poison statistics: National data 2014. Poison Statistics National Data 2014. See www.poison.org/poison-statistics-national (accessed December 2016).

2. Defendi GL. Acute salicylate toxicity in children: Diagnosis and treatment of over ingestion. *CPF* 2013; 12: 547–52.

3. O'Malley GF. Emergency department management of the salicylate-poisoned patient. *Emerg Med Clin N Am* 2007; 25: 333–46.

4. Frithsen IL, Simson WM. Recognition and management of acute medication poisoning. *Am Fam Phys* 2010; 81: 316–23.

5. Dargan PI, Wallace CI, Jones AL. An evidence-based flowchart to guide the management of acute salicylate (aspirin) overdose. *Emerg Med J* 2002; 19: 206–9.

Case 8

Contributing Author: Rebecca Jeanmonod

History

A 20-month-old girl is brought to the ED by a panicked father with concern for her temperature. Dad was supposed to drop the child at daycare this morning, which is a break in his usual routine. Typically, the child is brought by her mother, but her mother is out of town on a business trip. Dad put the child in the car, but in the course of his drive, the child fell asleep, and he forgot she was there. He went to work and left her in the car. His wife called his office about 2 hours into his workday to ask how he was doing as a "single dad," and he immediately realized his mistake. He ran out to the car to find his daughter still buckled into her front-facing car seat. The child was upset and crying. She had vomit on her shirt and car seat. She felt very warm to touch, so he brought her in for evaluation. The car has dark upholstery. It is July and the family lives in New

Jersey. The car was not left in the shade. The child has not had any recent illnesses, and was in her usual state of health this morning.

Past Medical History

- Inguinal hernia with repair shortly after birth. Immunizations are UTD.

Medications

- None.

Allergies

- Peanuts and red dye.

Physical Examination and Ancillary Studies

- *Vital signs*: 103.7 °F, HR 171, RR 36, BP 108/67, O_2 sat 100% on room air.
- *General*: The child is irritable and awake, consolable, and calling for her mother.
- *HEENT*: PERRL. Oropharynx with tacky mucous membranes. No tears.
- *Neck*: Supple and non-tender, with no adenopathy.
- *Cardiovascular*: Tachycardic and regular, no M/R/G.
- *Lungs*: Clear and equal, with no W/R/R.
- *Abdomen*: Soft and non-tender. No masses or guarding.
- *Skin and extremities*: Skin is clammy and diaphoretic. The child has gooseflesh.
- *Neurologic*: Irritable. Moves all four extremities symmetrically.

Questions for Thought

- What are appropriate ways to cool the child? Does the child need to be cooled?
- How do you determine which children require extensive laboratory evaluation and which can be observed and treated with supportive care?
- Do you need to contact CPS?
- How do you clinically distinguish among different kinds of heat illness?

Diagnosis

- Heat exhaustion.

Discussion

- *Epidemiology*: Although death from heat stroke is relatively rare, heat illness is common, accounting for approximately 325,000 ED visits each summer in the USA.[1] When heat stroke occurs, the case fatality rate is about 50 percent, but most patients with heat-related illness are discharged home from the ED.[1] The overall incidence of heat-related illness is likely much higher than these numbers indicate, as it is probable that many cases of more mild heat illness are treated in the field.

- *Pathophysiology*: The body produces heat continuously, and maintains a constant temperature gradient to allow for dissipation of that heat from the core to the periphery.[2] Sweating also allows for cooling through evaporation. Children have less efficient sweating and therefore have less ability to cool by this mechanism, although their larger surface areas allow for more heat dissipation through convection.[2,3] However, since sweating is the body's predominant cooling mechanism, children have less ability to cool. Additionally, children's large surface area allows them to increase their temperature more quickly than adults by the mechanism of convective warming when in a warm environment.[2] This combination of decreased ability to dissipate heat with an increased ability to absorb heat makes children more prone to heat-related illness. Heat illness occurs when the body's ability to cool is inadequate to match the environmental or endogenous heat burden and is overwhelmed.[2–4]

  Classic heat stroke (heat stroke from increased ambient temperature in a patient with normal endogenous heat production) and exertional heat stroke (heat stroke from increased production of heat secondary to activity, in addition to increased ambient temperatures) affect different pediatric populations. Classic heat stroke is more common in small children who cannot remove themselves from the hot environment and cannot access fluids on their own, such as our patient.[2,3] Children entrapped in cars are subjected to temperatures much higher than the outside temperature. As the sun warms the interior surfaces within the car, and subsequently the air in the car, the hot air cannot escape. The surfaces within the car can reach temperatures in excess of 180 °F, and the air temperature in the car can reach 150 °F within 15 minutes.[5] Leaving a car window open does not significantly alter this.

  Exertional heat stroke is most common in school-aged athletes who exercise excessively in warm environments, such as football practice during the summer months.[2,3] Regardless of the type of heat stroke, the end result is the same. As body temperature continues to rise and dehydration decreases sweat production, the child develops SIRS.[2] Heat-sensitive organs, such as the brain and the liver, become affected, and the child may develop cardiomyopathy and disseminated intravascular coagulopathy.[2] In fatal cases, diffuse serosal petechiae and pulmonary edema are common.[2,6] At temperatures above 107 °F, proteins denature and cell death occurs.

- *Presentation*: Heat illness includes prickly heat (a benign rash that is typically pruritic, which is secondary to keratin plugs blocking sweat ducts), heat-related edema (dependent edema from vasodilation), and heat-related syncope (orthostatic syncope related to vasodilation). These are not associated with elevated core temperature and are benign. More severe forms of heat illness include *heat cramps*, *heat exhaustion*, or *heat stroke*. Heat stroke can be further divided into *classic heat stroke* and *exertional heat stroke*.

  - *Heat cramps* are severe, typically lower extremity cramps that occur after exertion.[2,3] They are often attributed to hyponatremia secondary to sodium losses during sweating, and although they are painful, they typically do not occur in conjunction with elevated core temperature.[2,3]
  - *Heat exhaustion* is characterized by an inability to continue activities secondary to heat, often with increased temperature to < 104 °F.[2,4] Common presenting symptoms include increased thirst, irritability, nausea, vomiting, diarrhea, headache, tachycardia, weakness, and heavy sweating.[2,4] Patients may have piloerection from sympathetic stimulation.
  - *Heat stroke* is the most severe form of heat-related illness. It is characterized by a temperature > 104 °F and altered mental status.[2,4] Patients may lack sweating, but this is not a prerequisite to make the diagnosis. Since heat exhaustion and heat stroke exist on a continuum, patients may have some elements of heat exhaustion and some features of heat stroke. In these cases, the provider should err

on the side of treating the patient for heat stroke, as heat stroke has a high mortality and requires aggressive intervention. These patients may be obtunded or seizing, or may have subtle alterations in mental status. It is important to get a core body temperature on all patients with symptoms consistent with heat stroke, as other forms of temperature assessment have been found to be unreliable.

- *Diagnosis*: Diagnosis is clinical, based on history, core temperature, and presenting symptoms. It is not necessary to get further ancillary testing in patients with heat cramps or in patients with mild heat exhaustion. These patients generally have normal or near-normal laboratory findings, and there is no role for imaging. In patients with severe heat exhaustion in whom heat stroke is a diagnostic consideration and in those with heat stroke, extensive laboratory testing is indicated. These patients can develop rhabdomyolysis, renal failure, and disseminated intravascular coagulopathy. Therefore, they should have CBC, electrolytes, coagulation studies, calcium, magnesium, phosphorus, creatine kinase, and lactate levels checked. In patients in whom the diagnosis is not clear, toxic causes (for example, sympathomimetics, anticholinergics, aspirin, psychiatric medications, serotonergic medications), infectious causes, endocrine causes (such as thyroid), drug withdrawal, and neurologic causes should be considered.[2] These patients may require further ED testing such as neuroimaging, toxicologic screening, and LP to define the source of the symptoms.

- *Treatment*: Mild disease requires little more than supportive care and provision of oral rehydration fluids. This will typically improve symptoms from heat-related syncope as well as heat cramps.

The major goals of treatment for patients with more severe disease are to rapidly cool the patient and to restore circulating volume, as most of these patients are hypovolemic. Initial resuscitative measures should begin with the ABC algorithm, as in any sick patient. IV access should be established, and the patient should be volume resuscitated with room-temperature normal saline. This by itself will assist in cooling the patient's core. Excess clothing should be removed. Ice packs may be placed at the patient's axillae,

neck, and groin to assist in cooling.[2] Although it is impractical in most institutions to submerge heat stroke patients in cold water, this is probably the best way to cool a patient.[2,4] A realistic option is to spray the patient down with water from a spray bottle and use a large fan to assist in evaporative cooling. Patients who have cooling measures provided within 30 minutes of recognition of heat stroke have lower mortality than those with a delay to cooling, and therefore EMS providers should be educated and should begin cooling measures in the field when possible.[2] Patients with heat stroke who develop multi-system organ failure may require intubation and more aggressive supportive measures.

In patients with a disease that is unclear in severity, attempts may be made at oral rehydration and supportive care. If the patient's symptoms are not improved at 30 minutes, more aggressive evaluation and treatment should be undertaken.

- *Disposition*: Patients with mild illness (heat cramps or heat exhaustion with elevated core temperature but no altered mental status) may be treated and observed in the ED for symptom resolution, and discharged home. Most patients with heat stroke require admission to the hospital, and those with laboratory derangements will often require ICU-level care. For children who are left in vehicles or who are playing unattended and become entrapped in vehicles, CPS should be consulted for concern of neglect.

Historical clues	Physical findings
• Left in vehicle • Vomiting	• Fever • Tachycardia • Irritability • Clammy skin with gooseflesh

Follow-Up

IV access was established and the child received a total of 30 cc/kg normal saline. Her clothing was removed, she was sprayed with water, and a fan was brought into the room to aid with cooling. She received IV ondansetron for her nausea. Because the child was irritable and it was unclear if she had altered mental status, she had laboratory testing performed including CBC, electrolytes and renal function, glucose, creatine kinase, calcium, magnesium, and phosphorus.

The child had mild hyponatremia and a slightly low bicarbonate, but the remainder of her laboratory values were unremarkable. Her symptoms improved over the course of 2 hours in the ED. CPS were contacted because of the nature of the child's presentation, and they planned to follow up with the family within 24 hours. The child was discharged home with her father after her ED stay.

References

1. Hess JJ, Saha S, Luber G. Summertime acute heat illness in U.S. emergency departments from 2006 through 2010: Analysis of a nationally representative sample. *Environ Health Perspect* 2014; 122: 1209–15.

2. Atha WF. Heat-related illness. *Emerg Med Clin N Am* 2013; 31: 1097–108.

3. Bytomski JR, Squire DL. Heat illness in children. *Curr Sports Med Rep* 2003; 2(6): 320–4.

4. Becker JA, Stewart LK. Heat-related illness. *Am Fam Phys* 2011; 83: 1325–30.

5. Ferrara P, Vena F, Caporale O, et al. Children left unattended in parked vehicles: A focus on recent Italian cases and a review of literature. *Ital J Pediatr* 2013; 39: 71.

6. Adato B, Dubnov-Raz G, Gips H, et al. Fatal heat stroke in children found in parked cars: Autopsy findings. *Eur J Pediatr* 2016; 175: 1249–52.

Case 9

Contributing Authors: Keel Coleman and Khalief Hamden

History

The patient is a 17-year-old male who presents with a complaint of headache. The patient reports a fever (103 °F) at home, starting yesterday, that improved with acetaminophen. The onset of the headache was 3 days ago, and is associated with blurred vision, vomiting (one episode this morning), sore throat, and neck pain. He also complains of back pain after hitting a deer in his vehicle last week. The patient denies diarrhea, difficulty breathing, abdominal pain, ear pain, sinus symptoms, or chest pain. The patient reports a history of recurrent migraines in the past.

Past Medical History

- Migraine headaches.

Medications

- None.

Allergies

- Seasonal allergies.
- Sulfonamide antibiotics – nausea only.

Physical Examination and Ancillary Studies

- *Vital signs*: T 100.5 °F, HR 99, RR 20, BP 124/79, O_2 sat 98% on room air.
- *General*: Well-developed and well-nourished. No obvious distress.
- *HEENT*: PERRL. No signs of trauma. Moist mucous membranes. Clear oropharynx.
- *Neck*: Supple neck, with no Brudzinski's sign. No nuchal rigidity. He has tenderness to the posterior c-spine with bilateral paraspinal tenderness and pain with range of motion.
- *Cardiovascular*: Regular tachycardia. No M/R/G.
- *Lungs*: Normal work of breathing, lungs are clear, with normal breath sounds.
- *Abdomen*: Soft, with normal bowel sounds. No tenderness, distension, guarding, or rebound.
- *Extremities and skin*: Normal range of motion, with warm and perfused extremities. Normal capillary refill.
- *Neurologic*: Cranial nerves intact, alert and oriented, non-focal examination.
- *Pertinent laboratory values*: WBC 7,700, Hb 13.6, rapid strep positive, monospot positive. Electrolytes and LFTs normal.
- *Pertinent imaging*: EKG shown in Figure 4.1.

> **Questions for Thought**
> - How do patients typically present with this illness?
> - What laboratory findings would support this diagnosis?
> - What EKG changes are typically found in patients with this disease?
> - What treatments should be initiated in the ED?
> - What is the definitive treatment of this condition?

Diagnosis

- Acute viral perimyocarditis.

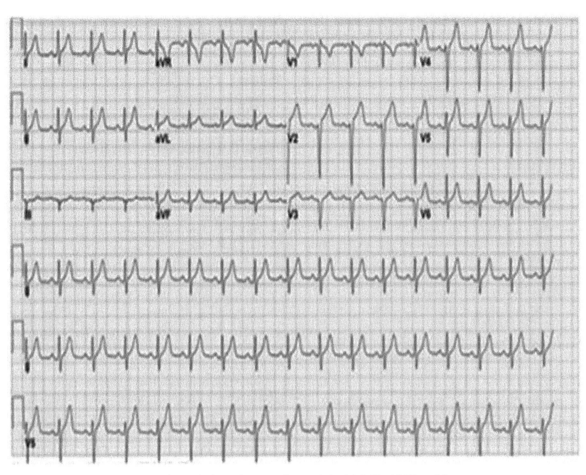

Figure 4.1 EKG demonstrating normal sinus rhythm with J-point elevation in leads I, II, aVL, aVF, V2, and V3.

Discussion

- *Epidemiology*: Pericarditis is responsible for up to 5 percent of all non-ischemic chest pain presenting to EDs in developed countries.[1,2] In patients with ST elevation, pericarditis is identified as the etiology of the EKG findings in 1 percent of cases.[3] The actual incidence of pericarditis is likely much higher, but is difficult to diagnose. Subacute cases may go unrecognized due to the lack of clinical significance, and acute cases may present non-specifically.[1,2,4] The majority of recorded cases in developed countries (40–90 percent) are idiopathic; however, it is postulated that many idiopathic cases actually have a viral etiology.[1,2] When an infectious agent is identified, viral is more common than bacterial. Non-infectious causes of pericarditis include autoimmune diseases (3–5 percent),

malignancy-related diseases, metabolic and endocrine disease, trauma, and iatrogenic causes.[1,2] Malignancy-related pericardial disease is the most frequent causative factor of tamponade from effusion in developed countries.[5] Uremia accounts for up to 10 percent of cases reported in patients with advanced renal failure prior to initiation of dialysis. Although rare in North America, in developing countries tuberculosis-induced pericarditis is a significant source of mortality and morbidity.[1,2] Pericarditis is more common in men than women, and is predominantly an adult disease. However, in children, there is a bimodal age distribution affecting primarily young children under 2 years of age and adolescents (14–18 years).[4]

- *Pathophysiology*: Inflammatory cell infiltration of the pericardium is the primary mechanism of injury in pericarditis. There are three inflammatory subtypes found along the spectrum of disease: (1) dry, (2) serous, and (3) fibrinous. Dry pericarditis involves inflammation of pericardial tissue that does not include epicardial vessel permeability. In contrast, serous pericarditis results when a protein-rich exudate is deposited along the pericardial wall, with resultant effusion. Fibrinous pericarditis follows serous pericarditis as the fibrinogen in the exudate is converted to fibrin, resulting in deposits along the normally smooth visceral–parietal interface.

- *Presentation*: Chest pain is the most commonly identified complaint in the patient suffering with pericarditis.[1,2,4] The pain is often pleuritic, but may be described as pressure, aching, sharp, or dull. Radiation is not common but referred pain to the trapezius, arm, or jaw may be present. The pain may be worsened by reclined positioning or swallowing. Improvement is often noted when the patient is positioned to lean forward. In the setting of effusion, dyspnea is frequently reported.[1-4] Cough, dysphagia, and low-grade fever frequently accompany the complaint of chest pain.[1,2] Night sweats and weight loss may be reported by those afflicted by malignancy or tuberculosis. On physical examination, children are often ill-appearing and tachycardic.[1,2,4] A careful examination to evaluate for signs of heart failure is imperative as this may indicate constrictive pericarditis or pump failure from perimyocarditis. The astute physician should also keep in mind that the presence of a friction rub may indicate the presence of a pericardial effusion while muffled heart sounds associated with jugular venous distention and hypotension increases the likelihood of a large effusion and pericardial tamponade.

- *Diagnosis*: The European Society of Cardiology guidelines are the only international guidelines assembled for the diagnosis of pericarditis.[1] The criteria for the diagnosis of acute pericarditis include at least two of the following:[1]

  · Chest pain (sharp and or pleuritic, worsened by supine position improved by sitting up and leaning forward);
  · Pericardial friction rub;

  · Suggestive changes on electrocardiography (widespread ST-segment elevation or PR depression);
  · New or worsening pericardial effusion.

  Additional supportive criteria may include:

  · Elevation of markers of inflammation (e.g. ESR, CRP, or WBC);
  · Evidence of pericardial inflammation by an imaging technique (CT or MRI).

  Perimyocarditis may be discernible by the elevation of injury markers (e.g. troponin or creatine kinase).

- *Treatment*: The complaint of chest pain or diagnostic tests revealing potential cardiac instability warrants a thorough evaluation for life-threatening causes. When there is diagnostic certainty that the entity being evaluated is in fact pericarditis, the mainstay of treatment remains NSAIDs.[1,2,4,6] Ibuprofen is considered first-line therapy and a weight-based dose should be given every 6 hours (up to 3,200 mg/d). Acetylsalicylic acid (2–4 g/d) and indomethacin (75–150 mg/d) are considered second-line. Indomethacin has specific drawbacks of reducing coronary flow and a poor side-effect profile. Colchicine (0.5 mg/d) has also been used in addition to NSAIDs in children, but support for doing so is limited to several case series and expert opinion.[4] In adults, there is convincing evidence that the use of colchicine can prevent recurrent pericarditis.[1,2] Low-dose corticosteroids (0.25–0.5 mg/kg per day) are recommended only for cases that are refractory to NSAIDs.[1,2]

- *Disposition*: Clinical decision tools to grade the degree of illness may be of assistance in treatment and disposition. Absence of all of the following complicating factors increases the likelihood that a patient is safe for outpatient treatment and discharge: fever greater than 100.4 °F, subacute onset, immunosuppression, trauma, oral anticoagulation therapy, NSAID treatment failure, perimyocarditis, and severe effusion or tamponade.[1,6]

Historical clues	Physical findings	Ancillary studies
• Fever	• Tachycardia	• Abnormal EKG
• Non-specific symptoms	• Fever	• Positive troponin
• Recent viral illness		

Follow-Up

The child had a troponin drawn, which showed an elevated level of 0.25 (reference range <0.08). A repeat level was 0.41. Because this patient had the combination of an abnormal EKG and elevated troponins and the diagnosis was uncertain, he was given a single dose of acetylsalicylic acid (325 mg) as thrombosis prevention for the concern of myocardial infarction. The patient was transferred to a tertiary care facility, where he was admitted to the PICU. The patient was started on IV fluid therapy, antipyretics for fever and antibiotics for streptococcal pharyngitis. His troponins were trended every 6 hours and peaked at 1.88 ng/mL after about 24 hours. He had an echocardiogram which was found to be normal. The patient was evaluated by pediatric cardiology who felt the diagnosis was a mild case of perimyocarditis due to the lack of chest pain and characteristic changes on the EKG. The patient was discharged home to follow up with pediatric cardiology to ensure the return to baseline of his troponins and to clear him to resume physical activity. On follow-up, the patient continued to improve and his EKG returned to normal.

References

1. Adler Y, Charron P, Imazio M, et al. 2015 ESC guidelines for the diagnosis and management of pericardial diseases: The Task Force for the Diagnosis and Management of Pericardial Diseases of the European Society of Cardiology (ESC) endorsed by The European Association for Cardio-Thoracic Surgery (EACTS). *Eur Heart J* 2015; 36: 2921–64.

2. Imazio M, Gaita F, LeWinter M. Evaluation and treatment of pericarditis: A systematic review. *JAMA* 2015; 314: 1498–506.

3. Brady WJ, Perron AD, Martin ML, et al. Cause of ST segment abnormality in ED chest pain patients. *Am J Emerg Med* 2001; 19: 25–8.

4. Bergmann KR, Kharbanda A, Haveman L. Myocarditis and pericarditis in the pediatric patient: Validated management strategies. *Pediatr Emerg Med Pract* 2015; 12: 1–22.

5. Mercé J, Sagristà Sauleda J, Permanyer Miralda G, et al. Pericardial effusion in the elderly: A different disease? *Rev Esp Cardiol* 2000; 53: 1432–6.

6. Imazio M, Demichelis B, Parrini I, et al. Day-hospital treatment of acute pericarditis: A management program for outpatient therapy. *J Am Coll Cardiol* 2004; 43: 1042–6.

Chapter

5

Eye, Ear, Nose, and Throat Complaints

Case 1

Contributing Authors: Jason Schwaber, Taylor R. Spencer, and Rebecca Jeanmonod

History

The patient is a 6-year-old boy who is brought in by his mother, stating: "I put a pencil in my ear," while at school. He denies any headache, dizziness, bleeding, hearing changes, discharge, or vomiting. His mother reports that he had tympanostomy tubes at age 2, but "they fell out years ago."

Past Medical History

- Seasonal allergies.

Medications

- Fluticasone 50 mcg intranasal.

Allergies

- NKDA, has tree pollen allergies.

Physical Examination and Ancillary Studies

- *Vital signs*: T 98.4 °F, HR 98, BP 104/74, RR 22, O$_2$ sat 98% on room air.
- *General*: Well-developed, well nourished school-aged child sitting in bed. He is anxious but consolable.
- *HEENT*: PERRL. Nares are clear bilaterally, oropharynx with moist mucous membranes. Teeth O and P are missing. Tonsils have no exudate. Right ear with pencil core in external canal 2 mm from tympanic membrane. Mild superficial laceration of canal. Tympanic membrane is translucent with an area of tympanosclerosis. Left ear with normal tympanic

membrane and no foreign body. Hearing is symmetric.
- *Neck*: Supple, with no lymphadenopathy.
- *Cardiovascular*: Regular, with no M/R/G. Good perfusion and normal capillary refill.
- *Lungs*: Normal work of breathing, CTA bilaterally, with no W/R/R.
- *Abdomen*: Soft, without tenderness. No masses. Normal bowel sounds.
- *Skin and extremities*: No rashes, full range of motion, warm, and well-perfused.
- *Neurologic*: Alert and interactive. Cranial nerves II–XII intact. Normal for age.

> **Questions for Thought**
> - What dictates the urgency of foreign-body removal?
> - What other structures can be damaged during foreign-body placement and removal?
> - When should ENT be consulted or the patient referred?
> - What other body areas should be examined for foreign bodies?

Diagnosis

- Foreign body in external auditory canal.

Discussion

- *Epidemiology*: Children presenting with foreign bodies in the ear have a median age of 8, slightly older than those with nasal foreign bodies.[1] Older children and adults will sometimes present with objects in their ears, as well. They are more often found in the right ear, perhaps because of handedness.[1] Multiple objects have been found in ear canals, including insects, beads, paper,

95

pebbles, organic material, small batteries, and hearing aids.[1] Nasal foreign bodies are also commonly seen in children. Common items include food, beads, buttons, paper, cloth, and candle wax.[1] Esophageal foreign bodies are commonly coins, but batteries, sharp objects, and food objects can be seen.

- *Pathophysiology*: The extent of harm depends on the object involved, its location, and its duration. In the ear, sharp materials can lacerate the fragile skin of the external auditory canal or tympanic membrane.[1] Drainage of cerumen from the ear can be blocked by organic materials that swell with moisture.[1] Insects cause irritation and local tissue reaction as well as vertigo.[1] Button batteries that leak contents cause necrosis of the surrounding tissues and can be very destructive.[1] Any foreign body that is present for a long period of time can cause infection and tympanic membrane perforation.

  The nose consists of two nasal fossae separated by a vertical septum and subdivided into three passages by the nasal turbinates. Nasal foreign bodies are usually lodged below the inferior turbinate, or anterior to the middle turbinate. In the nose, foreign bodies may cause similar complications to those in the ear. Sharp objects may cause direct trauma, and large objects, those which have expanded from absorbing moisture, can prevent sinus drainage and lead to secondary sinus infection.[1] Button batteries may cause septal erosion and subsequent saddle nose deformity or may lead to necrosis of other facial structures.[1] They can produce nasal or choanal stenosis. Obstruction of the sinuses by swelling can lead to secondary rhinosinusitis. Other infectious complications reported from nasal foreign bodies have been reported including otitis media, periorbital cellulitis, and meningitis. Nasal foreign bodies also pose the risk of object aspiration into the pulmonary tree. For further discussion of foreign-body aspiration, please see Chapter 3, Case 1.

  In the esophagus, foreign objects may be lodged at any of the three narrowings within the esophagus: proximal esophagus at the thoracic inlet, mid esophagus at the carina and aortic arch, or distal esophagus at the gastroesophageal junction. Although most esophageal foreign bodies pass without incident into the stomach, sharp objects, long objects, and large objects may all get stuck.

- *Presentation*: In the majority of cases, the child is brought in by a caregiver who witnessed the child place the foreign body. For ear foreign bodies, children may also report pain, bleeding, hearing loss, or ear discharge.[1] Less commonly, the child may present with cellulitis or other evidence of infection. Some foreign bodies are found during routine medical care for another issue.

  Nasal foreign bodies are also commonly witnessed. Children may also present with pain or bleeding. They may also present with a voice change (a nasal voice), unilateral nasal drainage, a foul odor from the child's nose, or evidence of infection.[1] Up to 25 percent of nasal foreign bodies present greater than 24 hours after placement and are unsuspected by the caregiver. In these cases, if the foreign body is not visualized, the diagnosis is often made by ENT when the child is referred for examination to rule out tumor, mass, or anatomic abnormality causing chronic nasal drainage.

  Esophageal foreign bodies may be asymptomatic or may cause respiratory compromise or drooling and pain. They are sometimes diagnosed incidentally during evaluation for cough or pneumonia. In children with lodged button batteries, the presentation may be dramatic and rapidly progressive, with esophageal perforation and fulminant collapse.

- *Diagnosis*: The diagnosis of ear or nasal foreign body is made by history and physical examination. The provider should use an otoscope to detect ear foreign body or a nasal speculum to assess for nasal foreign body. Children should have both ears and nose evaluated, since some children may have several foreign bodies. The provider should assess for presence of infection as well as complications of foreign body, such as tympanic membrane perforation. The provider should also test and document cranial nerves as well as conductive vs. sensorineural hearing with the Rinne test with a 512 hertz tuning fork.

  Esophageal foreign bodies are also typically diagnosed by history. In the case of swallowed metallic objects, radiography is quite helpful. Coins in the esophagus will appear en fasse on

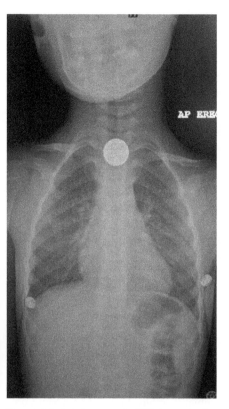

Figure 5.1 Anterior–posterior CXR demonstrating a penny stuck in the esophagus at the level of the thoracic inlet.

anterior–posterior film, whereas those in the trachea will appear edge-on (Figure 5.1). Button batteries can be identified by their size and often by their rounded edge, which distinguishes them from coins. Food boluses which are impacted are typically diagnosed by history, followed by endoscopy.

- *Treatment*: For any foreign-body removal, the goal is to remove the foreign body with minimal risk to the patient while maximizing patient comfort. It is important that you make your first attempt at foreign-body removal your best attempt, as success in foreign-body removal decreases with subsequent attempts. Emergency medicine providers are commonly successful at foreign-body removal, but round ungraspable objects increase the rate of failure.[2] The method of retrieval depends on both the object location and the physical characteristics of the object.[1,2]

For live insects in the ear, the provider should begin by killing or immobilizing the insect with mineral oil or lidocaine.[1] The insect can then be irrigated out of the ear.[1] Although forceps can be used to pull out beetles, for insects such as spiders forceps may simply serve to dismember the insect, resulting in multiple foreign bodies.

For inorganic firm smooth objects in ears, suction or irrigation may be successful. Occasionally, a right-angle hook can be advanced just distal to the object and used to dislodge the object from the canal. In the nose, a small catheter with a balloon may be advanced past the object, the balloon inflated, and the object pulled out.[1] A single positive pressure breath through the mouth with occlusion of the unaffected nostril or positive pressure oxygen directly into the unaffected nostril can also dislodge the object, particularly if the object is filling much of the nasal canal, such as in cases of crayon foreign body.[1] Round smooth objects in ears have a high rate of removal failure in the ED, and are more likely to require specialist care or sedation.[2]

Organic foreign bodies, such as popcorn in either the nose or the ear, may be removed with forceps. These should not be irrigated, as irrigation may cause them to swell and become more difficult to remove.[1]

Batteries pose a true emergency. They can cause low-voltage electrical currents and destruction of tissue. They can leak at any time after placement, causing irreversible tissue destruction from sodium hydroxide and chlorine gas, or they can cause liquefactive necrosis from their alkaline contents. Therefore, although it is reasonable for the provider to attempt to remove them (taking great care not to crush the battery), the child should be seen by ENT for immediate removal if the provider fails. Batteries should NOT be irrigated out of ears.

Magnetic foreign bodies in the nose create a risk for pressure necrosis and septal perforation, and also require prompt removal.

Esophageal foreign bodies are usually removed by a gastroenterologist by endoscopy if the foreign body is in the lower portion of the esophagus, but are sometimes removed by ENT or pulmonology if they are high up. You should become familiar with the regional differences or particular practices of your hospital. For rounded items that are not batteries, it is within the standard of care to allow the item 24 hours to pass spontaneously so long as the child has reliable follow-up and can handle his or her secretions. These children may be admitted for observation or may be discharged to return in a day for a repeat CXR to track progress. Once the object passes the pylorus, it is likely to continue on through the GI tract. Batteries and long, sharp objects should be removed emergently. Since some parents lack the means to bring their child back to the hospital promptly, it is appropriate to remove objects that are lodged at the time of presentation where services are immediately available, even if the object is rounded and lower risk, as many will still remain lodged.

After removal, the child should be examined again to ascertain any injury that was masked by the foreign-body presence, or that occurred secondary to its removal. Potential complications of ear foreign-body removal include laceration of the thin skin of the external auditory canal, formation of a hematoma, facial nerve palsy, perforation of the tympanic membrane, disruption of the ossicular chain, and movement of the foreign body proximally. For noses, complications include bleeding, pushing the object deeper, or inadvertent dislodgement into the airway.

- *Disposition*: Patients with ear foreign bodies that are successfully removed without complications can be discharged home. Patients with laceration to the canal or tympanic membrane perforation require otic antibiotics such as ciprofloxacin-dexamethasone and outpatient follow-up.[1] Those with objects that cannot be removed require ENT consultation or referral for removal with microscopy or in the OR. Button batteries need emergency removal. Esophageal foreign bodies may be removed endoscopically, after which the child may be discharged home.

Historical clues	Physical findings
• Report of child placing object in ear	• External auditory canal foreign body • Laceration

Follow-Up

After discussion of the risks and benefits with the parent and the patient, the pencil core was grasped with alligator forceps under direct visualization and retrieved in a single attempt. Examination after removal demonstrated a small laceration to the external auditory canal. The patient was prescribed otic ciprofloxacin–dexamethasone solution twice a day and referred to his PCP for follow-up in the next 5–7 days.

References

1. Heim SW, Maughan KL. Foreign bodies in the ear, nose and throat. *Am Fam Phys* 2007; 76: 1185–9.

2. Thompson SK, Wein RO, Dutcher PO. External auditory canal foreign body removal: Management practices and outcomes. *Laryngoscope*, 2003; 113: 1912–15.

The Academic Life in Emergency Medicine blog has multiple articles on particular techniques for particular types of foreign objects. See www.aliem.com.

Case 2

Contributing Author: Edwin Layng

History

An 8-year-old girl presents to the fast track area of your ED with a complaint of bleeding from her right nostril for the past 3 hours. Her mother tells you that she has recently recovered from a URI, in which she had a low-grade fever as well as coryza for the past week. Upon questioning, the patient admits to picking her nose earlier in the day and that the bleeding began shortly after that. The mother has tried putting tissue paper under the bleeding nostril as well as instructing the child to "tilt her head back," but neither of those techniques were able to stop the bleeding. The child has no complaints of dyspnea, swallowing blood, nausea, vomiting, diarrhea, fever, or chills. She denies any recent trauma. This is the child's first nosebleed and there is no family history of bleeding diathesis.

Past Medical History

- Asthma.
- Eczema.

Medications

- Albuterol inhaler.

Allergies

- Pollen, dust, and mold.

Physical Examination and Ancillary Studies

- *Vital signs*: T 99.2 °F, HR 95, BP 100/60, RR 20, O$_2$ sat 99% on room air.
- *General*: Uncomfortable-appearing child, awake and alert, leaning forward in bed.
- *HEENT*: There is a moderate amount of blood flowing from the right nostril. Upon examination with a nasal speculum, bleeding is seen in the antero-inferior part of the right nasal septum. There is no bleeding from the left side. No septal hematoma. No blood in the oropharynx. Mucous membranes are moist.
- *Neck*: Supple, with a midline trachea and no adenopathy.
- *Cardiovascular*: Regular rate and rhythm, with no M/R/G. Good capillary refill.
- *Lungs*: CTA bilaterally, with no W/R/R.
- *Abdomen*: Soft with no tenderness, no masses, no distension.
- *Skin and extremities*: No edema, clubbing, or cyanosis. No bruising or petechiae.

Questions for Thought

- What is the most common location of bleeding in pediatric epistaxis?
- What is the treatment algorithm for pediatric epistaxis?
- Are prophylactic antibiotics indicated, and if so, which?
- What are other diagnoses that should be considered in young infants and neonates with epistaxis?

Diagnosis

- Anterior epistaxis.

Discussion

- *Epidemiology*: Epistaxis is very common in children and the vast majority of cases are self-limited.[1-3] The lifetime incidence of epistaxis is 60 percent, with most first occurrences in childhood or adolescence.[1,2] The incidence of pediatric epistaxis is highest during the winter, and this is thought to be secondary to increased frequency of URIs as well as drying of the nares due to low ambient humidity from indoor heating. Epistaxis is rare in patients less than 2 years old,

and should prompt consideration of trauma or serious illness.[4] Resolved nosebleeds in infants may be secondary to attempted smothering or suffocation. Roughly 10 percent of epistaxis in children is caused by bleeding diatheses, including blood-clotting disorders, telangiectasis, juvenile angiofibroma, von Willebrand's disease, and idiopathic thrombocytopenia purpura. Children with systemic predisposing factors rarely present with self-limited bleeds.

- *Pathophysiology*: The nose functions to humidify and warm air as it passes through to the lungs as well as to filter allergens, irritants, and pathogens. As such, it has a large surface area with a thin, highly vascular mucosa that provides little support or protection to the underlying blood vessels. These characteristics predispose the nasal mucosa to bleeding. The major source of bleeding in most patients is Kesselbach's plexus, a highly vascular area in the anterior nasal septum formed by the anastamosis of the anterior ethmoidal artery, the lateral nasal branch of the sphenopalatine artery, and the superior labial artery. Posterior bleeds arise from branches of the sphenopalatine or posterior ethmoidal arteries that supply the posterolateral wall and the posterior choanae.
- *Presentation*: The majority of children present with self-limited bleeding from one or both nares. Anterior bleeds are more commonly unilateral, although it is possible to have bilateral anterior bleeding or reflux of blood from an anterior bleed into the nasopharynx with subsequent leakage out the other side. Digital trauma from nose-picking is by far the most common cause of anterior nosebleeds in children. Other types of trauma to the face are also commonly encountered. If there is purulent discharge associated with the nasal bleeding, one should consider a nasal foreign body.

  Posterior nosebleeds are more often bilateral, heavier, and associated with back-bleeding (blood leaking down the pharynx and into the esophagus or even into the airway). Rarely, posterior bleeding may present with catastrophic exsanguination from an arterial aneurysmal source.
- *Diagnosis*: The EM provider should seek historical clues that might point to any condition that might predispose the child to bleeding. Family and personal history of coagulopathy or bleeding

disorder should be sought. The provider should query the family regarding night sweats, easy bruising, bleeding on toothbrushing, hemarthroses, fevers, weight loss, or any historical or physical examination elements that suggest underlying malignancy or medical disorder. Recent trauma, surgery, and anticoagulant use should be reviewed. Over-the-counter and prescription medications such as intranasal decongestants could be a possible cause. Cocaine and other inhaled illicit substances can also cause epistaxis. The provider should make certain to ascertain that the bleeding is in fact nasal, and not hematemesis or hemoptysis. The provider should do a careful head and neck examination using a nasal speculum and a good light source to attempt to determine the source of bleeding.[1] Anterior epistaxis is diagnosed on examination, with either a fresh clot or active bleeding indicating the location of hemorrhage. If bleeding is determined to be nasal in origin and an anterior site cannot be visualized, posterior bleeding should be presumed to be present.

In well children over the age of 2 without a concerning history or examination, laboratory or imaging evaluation is generally not indicated for a single episode of anterior epistaxis.[3,5] Coagulation studies should be ordered for patients with a known or suspected coagulopathy or bleeding diathesis. In children with recurrent unilateral epistaxis, referral to ENT for assessment for a mass is appropriate.[3,5] In very young children with nosebleeds, consideration should be given for non-accidental trauma as well as for hematologic malignancy, and work-up for these entities is appropriate.[4] ENT should be consulted for all cases of posterior nosebleeds in children.

- *Treatment*: When treating epistaxis, it is important to use personal protective equipment, including a face mask, gloves, and a gown, as the patient sneezing or coughing can lead to an exposure risk. Since some nosebleeds may interfere with airway and breathing, initial assessment of airway patency and vital signs is necessary. If the patient is hemodynamically unstable or unable to protect his or her airway, proceed to resuscitation algorithms. Severe bleeding, signs of anemia, or hemodynamic instability require IV access, a stat Hb/HCT test, and blood crossmatching.

For the initial tamponade, the patient is instructed to blow out blood and clots. Application of a topical vasoconstrictor/anesthetic such as oxymetazoline and 1% lidocaine into the nares, either using a spray bottle, atomizer, or applying cotton-soaked pleats, will aid in examination.[1] Cocaine can also be used. Next, use a nasal speculum to find the source of bleeding by first inspecting Kesselbach's plexus. It is important also to assess for the presence of a septal hematoma. Next, inspect the oropharynx for bleeding. Have the patient pinch the alae together and hold for roughly 10 minutes. If the patient is too young to reliably pinch his/her nose closed, the parents or clinical personnel can perform the compression maneuver. During the initial compression, the child should be sitting up and bent forward at the waist to minimize bleeding into the oral cavity and hypopharynx, as this predisposes to vomiting.

If the bleeding is able to be stopped after direct pressure and/or chemical cautery, the patient should be prescribed a topical antibiotic ointment, such as bacitracin.[5] This may be applied three times per day. Patients should also be educated about the use of humidifiers to help keep the nasal mucosa moist and the importance of not picking the nose to prevent against future bleeds. For chronic or recurrent epistaxis, one can use hydrocortisone ointment 1%, applied topically to the anterior septal mucosa (twice per day for 10 days, limited to no longer than 2 weeks to prevent thinning of the mucosa).

If the nasal bleeding is refractory to direct pressure, but slows or stops temporarily and an anterior source is clearly visualized, proceed to chemical cautery with 75% silver nitrate.[1,3] Dab the applicator gently around the suspected source of bleeding. Avoid prolonged cautery and bilateral cautery to prevent septal perforation.[1] Do not attempt to cauterize an actively bleeding vessel.

If the bleeding is swift after direct pressure or attempts at cautery are unsuccessful, topical prothrombotic agents such as topical thrombin or gelatin-impregnated products can be attempted. If this fails or is unavailable, the provider should proceed to nasal packing. Nasal packing may be achieved using strips of petroleum-impregnated gauze, applied in layers to fill the entire nasal cavity, or with a commercial nasal tampon designed for this purpose. Coat the nasal tampon with bacitracin ointment, then insert it directly back into the nasal cavity with constant pressure. It is important to apply constant pressure and not delay advancing the nasal tampon, as it begins to expand once exposed to the moist environment of the nare. Expand the tampon with the remaining oxymetazoline and 1% lidocaine or a normal saline flush. Non-absorbable packs are typically left in place for 1 to 5 days and then removed by ENT as an outpatient. While the pack is in place, and even after its removal, there may be a potential risk of staphylococcal toxic shock syndrome. Neither prophylactic systemic antibiotics nor impregnation of nasal packing with antibiotic ointment eradicate nasal carriage of staphylococcus or reliably prevents against toxic shock syndrome.[2,6] Thus, antibiotics are not routinely recommended. However, antibiotics may be prescribed if there is evidence of an underlying sinus infection or if follow-up is anticipated to be more than 48 hours. Commonly used antibiotics include amoxicillin–clavulanate or clarithromycin.

One should suspect a posterior bleed if the patient reports swallowing blood after anterior nasal packing or if bleeding is refractory to anterior packing. Posterior bleeds are much more serious as they tend to bleed more, their location makes them more difficult to tamponade, and the risk of airway compromise from bleeding into the posterior oropharynx is increased. Posterior bleeds require an ENT consultation and inpatient admission. These are treated with the insertion of a balloon catheter. A 10 or 14 French Foley catheter can be used if a standard balloon catheter designed for nasal packing is unavailable. The tip of the Foley catheter is cut off and advanced until it can be seen in the posterior oropharynx. The balloon is then inflated and tugged back until it is seated just above the soft palate. It is further inflated until the soft palate begins to bulge or the patient complains of pain. It is then fixed in place with a Kelly clamp and tape, taking care not to apply pressure to the alar rim. This can be an uncomfortable procedure. As a last resort, operative management or endovascular treatment of refractory bleeds can be considered if a patient is critically ill or if the bleeding cannot be stopped.

- *Disposition*: Patients with resolved or treated anterior nosebleeds may be discharged home. Those with packing in place should have it removed in 2–5 days. Patients with posterior nosebleeds or concerns for underlying serious pathology should be admitted to the hospital for observation.

Historical clues	Physical findings
• Recent URI • History of epistaxis • History of nose-picking	• Bleeding from left nare from Kesselbach's plexus • No other abnormalities on examination to suggest underlying pathology

Follow-Up

This patient had anterior epistaxis caused by digital trauma. Her recent URI and being in a low-humidity environment during the winter put her at a greater risk of developing epistaxis. After compressing the nares for roughly 15 minutes, the bleeding stopped. Chemical cautery was applied with 75% silver nitrate and the patient was prescribed a topical antibiotic ointment to apply three times each day. She was educated about the use of humidifiers to help keep the nasal mucosa moist and the importance of not picking the nose to prevent against future bleeds.

References

1. American College of Emergency Physicians. Focus on: Treatment of epistaxis. See www.acep.org/Clinical—Practice-Management/Focus-On–Treatment-of-Epistaxis/ (accessed August 23, 2016).
2. Cohn B. Are prophylactic antibiotics necessary for anterior nasal packing in epistaxis? *Ann Emerg Med* 2014; 65: 109–11.
3. Qureishi A, Burton MJ. Interventions for recurrent idiopathic epistaxis (nosebleeds) in children. *Cochrane Database Syst Rev* 2012; 9: CD004461.
4. McIntosh N, Mok JYQ, Margerison A. Epidemiology of oronasal hemorrhage in the first 2 years of life: Implications for child protection. *Pediatrics* 2007; 120:1074–8.
5. Patel N, Maddalozzo J, Billings KR. An update on management of pediatric epistaxis. *Int J Pediatr Otorhinolaryngol* 2014; 78: 1400–4.
6. Biggs TC, Nightingale K, Patel NN, et al. Should prophylactic antibiotics be used routinely in epistaxis patients with nasal packs? *Ann R Coll Surg Engl* 2013; 95: 40–2.

Case 3

Contributing Author: Shellie Asher

History

The patient is a 12-year-old boy who was playing with a stretchy rubber action figure when it snapped back, striking him in the left eye. He complained of eye pain and presented to the school nurse who examined his eye and referred him to the ED for further evaluation. The patient currently complains of 8/10 left eye pain, tearing, and blurry vision. He has no other complaints or injuries.

Past Medical History

- None.

Medications

- None.

Allergies

- No known food or drug allergies.

Physical Examination and Ancillary Studies

- *Vital signs*: T 98.6 °F, HR 82, RR 16, BP 98/52, O_2 sat 100% on room air.
- *General*: Appears well-developed and well-nourished, resting on the stretcher, in no acute distress.
- *HEENT*: The right pupil is round and reactive to light. The globe appears normal, the anterior chamber and cornea are clear. Right eye visual acuity is 20/20. The left pupil is irregularly shaped and minimally reactive to light. The anterior chamber and cornea are clear. Visual acuity is 20/200. Visual fields are full to confrontation, and extraocular movements are intact. The conjunctivae are diffusely injected, with no limbic sparing. In the two o'clock position there is noted an extruded portion of iris through a full-thickness corneal laceration (Figure 5.2).

> **Questions for Thought**
>
> - What historical elements are important in the assessment of eye trauma?
> - What physical examination elements are important in the assessment of eye trauma?
> - What are other traumatic eye injuries?
> - What is the appropriate evaluation and management for this condition?

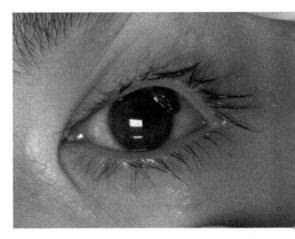

Figure 5.2 Photograph of patient's left eye, demonstrating an irregular pupil and extruded iris. For the color version, please refer to the plate section.

Diagnosis

- Globe rupture due to penetrating trauma.

Discussion

- *Epidemiology*: Globe injuries are commonly encountered in EDs, and may result from blunt or penetrating trauma. The annual incidence of globe rupture or laceration is approximately 3.5 per 100,000 worldwide.[1] In the USA, 2.4 million eye injuries occur annually, with over a third of these occurring in children.[2] The majority of patients presenting with globe injury are young and male. In younger children, injuries tend to be related to running or walking with sharp objects such as scissors or pens, whereas older patients tend to have work-related injuries or injuries sustained in motor vehicle crashes.[1-3] Intraocular foreign bodies are common in patients with globe rupture.[1-4] Children also commonly present with other ocular traumatic injuries, such as corneal foreign body, hyphema, corneal or scleral laceration, corneal abrasion, corneal ulcer, traumatic iritis, traumatic glaucoma, vitreous hemorrhage, retinal trauma, optic nerve injury, lens dislocation, or injuries to the lids or surrounding bony structures.
- *Pathophysiology*: Open globe injuries are characterized as globe rupture (caused by blunt injury) or globe laceration (caused by penetrating injury). The globe is relatively protected from blunt injury by the surrounding bony structures. High-impact blunt trauma with enough force to

injure the bony structures may also result in globe injury. In blunt trauma, globe rupture typically occurs behind the insertion of the rectus muscle, where the sclera is weakest. Penetrating injury is more common in children.[2] In the setting of penetrating injury, lacerations typically occur in the cornea, followed by scleral or limbal lacerations. Intraocular foreign bodies should be considered and may be found in any chamber of the eye. Extrusion of intraocular contents may occur secondary to penetrating trauma or due to increased intraocular pressure after blunt trauma.

- *Presentation*: Patients may present with an isolated globe injury or with a globe injury in the setting of a multi-system trauma. In the setting of multi-system trauma, life-threatening injuries must be addressed prior to the globe injury. In any patient with head or facial trauma, the globe should be inspected carefully. High-risk mechanisms of injury include high-velocity projectiles, injuries from sharp objects, and high-force blunt trauma. Patients may present with eye pain, blurry vision, tearing, or a paucity of symptoms, particularly in penetrating, small, high-velocity injuries. The clinician should have a high index of suspicion and perform a complete eye examination in any patient with a concerning history (for example, hammering metal on metal without eye protection).

- *Diagnosis*: Diagnosis of globe rupture and differentiation of this entity from other ocular emergencies is made with a careful history and physical examination.

  - Important elements of history include time and mechanism of injury, complaints of pain, visual disturbances, and associated injuries.
  - Physical examination should include a complete slit-lamp examination as well as visual acuity. In globe rupture, findings may include decreased visual acuity, an irregularly shaped pupil, hyphema, visible laceration of the cornea and/or sclera, extrusion of ocular contents, and gross deformity of the globe. If the provider is concerned globe rupture exists, he or she should avoid any maneuvers which may increase intraocular pressure, such as direct pressure on the globe, tonometry, or eyelid retraction, as these may result in further extrusion of ocular contents. Visual acuity

should be assessed in each eye independently. Structures surrounding the eye should be carefully assessed for associated injury.

  - Fluorescein staining may reveal Seidel's sign, which is a streaming away of fluorescein from the site of a corneal puncture from leaking aqueous humor. This is pathognomonic for globe rupture. Fluorescein uptake may be seen in corneal abrasions or ulcers, and may help delineate a corneal foreign body. Vertical abrasions may be evidence of a foreign body under the eyelid.
  - Slit-lamp examination may demonstrate inflammation in the anterior chamber (cell and flare) from traumatic iritis. Photophobia is also common in iritis due to pupillary spasm.
  - U/S is a helpful adjunct and may demonstrate vitreous hemorrhage, traumatic retinal detachment (which is rare), or traumatic lens dislocation.
  - CT imaging of the globe may be used as an adjunct to a thorough history and physical examination when globe rupture is suspected, and may be useful when intraocular foreign body is suspected. However, the sensitivity of a CT scan for globe rupture is 56–75 percent and thus should not be considered definitive when pre-test probability is high.[4]

- *Treatment*: Management of globe injury should occur in the setting of standard trauma management for other associated injuries. If globe injury is highly likely, the clinician should take care to avoid maneuvers that may increase intraocular pressure and therefore exacerbate the globe injury. The eye should be shielded, and the patient should be encouraged to rest quietly.[1,2] Associated vomiting should be treated, and the patient's pain should be managed appropriately. An ophthalmologist should be consulted emergently when globe rupture is diagnosed or highly suspected. Patients should be kept NPO and receive empiric antibiotic therapy and tetanus prophylaxis.[1,2] Definitive management of globe rupture is surgical intervention. Vision may be preserved in more than half of pediatric patients with appropriate, rapid evaluation and management.[2]

- *Disposition*: Patients with diagnosed or highly suspected globe injuries should be evaluated by an ophthalmologist or transferred to a facility where consultation is available. If examination is difficult, the patient should go to the OR for examination under anesthesia.

Historical clues	Physical findings
• History of eye trauma	• Irregular pupil
• Eye pain	• Decreased acuity
• Blurry vision	• Visualized laceration with extrusion of iris

Follow-Up

The patient was taken emergently to the OR by ophthalmology for surgical repair of his corneal laceration and reduction of extruded ocular contents. He did well post-operatively, with preserved vision in the affected eye.

References

1. Gelston CD. Common eye emergencies. *Am Fam Phys* 2013; 88: 515–19.

2. Li X, Zarbin MA, Bhagat N. Pediatric open globe injury: A review of the literature. *J Emerg Trauma Shock* 2015; 8: 216–23.

3. May DR, Kuhn FP, Morris RE, et al. The epidemiology of serious eye injuries from the United States Eye Injury Registry. *Graefes Arch Clin Exp Ophthalmol* 2000; 238: 153–7.

4. Yuan WH, Hsu HC, Cheng HC, et al. CT of globe rupture: Analysis and frequency of findings. *AJR Am J Roentgenol* 2014; 20: 1100–7.

Case 4

Contributing Author: Tom Dittrich

History

The patient is a 2-year-old girl with history of recurrent otitis media, who presents with left-ear pain and yellow drainage from the ear canal for the past 3 days. The child has been fussier than usual and is pulling at the left ear, which is when mom "knows there's going to be another ear infection." She noticed yellow drainage from the ear canal today and was referred to the ED. Mom notes she has had fever of 102.2 °F by rectal thermometer for the past 2 days. She has been using ibuprofen and acetaminophen appropriately. Mom is more concerned about this episode because she feels that her daughter's ear is bulging forward and doesn't match the opposite side, which is new for her. She also

reports she has been falling over more frequently and not responding to her name as she normally would. She has been tolerating PO without difficulty although she is drinking less than usual. She is wetting diapers and passing stool normally. There are no rashes. Her mother called her pediatrician to ask for a prescription for amoxicillin, which typically works for her, but the pediatrician referred her to the ED for evaluation.

Past Medical History

- Recurrent episodes of otitis media.
- Immunizations are UTD.

Medications

- None.

Allergies

- NKDA.

Physical Examination and Ancillary Studies

- *Vital signs*: T 102.2 °F, HR 132, RR 26, BP 90/50, O_2 sat 99% on room air.
- *General*: Well-developed child, fussy and crying throughout examination.
- *HEENT*: PERRL, extraocular movements intact. Left ear appears to be "bulging" forward and is asymmetric compared to the right ear. The left external ear canal is erythematous and swollen, with mucopurulent drainage, the tympanic membrane is difficult to visualize but appears erythematous with bulging and appears opaque with no bones visible. Posterior to the auricle there is swelling, redness, induration, and tenderness over the mastoid process. No lymphadenopathy present. No depressions or elevations in the skull. The left eye appears grossly unremarkable and the orbit is without swelling or erythema. The neck has no decreased range of motion nor tenderness on examination.
- *Cardiovascular*: Tachycardic and regular, without M/R/G, S1 and S2 appeciated. < 2 second capillary refill.
- *Lungs*: CTA bilaterally, with no W/R/R.
- *Abdomen*: Soft and non-tender throughout, normal bowel sounds.
- *Extremities and skin*: Warm and well perfused, 2+ radial and dorsalis pedis pulses.
- *Neurologic*: Awake, symmetric face, normal level of alertness, moves all four extremities spontaneously.

- *Pertinent laboratory values*: WBC 17,600, all other laboratory tests are unremarkable.
- *Pertinent radiologic studies*: Head CT demonstrates fluid-filled mastoid air cells, with destruction of the bony septae normally found there.

Questions for Thought

- What is the differential diagnosis for this child's symptoms?
- What are the indications for obtaining an imaging study for this patient?
- How should treatment be approached?
- What should this patient's disposition be from the ED?

Diagnosis

- Acute mastoiditis.

Discussion

- *Epidemiology*: The vast majority of cases of mastoiditis occur in the same age group as cases of acute otitis media, usually 6 months to 2 years of age.[1] The disease process does occur in older children but the incidence drops off as the child gets older. This is thought to be secondary to the anatomy of the eustachian tube and an immature immune system.[1] Generally, risk factors for acute mastoiditis parallel those for acute otitis media, which include age, tobacco-smoke exposure, non-breast-fed infants, daycare, and family history of acute otitis media.[1]
- *Pathophysiology*: Acute mastoiditis is a complication and an extension of otitis media.[2] The mucosa that lines the inner ear extends to the lining of the mastoid air cells. When bacteria induce inflammation in this lining, the bacteria can take hold within the mastoid air cells. If the inflammation destroys the thin walls of bone between air cells, called coalescent mastoiditis, then tiny pockets of abscess may form and may spread to nearby areas.[2] The direction of the bacterial extension will determine the patient's symptoms. If the bacteria travel to the outer cortex of the bone, then an abscess may form there, called a sub-periosteal abscess, marked by induration and fluctuance. If there is extension into the round window, leading to the vestibular labyrinths, then suppurative labyrinthitis develops giving vertigo, hearing loss, and tinnitus. If the

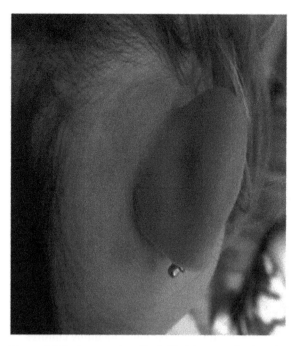

Figure 5.3 Erythema and swelling behind the pinna. For the color version, please refer to the plate section.

infection encompasses the facial nerve, than a facial nerve palsy can be the result. Extension into the inner cortical bone yields bacteria in the cranial fault, which can lead to meningitis, sinus venous thrombosis, or intracranial abscess. The bacteria most commonly implicated are *Streptococcus pneumoniae, S. pyogenes,* or *Staphylococcus aureus.*[3-5]

- *Presentation*: Children may present with a range of complaints depending on the progression of the disease and the direction of bacterial extension. The child may complain of otalgia, otorrhea, fever, headache, malaise, or vertigo. Examination findings may include mastoid tenderness, erythema, and swelling (see Figure 5.3), protrusion of the auricle, meningeal findings, abnormal tympanic membrane, obtundation, or sepsis.
- *Diagnosis*: The diagnosis can be made clinically by historical and physical examination features. CT imaging of the head is not always indicated. CT imaging can be helpful to investigate cases without classic findings, evaluate for complications such as an abscess, which will require further intervention beyond antibiotics, or to determine the extent and severity of the disease. CT findings include fluid

in the middle ear and air cells of the mastoid bone, abnormal densities of the mastoid bone, thickening of the periosteum, or findings of complications such as extra-axial fluid collections. MRI with gadolinium is an alternative option to CT but is generally more difficult to obtain.

- *Treatment*: Broad-spectrum antibiotic treatment should be initiated for all pediatric patients suspected to have acute mastoiditis. Generally, coverage for Gram-positive organisms, including MRSA, are of greatest importance as these organisms are the most common.[3-5] For those with recurrent acute otitis media, which is a common occurrence, coverage for Gram-negative organisms, including *Pseudomonas aeruginosa* coverage, should be provided.[3-5] Generally, vancomycin and piperacillin–tazobactam is typically the first-line recommended antibiotic therapy. For penicillin-allergic patients, aztreonam or cefepime are reasonable alternatives to piperacillin–tazobactam. Obtaining cultures from the middle ear, an abscess, blood, or CSF (if clinically indicated) can help identify the pathologic organism. Broad-spectrum IV antibiotics should be given for a minimum of 7 days or until clinical improvement. Coverage may continue as an outpatient with oral antibiotics to complete a 4-week course.

  As mastoiditis represents an abscess, drainage is an integral aspect to the treatment. Myringotomy, with or without tympanostomy tube placement, should occur in all patients suspected of mastoiditis, to allow for drainage of the infection and for collection of culture specimens.[4] Patients with infections refractory to treatment with IV antibiotics and tympanostomy tube placement may require resection of the mastoid bone (mastoidectomy) in order to help eradicate the infection. All patients with mastoiditis should be referred for consultation by ENT for further evaluation.

- *Disposition*: Patients with mastoiditis will require broad-spectrum IV antibiotic therapy and therefore will universally require admission to the hospital. If there are symptoms of meningeal involvement or intracranial extension, then children may require ICU level of care for monitoring of neurologic examinations. Once clinical improvement has occurred, patients should be discharged to follow up with ENT.

Historical clues	Physical findings	Ancillary studies
• History of otitis media • Fever • Complaints of ear pain and drainage	• Protruding pinna • Tender, red postauricular space • Otorrhea • Fever	• Leukocytosis • CT with fluid coalescing within mastoid air cells

Follow-Up

The patient's head CT demonstrated signs consistent with acute mastoiditis with periosteitis. A myringotomy was performed, yielding white purulent fluid which was sent for Gram's stain and culture. Blood cultures were obtained. The patient was started on vancomycin and piperacillin–tazobactam per recommendation from ENT. She was admitted to the hospital and demonstrated improvement. Cultures returned positive for *S. pyogenes* sensitive to amoxicillin–clavulanate. The patient was transitioned to oral antibiotics to complete a 4-week course and had a full recovery.

References

1. Uhari M, Mantysaari K, Niemela M. A meta-analytic review of the risk factors for acute otitis media. *Clin Infect Dis* 1996; 22: 1079–83.

2. Lin HW, Shargorodsky J, Gopen Q. Clinical strategies for the management of acute mastoiditis in the pediatric population. *Clin Pediatr (Phila)* 2010; 49: 110–15.

3. Bilavsky E, Yarden-Bilavsky H, Samra Z, et al. Clinical, laboratory, and microbiological differences between children with simple or complicated mastoiditis. *Int J Pediatr Otorhinolaryngol* 2009; 73: 1270–3.

4. Luntz M, Brodsky A, Nusem S, et al. Acute mastoiditis – the antibiotic era: A multicenter study. *Int J Pediatr Otorhinolaryngol* 2001; 57: 1–9.

5. Nussinovitch M, Yoeli R, Elishkevitz K, et al. Acute mastoiditis in children: epidemiologic, clinical, microbiologic, and therapeutic aspects over past years. *Clin Pediatr (Phila)* 2004; 43: 261–7.

Case 5

Contributing Authors: Jonathan R. Morgan and Melanie K. Prusakowski

History

The patient is a 13-year-old boy who was hit in the left eye with a baseball. He reportedly lost consciousness for a few seconds, which prompted transport to the ED. Per EMS, he had one bout of vomiting en route. He presents with eye pain, blurred vision, nausea, and vomiting. He has severe pain with eye movement and throbbing pain when not moving the eye. Upon questioning, he also complains of numbness under the left eye. There is no headache or neck pain.

Past Medical History

- Eczema.

Medications

- No medications.

Allergies

- NKDA.

Physical Examination and Ancillary Studies

- *Vital signs*: T 98.6 °F, HR 44, RR 16, BP 120/70, O_2 sat 99% on room air.
- *General*: Well-developed, well-nourished teenager, who is alert and oriented, in moderate distress secondary to pain.
- *HEENT*: PERRL. Decreased visual acuity in left eye (20/30); diplopia and limited upward gaze in the left eye. Appreciable orbital dystopia and hyphema in the left eye. No periorbital ecchymosis. Palpable tenderness and crepitus of the left zygomatic arch.
- *Neck*: Supple and non-tender, with full range of motion.
- *Cardiovascular*: Bradycardia, normal S1, S2, no audible M/R/G.
- *Lungs*: Clear and equal, with no W/R/R.
- *Abdomen*: Soft and non-tender, with no signs of trauma.
- *Extremities and skin*: Warm and well-perfused, with no signs of trauma and good pulses.
- *Neurologic*: GCS 15. Speech fluent. Strength is 5/5 in all extremities. Sensation is intact. Deep tendon reflexes are 2+ and symmetric.

Questions for Thought

- What is the differential diagnosis for this child's symptoms?
- What other injuries are potentially associated with this condition?

- What signs and symptoms on this child's examination give away the diagnosis?
- What are common associated complications?
- What is the management of this condition?

Diagnosis

- Fracture of the left orbital floor with inferior rectus entrapment.

Discussion

- *Epidemiology*: Facial fractures have an incidence of 5–15 percent in the pediatric population. Nasal fractures are the most common, and are generally handled in a conservative fashion. Orbital fractures represent the third most common type of pediatric facial fracture.[1] The orbital floor and medial wall are the most common sites for orbital fractures.[2-4] The primary mechanism of injury is blunt trauma, often with a direct blow to the periorbital region, and is most frequently related to sports activity or motor vehicle collisions.[2-4]
- *Pathophysiology*: Controversy surrounds the causative mechanism of fractures to the orbital floor and/or medial wall, commonly referred to as blow-out fractures. There are three current theories: the bone conduction theory, the globe to wall theory, and the hydraulic theory. The bone conduction theory states that the transmission of force from the strong orbital rim causes the thin internal orbital bones to buckle.[2] The globe to wall theory proposes that, under a force, the globe contacts the floor and results in an orbital floor fracture.[2] The hydraulic theory attributes the fracture to an increase in indirect pressure from the globe.[2] There is evidence to support each theory, and the actual cause is likely to be a combination or interaction of all three theories.

  Although blow-out fractures are the most common orbital fracture, children can suffer other forms of orbital and facial fracture. Nasoethmoid fractures result from the collapse of the nasal bones into the skull base and accompanying fractures that displace paired nasal, lacrimal, and ethmoid bones. Orbital roof fractures in children commonly have a fracture pattern that extends from the orbital roof through the supraorbital foramen and along the frontal bone.[4] An orbital blow-in fracture refers to the collapsing of the orbital roof from an inferior supraorbital impact. The zygomatic complex is a quadripod structure consisting of the lateral orbital wall, the lateral orbital rim, the inferior orbital rim, the zygomatic-maxillary buttress, and the zygomatic arch. Orbital zygomatic fractures commonly occur along the three buttress-related sutures.

Orbital fractures can result in entrapment of orbital tissues, especially fat or extraocular muscles.[2,5,6] Children, whose bones are less calcified and therefore more pliable with external force, can develop a trapdoor variant of a blow-out fracture that results in extreme external ophthalmoplegia.[5,6] Another pediatric-specific variant is the "white-eyed blow-out," where a lack of typical signs of surrounding periorbital trauma belies underlying significant bony trauma.

The oculocardiac reflex may be seen in patients with orbital bone injuries. This reflex occurs when eye pain/pressure causes a drop in blood pressure or heart rate. Activation of the oculocardiac reflex is associated with nausea, bradycardia, and, potentially, syncope.[5,6] The ophthalmic division of the fifth cranial nerve controls the afferent limb of the oculocardiac reflex. Impulses pass to the vagus nerve, then travel through the spinal cord to vagal nerves that deliver the signal to the heart and stomach. Orbital fractures present a sufficient opportunity for activation of the oculocardiac reflex, which results in physiologic responses.

- *Presentation*: Orbital fractures in children have varying presentations. Typical signs of an orbital fracture include pain, periorbital swelling, and periorbital ecchymosis.[1,2] Numbness, decreased visual acuity, diplopia, limited extraocular motility, orbital dystopia, and enophthalmos may also be seen.[1-6] Children may experience vomiting, bradycardia, and syncope with orbital fractures, due to entrapment of extraocular muscles.[5,6] Entrapment most commonly results in double vision on directed gaze. Palpable tenderness, crepitus, and/or step-off of the facial bones suggest an underlying fracture. Signs of a possible displaced fracture include proptosis, widened intercanthal distance, subconjunctival emphysema, and CSF leak.[1,2] Children may also present with signs of globe rupture (irregular pupil), corneal abrasions, lens dislocation, hyphema, lacrimal injuries, or retinal detachment.

- *Diagnosis*: Patients with a history of blunt orbital trauma should be promptly evaluated for traumatic injuries to the eye. The physical examination should include assessment of the facial bones, surrounding soft tissues, and the eye itself. A complete ophthalmologic examination should occur quickly as periorbital swelling may progress. The child may need help retracting a swollen lid so that visual acuity, pupillary function, and extraocular motility can be assessed. Eyelid retractors (Desmarres) may be needed. When feasible, a slit-light lamp examination should be completed.

  A thin-cut coronal CT scan of the orbit should be performed in patients with a history of orbital trauma combined with any of the following findings: palpable crepitus or step-off, severe pain, limited extraocular motility, decreased visual acuity, enophthalmos, proptosis, widened intercanthal distance, activation of the oculocardiac reflex, or extrusion of intraocular contents. CT imaging can also provide necessary information when the child cannot cooperate with a full examination due to pain.

  As with any trauma to the head, a complete neurologic examination and c-spine assessment should be performed. Pediatric facial injuries commonly occur with concomitant injury to the skull and brain, and therefore a high index of suspicion for associated injuries should be maintained.[1]

- *Treatment*: A conservative treatment plan is recommended for orbital fractures in children to prevent disruptions in growth and the formation of periosteal bone. Patients with associated globe injuries, severe vagal symptoms, or visual impairment require immediate ophthalmologist evaluation.[2] Muscle entrapment, enophthalmos, orbital dystopia or injury to the lacrimal apparatus, and/or medial canthal ligament also need emergent consultation with an ophthalmologist.[2] Nausea, vomiting, and pain may also need to be controlled. There is limited evidence to support or refute the use of prophylactic antibiotics covering sinus pathogens for patients with fractures into a sinus. An effort should be made to reduce local swelling with cold packs.

- *Disposition*: Patients with an orbital wall fracture not associated with decreased vision, globe

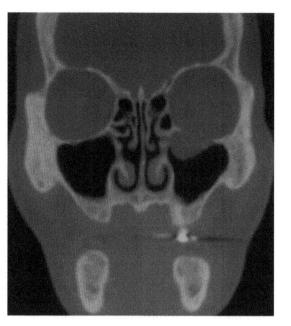

Figure 5.4 Coronal section of CT face demonstrating an inferior orbital wall fracture with herniation of orbital contents into the left maxillary sinus.

trauma, or extraocular muscle entrapment may be suitable for discharge. Such children should be instructed to use cold compress for 48 hours, keep the head elevated during sleep, use nasal decongestants (if age appropriate), and avoid nose blowing. Follow up can be arranged with ophthalmology or oromaxillofacial surgery, depending on regional practices.

Historical clues	Physical findings
• History of eye trauma	• Decreased visual acuity
• Blurry vision	• Limited extraocular motility
• Numbness to cheek	• Orbital dystopia
• Pain with eye movement	• Hyphema
	• Zygoma tenderness and crepitus

Follow-Up

The child underwent CT scanning of his facial bones, which revealed a left orbital blow-out fracture with entrapment (Figure 5.4). He was admitted to the pediatric service due to intermittent bradycardia. He received surgical reduction of the left orbital wall fracture and the entrapment of his inferior rectus muscle. He remained in the hospital one night for control of pain and swelling. At discharge he had no residual vision deficits.

References

1. Chao MT, Losee JE. Complications in pediatric facial fractures. *Craniomaxillofac Trauma Reconstr* 2009; 2: 103–12.

2. Bord SP, Linden J. Trauma to the globe and orbit. *Emerg Med Clin N Am* 2008; 26: 97–123.

3. Gerber B, Kiwanuka P, Dhariwal D. Orbital fractures in children: A review of outcomes. *Br J Oral Maxillofac Surg* 2013; 51: 789–93.

4. Hatton MP, Watkins LM, Rubin PA, et al. Orbital fractures in children. *Ophthal Plast Reconstr Surg* 2001; 17: 174–9.

5. Wei LA, Durairaj VD. Pediatric orbital floor fractures. *J AAPOS* 2011; 15: 173–80.

6. Cohen SM, Garrett CG. Pediatric orbital floor fractures: Nausea/vomiting as signs of entrapment. *Otolaryngol Head Neck Surg* 2003; 129: 43–7.

Case 6

Contributing Authors: Denis R. Pauzé and Daniel K. Pauzé

History

The patient is a 14-year-old male who presents to fast track with a sore throat. Ten days prior to arrival he developed a sore throat with fever. He was seen by his PCP and had a negative rapid strep test. His symptoms persisted, and 5 days prior to arrival he again saw his PCP, this time with swelling of the left side of the neck. He was diagnosed with lymphadenitis and started on amoxicillin–clavulanate. The pain and swelling in the neck persisted, and he again saw his PCP. Blood work was checked, and he was found to have WBC of 25,000. He was told to go to the ED.

His family decided to "wait it out" for 2 more days and show up to the ED today. The child arrives with persistent sore throat, neck pain, and neck swelling. On review of systems, there is no trauma, recent dental work, chest pain, or shortness of breath. He does have an occasional cough. The triage nurse states that "it is just a fast-track sore throat patient."

Past Medical History

• None.

Medications

• Amoxicillin–clavulanate; acetaminophen as needed for pain or fever.

Allergies

- NKDA.

Physical Examination and Ancillary Studies

- *Vital signs*: T 101.3 °F, HR 97, BP 157/68, RR 16, O_2 sat 97% on room air.
- *General*: Awake and non-toxic in appearance, in no acute distress.
- *HEENT*: PERRL. Extraocular movements intact. Oropharynx clear, posterior pharynx, with mild erythema. No exudates, lesions, petechiae, or masses.
- *Neck*: Decreased range of motion. Left side of neck is tender and warm. There is anterior cervical adenopathy. Non-erythematous, no crepitus.
- *Cardiovascular*: Normal S1, S2. No M/R/G. Brisk capillary refill.
- *Lungs*: CTA bilaterally, with no W/R/R.
- *Abdomen*: Non-tender. No splenomegaly.
- *Extremities and skin*: No rashes or joint swelling. Warm and well-perfused.
- *Neurologic*: Awake, alert, and age appropriate, with no focal deficits.
- *Pertinent laboratory values*: WBC 23,000; HCT 37, Plt normal. CRP 11, ESR 59. Na 129, K 3.3, Cl 88, bicarbonate 31. BUN, Cr, and LFTs normal.

Questions for Thought

- Should you have any concerns for airway involvement or compromise?
- Does the child's vaccination status matter?
- What are common complications of this entity?
- What imaging study, if any, is warranted?

Diagnosis

- Lemierre syndrome (septic thrombophlebitis of the internal jugular vein).

Discussion

- *Epidemiology*: The first case description of sore throat and jugular vein thrombosis came in 1900 by Courmont and Cade. In 1936, Dr. Lemierre reported a case series of 20 patients with similar findings. In this article, Dr. Lemierre stated: "...*the appearance and repetition several days after*

the onset of a sore throat of severe pyrexial attacks with an initial rigor, ... the occurrence of pulmonary infarcts and arthritic manifestations, constitute a syndrome so characteristic that mistake is almost impossible..."[1]

Sore throat is a commonly encountered complaint, with at least 10 million annual healthcare encounters. Pharyngitis is the most common cause of sore throat, and is usually found to be viral or bacterial in nature. Group A beta-hemolytic *Streptococcus* is the most common bacterial etiology (see Chapter 7, Case 9 for a detailed discussion of this entity). Although usually self-limiting, life-threatening causes of sore throat and pharyngitis do exist, and include deep space infections such as parapharyngeal abscess or retropharyngeal abscesses (discussed in detail later in this chapter). Unvaccinated children are at additional risk for life-threatening causes of sore throat, as they are at higher risk for diphtheria or *Haemophilus influenzae* infections, such as epiglottitis.

Lemierre syndrome is another rare cause of life-threatening pharyngitis. Fortunately, this entity is rare. There is an estimated annual incidence of approximately five cases per million people.[2,3]

- *Pathophysiology*: Lemierre syndrome is classically caused by normal oropharyngeal bacteria, most commonly *Fusobacterium necrophorum*.[4–6] *Fusobacterium* are Gram-negative anaerobes and are part of the normal mucosal flora. As an anaerobe, they can invade tissue and act as a pathogen. They produce an endotoxin that destroys cells and causes platelet aggregation. Other causative organisms may include *Eikenella*, *Bacteroides*, *Peptostreptococcus*, and *Streptococcus*.[4,5] These organisms migrate from the oropharynx into the adjacent parapharyngeal space, where they subsequently infiltrate the nearby carotid sheath. From there, they infiltrate the internal jugular vein and gain access to the vascular system. Once in the vascular system, infection can spread to the lungs, brain, joints, liver, or heart valves.[2–6] Local infectious spread can result in an expanding neck abscess, compromising the upper airway.
- *Presentation*: Patients are usually teenagers or young adults, although cases in toddlers and young children have been described.[6] Sore throat

and pharyngitis are common initial complaints.[1,2-5] Patients may be on antibiotics and complain of "not getting better." Commonly, the pain expressed by the child seems in excess of the physical findings on oropharyngeal examination. Vital signs may reveal fever, tachycardia, and, with advanced illness, hypotension. Examination may (but will not always) show abnormalities of the oropharynx, such as erythema, fluctuance, and/or petechiae.[2,3] Tenderness overlying the jugular vein/sternocleiodomastoid muscle may be observed. This tenderness is sometimes impressive and prominent, and is often accompanied by a palpable mass. Children may also present with late complications, such as septic emboli to the lung, septic joint, or a brain abscess.[2,3] Children who are on antibiotics may have attenuated symptoms, but many children with Lemierre syndrome are toxic-appearing.

- *Diagnosis*: Blood cultures usually reveal normal oropharyngeal flora pathogens, with the most common being *F. necrophorum*. *F. necrophorum* is a fastidious organism and cultures can be falsely negative. *F. necrophorum* is also rarely cultured from the oropharynx, as it requires a special medium that is not routinely used.[4] A CT scan of the neck with IV contrast reveals a thrombus in the internal jugular vein, and an extension of the CT into the lungs commonly demonstrates septic pulmonary emboli. U/S can also evaluate for thrombosis of the internal jugular vein.

- *Treatment*: Treatment regimens start with prompt antibiotic use. Antibiotic therapy should include a beta-lactamase-resistant beta-lactam antibiotic.[4,5] Options include ampicillin–sulbactam or piperacillin–tazobactam. Carbapenems such as imipenem or meropenem may also be used. Metronidazole is an option, as it also has bacteriocidal activity against *F. necrophorum*. Antibiotic treatment is indicated for several weeks.

Anticoagulation therapy for jugular vein thrombosis is debated and remains somewhat controversial.[2] Currently, there is not enough evidence to support the use of anticoagulation for isolated thrombosis. Some clinicians advocate for anticoagulation when there is extension of the thrombus.

Surgical intervention may be needed for drainage of abscesses. Surgical intervention on the jugular vein also remains debatable, and may be utilized when the patient does not respond to IV antibiotic therapy.

- *Disposition*: All patients with a diagnosis of Lemierre syndrome should be admitted to the hospital. Patients with hemodynamic compromise or airway involvement should be admitted to the ICU.

Historical clues	Physical findings	Ancillary studies
• Sore throat with no improvement on antibiotics • Unilateral neck swelling • Ongoing fever	• Pain out of proportion to examination • Neck mass • Fever • Tachycardia	• Elevated WBC • Elevated ESR

Follow-Up

The patient was diagnosed with Lemierre syndrome. He was evaluated by vascular surgery, hematology, and infectious disease specialists and was started on IV ampicillin–sulbactam. After a week of hospitalization, with significant clinical improvement, he was transitioned to a PICC line and completed a 6-week course of IV antibiotics with no significant sequelae.

References

1. Lemierre A. On certain septicemias due to anaerobic organisms. *Lancet* 1936; 227: 701–3.

2. Phua CK, Chadachan VM, Acharya R. Lemierre syndrome: Should we anticoagulate? A case report and review of the literature. *Int J Angiol* 2013; 22: 137–42.

3. Tromop-van Dalen C, Mekhail A-M. Lemierre syndrome: Early recognition and management. *CMAJ*. 2015; 187: 1229–31.

4. Goldenberg NA, Knapp-Clevenger R, Hays T, et al. Lemierre's and Lemierre's-like syndromes in children: Survival and thromboembolic outcomes. *Pediatrics* 2005; 116: e543.

5. Ramirez S, Hild TG, Rudolph CN, et al. Increased diagnosis of Lemierre syndrome and other *Fusobacterium necrophorum* infections at a children's hospital. *Pediatrics* 2003; 112: e380.

6. Garcia-Salido A, Unzueta-Roch JL, Garcia-Teresa MA, et al. Pediatric disseminated Lemierre syndrome in 2 infants: Not too young for an ancient disease. *Pediatr Emerg Care* 2017; 33: 490–3.

Case 7

Contributing Authors: Dorota Pazdrowska and Melanie K. Prusakowski

History

The patient is a 30-month-old female who presents with drooling for one day. One week ago she developed a URI, which subsequently resolved. Four days prior to arrival she developed fevers, with a maximum temperature of 102.6 °F yesterday. During the previous 24 hours, she refused all oral intake. When mom noticed that she had difficulty moving her neck, she was taken to the pediatrician, who diagnosed her with viral meningitis. She was prescribed hydroxyzine to help with sleep. There was no travel history or sick contacts. The patient has had multiple mosquito bites throughout the summer and the family dog had a tick removed 2 weeks ago.

Past Medical History

- Concussion at 27 months.
- Eczema.

Medications

- Hydroxyzine for the last 2 days.

Allergies

- NKDA.

Physical Examination and Ancillary Studies

- *Vital signs*: T 100.2 °F, HR 150, RR 48, BP 132/72, O_2 sat 97% on room air.
- *General*: Awake and alert. Child appears fussy and intermittently irritable.
- *HEENT*: PERRL. No injection. Atraumatic head, tympanic membranes clear bilaterally. Erythematous oropharynx, without exudates. Left tonsil enlarged, no petechiae.
- *Neck*: No adenopathy, midline trachea, child resists movement.
- *Cardiovascular*: Regular tachycardia, normal S1, S2, no murmurs, femoral pulses 2+ bilaterally.
- *Lungs*: Breathing non-labored, CTA bilaterally, no W/R/R.
- *Abdomen and genitourinary*: Soft, non-tender, no organomegaly, bowel sounds present, normal female genitalia.

- *Extremities and skin*: No rashes or petechiae. Ruddy cheeks. No joint swelling or deformity.
- *Neurologic*: Normal mental status, fussy but consolable.
- *Pertinent laboratory values*: WBC 29,000, Plt 596,000, HCT normal.
- *Pertinent radiographs*: Soft-tissue lateral neck radiograph shows moderately prominent adenoidal soft tissues and prominent prevertebral soft tissues, which may be positional in nature.

Questions for Thought

- What is the differential diagnosis for decreased neck movement in a toddler?
- What is the utility of radiographic studies in confirming or ruling out the diagnosis?
- What are definitive treatments?

Diagnosis

- Left peritonsillar abscess.

Discussion

- *Epidemiology*: Peritonsillar abscess is the most common head and neck abscess in children, with an incidence of about 30 in 100,000 cases per year.[1,2] The disease coincides with periods of highest incidence of streptococcal pharyngitis.[1,2] Although it is most commonly seen in teenagers and young adults, it has been reported in infants and toddlers, as well.[2,3]
- *Pathophysiology*: Peritonsillar abscess is a collection of purulent fluid in the soft tissues surrounding the palatine tonsil. Most commonly, it develops between the tonsillar capsule and the pharyngeal muscles (superior constrictor and palatopharyngeus muscles).[1–4] It can be associated with cellulitis of the palatal tissues.[4] The infection tends to be polymicrobial, including group A streptococci, *Staphylococcus aureus*, and respiratory anaerobes.[1–5] These organisms can spread to the masseter and other nearby musculature, subsequently with infiltration of the carotid sheath. This can result in bacteremia, sepsis, and airway compromise.
- *Presentation*: Children with peritonsillar abscess may have a preceding diagnosis of exudative tonsillitis, or they may have their first presentation

of their illness with the abscess already present. About one-fifth have prior diagnosis of URI at the time of the diagnosis of peritonsillar abscess.[3] The time from the onset of symptoms to abscess formation ranges from 2 to 8 days. The most common initial complaint is a sore throat in the majority of children, which is typically unilateral, followed by fever.[3] They may complain of neck pain and neck stiffness, or the caregiver may have noted a neck mass. Although older children characteristically have a sore throat, about a third of children under the age of 12 will not have this complaint, and therefore a careful physical examination is always warranted.[3] Patients may have dysphagia and/or odynophagia. Trismus may be seen and is also a hallmark feature of peritonsillar abscess.[3] It results from irritation and reflex spasm of the internal pterygoid muscle. They may have a muffled voice, known as "hot potato" voice, or may report referred ear pain.

- *Diagnosis*: The diagnosis of peritonsillar abscess must be considered in patients with severe sore throat, especially when accompanied by odynophagia, dysphagia, fever, and trismus. Severe sore throats can also be caused by retropharyngeal abscess, tracheitis, epiglottitis, pharyngitis, parapharyngeal abscess, uvulitis, or tonsillitis. These entities can be distinguished from one another by direct visualization (in the case of uvulitis, tonsillitis, and pharyngitis), indirect visualization (in the case of epiglottitis), or diagnostic imaging (in the case of abscesses).

In physical examination of peritonsillar abscess in patients who can comply, there is edema and erythema of the affected tonsil and the overlying soft palate, uvular deviation to the contralateral side, trismus, and lymphadenopathy. Other etiologies of unilateral tonsillar enlargement, such as tumor infiltration or benign hypertrophy, and coexistent pathology, such as mononucleosis, palatal cellulitis, or local adenitis, should be considered.

In small patients without a complaint of sore throat and in whom a detailed physical examination is challenging, diagnosis is often made with imaging.[3] Peritonsillar abscess can be confirmed with intraoral or transcutaneous U/S.[4] A CT scan or MRI of oropharyngeal and neck tissues is usually reserved for patients with suspected spread of infection outside of the peritonsillar space. CT provides highly specific characterization of pediatric deep neck infections and masses.[4,5] MRI provides better soft-tissue definition than CT scan, without exposure to radiation, which may improve detection. In straightforward cases, diagnosis can be confirmed upon abscess drainage with no imaging at all.

- *Treatment*: Management of peritonsillar abscess begins with an airway evaluation and management of acute obstruction when present. IV fluid therapy may be required for patients with poor oral intake. In some instances, IV antibiotics may be the only treatment necessary.[4,5] More commonly, the definitive treatment is drainage of the abscess by needle aspiration, or incision and drainage.[4,5] Use of U/S to guide drainage improves diagnostic accuracy and outcomes.[4] Antibiotics are recommended following surgical intervention, to clear remaining and disseminated infection. Common antibiotic options for children are clindamycin (30 mg/kg per day, divided every 8 hours) and cefotaxime (150 mg/kg per day, divided every 8 hours). Routine culturing of the abscess is reported to be unnecessary, although some practitioners still adhere to this. Corticosteroids may hasten recovery by reducing edema and inflammation. A single dose of dexamethasone at 0.6 mg/kg, with a maximum dose of 10 mg, IV may improve pain.[5]

- *Disposition*: Outpatient treatment may be appropriate in children without airway compromise, who are not clinically dehydrated and can tolerate oral antimicrobials. Those requiring immediate surgical intervention benefit from consultation with ENT and admission for IV antibiotics. Patients who complete a course of antibiotics after drainage have good outcomes, and recurrence in children is rare. Late recognition and inadequate treatment can result in complications such as jugular vein thrombosis, extension of infection into tissues of the deep neck, posterior mediastinum, or lung, and hemorrhage from erosion into the carotid sheath.

Follow-Up

The child was given IV antibiotics and admitted to the hospital. Her blood and urine cultures were negative, and she underwent LP, which was also negative. An inpatient MRI was performed which revealed

Historical clues	Physical findings	Ancillary studies
• Recent URI • Decreased PO • Neck stiffness	• Unilateral tonsillar hypertrophy • Neck stiffness • Tachycardia	• Elevated WBC • Elevated Plt (acute phase reactant) • X-ray with large adenoids and generous prevertebral space

a 3.4-cm peritonsillar abscess. The child underwent drainage of the abscess in the OR by ENT. She completed her antibiotic course and had resolution of her symptoms.

References

1. Cirilli AR. Emergency evaluation and management of the sore throat. *Emerg Med Clin N Am* 2013; 31: 501–15.

2. Stoner MJ, Dulaurier M. Pediatric ENT emergencies. *Emerg Med Clin N Am* 2013; 31: 795–808.

3. Hsiao H-J, Huang Y-C, Hsia S-H, et al. Clinical features of peritonsillar abscess in children. *Pediatr Neonat* 2012; 53: 366–70.

4. Costantino T, Satz W, Dehnkamp W, et al. Randomized trial comparing intraoral ultrasound to landmark-based needle aspiration in patients with suspected peritonsillar abscess. *Acad Emerg Med* 2012; 19: 626–31.

5. Powel J, Wilson JA. An evidence-based review of peritonsillar abscess. *Clin Otolaryngol* 2012; 37: 136–45.

Case 8

Contributing Author: Rebecca Jeanmonod

History

A 4-year-old boy presents to the ED with his father with a chief complaint of right ear pain. The child has had a coarse cough and runny nose for the past 5 days, but has otherwise "been fine." Dad didn't check his temperature, but didn't think he felt particularly warm. The child had been eating and drinking well, but vomited one time yesterday. There has been no diarrhea. This morning, he began crying and complaining of right ear pain. Dad denies any trauma to the ear. The child has a history of two prior ear infections, the last one about 18 months ago. He has been meeting his developmental milestones and passed a hearing screen at preschool. He has a history of snoring, and has a sleep study scheduled in a month.

Past Medical History

- Two prior episodes of acute otitis media.
- Immunizations are UTD.

Medications

- None.

Allergies

- NKDA.

Physical Examination and Ancillary Studies

- *Vital signs*: T 100.4 °F, HR 115, RR 20, BP 98/60, O₂ sat 98% on room air.
- *General*: Well-developed and well-nourished, normal appearance, perfusion, and work of breathing.
- *HEENT*: PERRL, oropharynx with enlarged tonsils, and child with nasal voice. No trismus. Right tympanic membrane, with mild bulging and clouding. Left tympanic membrane normal. No mastoid tenderness or erythema. Moderate rhinorrhea.
- *Neck*: Supple, with shotty adenopathy. No masses.
- *Cardiovascular*: Regular rate and rhythm, with no M/R/G.
- *Lungs*: CTA bilaterally, with no W/R/R. No retractions, grunting, or flaring.
- *Abdomen*: Soft and non-tender, with no masses or organomegaly.
- *Skin and extremities:* Warm and well-perfused, good capillary refill, no rashes.
- *Neurologic*: Normal mental status, follows commands.

Questions for Thought

- Does this child have acute otitis media? Is his disease severe?
- Does this child require antibiotics?
- Which children with this disease entity require antibiotics?
- What role does pain management play in treatment of this disease?

Diagnosis

- Acute otitis media.

Discussion

- *Epidemiology*: Acute otitis media is exceedingly common in children, affecting 80 percent of children prior to entering school.[1] Most children have their first episode prior to age 3.[2] Many children have recurrent episodes during their childhoods. Risk factors for developing recurrent otitis media include allergy, craniofacial abnormalities, GERD, large adenoids, exposure to smoke, daycare attendance (or multiple siblings), lack of breastfeeding, and pacifier use.[3]

- *Pathophysiology*: Acute otitis media generally occurs secondary to eustachian tube dysfunction coincident with an acute URI.[1,4] It is defined by the presence of fluid in the middle ear with acute local or systemic illness, and is distinct from otitis media with effusion, which also consists of fluid in the middle ear but is in the absence of acute local or systemic illness. Otitis media with effusion is not a medical emergency, and children should be referred back to their pediatricians for monitoring for resolution of effusion or referral to ENT as necessary. In acute otitis media, the middle ear fluid may contain a variety of bacterial pathogens, with *Streptococcus pneumoniae* and *Haemophilus influenzae* historically the most common.[2,5] Since introduction of the *S. pneumoniae* vaccine in the USA, the relative proportion of cases of acute otitis media secondary to *S. pneumoniae* has decreased, and the relative proportion of those secondary to *H. influenzae* has increased.[1,2] Otitis media with effusion is more commonly associated with *H. influenzae*.[4]

  From the middle ear, acute otitis media can spread to involve other local structures, resulting in mastoiditis, meningitis, brain abscess, venous sinus thrombosis, labyrinthitis, osteomyelitis, or facial nerve paralysis. Otitis media with effusion does not have local or systemic inflammatory findings by definition, and therefore does not lead to the same complications as acute otitis media. The primary morbidity of otitis media with effusion is chronic effusion with hearing loss, which can disrupt speech development in young children.[4]

- *Presentation*: Most children present with ear pain and many have ear tugging, although neither of these complaints is very specific.[2] Small children often have fever, malaise, vomiting, and diarrhea, or may present with otorrhea from tympanic membrane perforation.[2] Older children often complain of headache and disrupted hearing, as well.[2]

- *Diagnosis*: Ear pain can be *primary* or *secondary* in etiology, and it is important for the medical provider to determine which. Primary ear pain, or pain arising from the ear itself, can be caused by acute otitis media, chronic otitis with effusion, otitis externa, bullous myringitis, trauma, or foreign body. Innervation to the ear arises from cranial nerves V, VII, IX, and X, as well as cervical nerves 1–3. Therefore, referred pain to the ear can be related to any structures innervated by these nerves, including the temporomandibular joint, the teeth, the brain or cranium, the thyroid, or the c-spine.

  To make the diagnosis of otitis media, then, the provider must take a history that helps to exclude other sources of ear pain. The history should not only include items related to the ear, but also to the neurologic and musculoskeletal system. The provider should ask about tongue function, including chewing and swallowing as well as speech, should inquire about dental symptoms or problems, and should consider trauma. Smoke exposure and alcohol use should also be reviewed.

  A complete examination for ear pain should include inspection of the external ear, speculum examination of the internal ear, assessment of the sinuses and nose, oropharyngeal examination, neurologic examination, neck examination, and skin examination. This will minimize the likelihood of the EM provider erroneously attributing ear pain to the wrong source.

  Per the AAP, the diagnosis of acute otitis media should only be made in children with moderate to severe bulging of the tympanic membrane or new otorrhea in the absence of otitis externa, or in children with mild bulging and recent onset of significant ear pain or intense erythema of the tympanic membrane.[6] A cloudy color to the tympanic membrane is common in acute otitis media and impaired mobility of the tympanic membrane also increases the predictive value of physical examination.[4] The most accurate way to assess tympanic membrane mobility is with pneumatic otoscopy or tympanometry, but these techniques are not always feasible in agitated small children, and tympanometry is not available in most EDs.

- *Treatment*: Acute otitis media may be viral in origin, and antibiotics do not benefit every case. The AAP recommends that children be assessed and treated for pain, as this is the most common reason for their presentation to the ED.[6] They recommend initiation of antibiotic therapy for all children 6 months of age or older with acute otitis media with severe signs or symptoms (severe or moderate pain for at least 2 days and a temperature $\geq$ 102.2 °F).[6] In children without severe signs or symptoms, antibiotics should be initiated in those less than 2 years of age with bilateral acute otitis media.[6] For unilateral non-severe disease in children less than 2, or unilateral or bilateral disease in children older than 2, the clinician can use deferred antibiotics ("watchful waiting") and close follow-up, or may prescribe antibiotic therapy.[6] Children with no improvement at 48–72 hours follow-up should receive antibiotics. The antibiotic of choice is currently high-dose amoxicillin (90mg/kg per day) in children without allergies who have not received a beta-lactam antibiotic in the prior 30 days.[6] In children whose disease is accompanied by purulent conjunctivitis, the pathogen is likely to be *H. influenzae*, and should be treated with amoxicillin–clavulanate, as it is resistant to amoxicillin alone.[4] Even with antibiotics, not every child shows improvement or a shortened course. For every 20 children prescribed antibiotics for acute otitis media, one will have decreased pain at day 3 of illness, and one will get a rash, diarrhea, or vomiting from the antibiotics.[7] Thirty-three children need to be treated to prevent a single tympanic membrane rupture.[7]

  Duration of therapy is a subject of debate in the literature, with the initial recommendation of 10 days of therapy stemming from literature for treatment of other *Streptococcus* infections. Longer courses appear more effective in younger children, so children less than 2 years of age should receive a 10-day course.[6] In children age 2–5, 7 days of therapy appear as effective as 10, and so it is reasonable to give these children a 7-day course of antibiotics.[6] In children older than 5, 5–7 days of antibiotics are sufficient.[6]

- *Disposition*: Non-toxic-appearing children can be discharged home with careful return precautions to follow up with their PCP within 48–72 hours.

Historical clues	Physical findings
• Recent viral illness • History of snoring (suggesting enlarged adenoids and possible eustachian tube dysfunction) • Ear pain	• Tympanic membrane clouding and mild bulging • Low-grade fever • Enlarged tonsils

Follow-Up

Dad was advised to give the child ibuprofen for ear pain, and was given a prescription for amoxicillin to be filled if the child was still complaining of pain at 48 hours after his index visit. The child was low risk, and deferred antibiotics are acceptable for this age group with non-severe disease. The child had improved symptoms when following up with his pediatrician 2 days later, and was referred to ENT. The child's sleep study was positive for apnea, and the child went on to have his tonsils and adenoids removed, with improved snoring and no further episodes of otitis.

References

1. Harmes KM, Blackwod RA, Cook JM, et al. Otitis media: Diagnosis and treatment. *Am Fam Phys* 2013; 88: 435–40.

2. Thomas JP, Berner R, Zahnert T, et al. Acute otitis media: A structured approach. *Dtsch Arztebl Int* 2014; 111: 151–60.

3. Lubianca Neto JF, Hemb L, Silva DB. Systematic literature review of modifiable risk factors for recurrent acute otitis media in childhood. *J Pediatr (Rio J)* 2006; 82: 87–96.

4. Conover K. Earache. *Emerg Med Clin N Am* 2013; 31: 413–42.

5. Ngo CC, Massa HM, Thornton RB, et al. Predominant bacteria detected from the middle ear fluid of children experiencing otitis media: A systematic review. *PLoS One* 2016; 11: e0150949.

6. Lieberthal AS, Carroll AE, Chonmaitree T, et al. The diagnosis and management of acute otitis media. *Pediatrics* 2013; 131: e964–99.

7. Venekamp RP, Sanders SL, Glasziou PP, et al. Antibiotics for acute otitis media in children. *Cochrane Database Syst Rev* 2015; 6: CD000219.

Case 9

Contributing Author: Khalief Hamden

History

The patient is a 3-year-old girl brought to the ED because she "will not turn her head." Mom reports that the child's symptoms started 3 days ago with a high fever, cough, and nasal congestion. The next day, mom took the patient to her pediatrician, where she was evaluated and diagnosed with a routine URI. She was started on azithromycin. That evening the patient started complaining of pain in the back of her neck and a sore throat. Mom noted that the fever had continued, and this morning the patient was unwilling to turn her head at all. Mom states that she only turns her shoulders in order to look to the side. This prompted a visit to an urgent care center where the patient was advised to come to the ED for evaluation of possible meningitis.

The patient has been tolerating fluids by mouth but has not been eating well. She has been making wet diapers. Her fevers have been well controlled with antipyretics, allowing her to play and interact at her baseline until today. There are no known sick contacts.

Past Medical History

- Full term, UTD on immunizations.

Medications

- Azithromycin.

Allergies

- NKDA.

Physical Examination and Ancillary Studies

- *Vital signs*: T 98.3 °F, HR 129, RR 25, BP 137/75, O_2 sat 98% on room air.
- *General*: The patient is non-toxic-appearing. There is no respiratory distress. She is interactive.
- *HEENT*: Normocephalic and atraumatic. Extraocular movements are normal. PERRL. Tympanic membranes normal bilaterally. Oral mucosa is moist with mildly enlarged tonsils, without significant erythema or exudate. Nasal congestion is present with some cobblestoning of the nasal mucosa.
- *Neck*: The patient has decreased mobility of her neck. She will not turn her head when tracking side to side, instead turning only her shoulders.

She resists side-to-side movement of the head. There is mild cervical adenopathy.

- *Cardiovascular*: Regular rate and rhythm, with no M/R/G. Peripheral pulses are palpable and symmetric.
- *Lungs*: Breath sounds are normal. No evidence of labored breathing. No W/R/R.
- *Abdomen*: Soft and non-tender with normal bowel sounds. No distension or tenderness. No organomegaly or palpable masses.
- *Skin and extremities*: There is a maculopapular, patchy, erythematous but blanching rash on the trunk.
- *Neurologic*: She is awake and alert. Face is symmetric. Speech and gait are normal. 5/5 upper extremity and lower extremity strength.
- *Pertinent laboratory values*: WBC 18,300, Hb, HCT, and Plt normal. ANC 12,900. Comprehensive metabolic panel with bicarbonate 18, anion gap of 20. U/A shows small amount of blood with occasional renal epithelial cells on microscopy but no other abnormalities. LP was performed and CSF is clear and colorless, WBC 2 and RBC 2 on cell count.
- *Pertinent radiographic findings*: Soft-tissue neck X-ray and soft-tissue neck CT were performed and are shown in Figures 5.5 and 5.6.

Questions for Thought

- How do patients typically present with this illness?
- What laboratory findings would support this diagnosis?
- What is the role of imaging studies in making the diagnosis?
- What findings on X-ray are considered abnormal?
- What treatments should be initiated in the ED?
- What is definitive treatment of this condition?

Diagnosis

- Acute retropharyngeal abscess.

Discussion

- *Epidemiology*: The incidence of retropharyngeal abscess in the USA has increased over the last decade. Using the Kid's Inpatient Database, Woods *et al.* report that the incidence of retropharyngeal abscess from 2003 to 2012 has

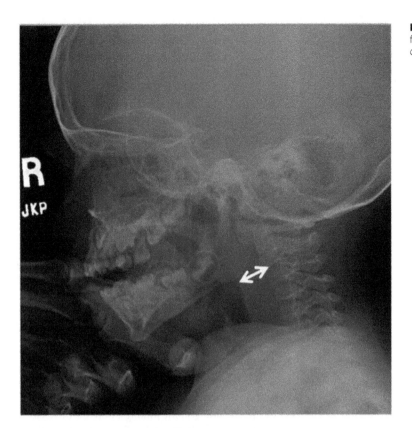

Figure 5.5 Lateral view of the c-spine. The film demonstrates prevertebral edema of 1.5 cm concerning for a retropharyngeal abscess.

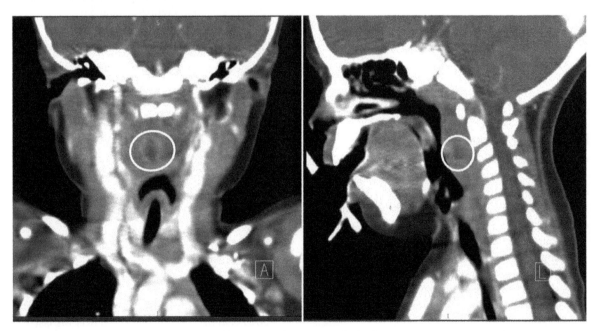

Figure 5.6 CT cervical soft tissue with IV contrast. These images demonstrate a fluid collection measuring approximately 9 x 8 x 11 mm at the level of C3 with prevertebral soft-tissue swelling from the skull base to approximately C6, consistent with a retropharyngeal abscess.

increased dramatically from 2.98 to 4.10 per 100,000 children.[1] The disease is more common in younger children under the age of 6 but can also afflict older children and even adults. Males are affected more commonly than females. The disease is also more commonly diagnosed in the winter and spring months.

- *Pathophysiology*: Retropharyngeal abscesses are an infrequent complication of URIs and ear infections. There are many potential bacterial culprits, including Gram-positive organisms, Gram-negative organisms, and species from the respiratory tract, particularly anaerobes. Thus, polymicrobial treatment is indicated.

  The lymphatic drainage of these tissues proceeds through the retropharyngeal space into a pair of paramedian lymph node chains between the base of the skull and the level of T1.[2] Suppuration of these lymph nodes may result in abscess formation, which subsequently allows for the spread of infection to adjacent structures such as the jugular vein, carotid artery, or distally into the mediastinum. In younger children, the retropharyngeal lymph nodes are quite prominent but usually regress and involute by early adolescence. This is a potential explanation for the decreased incidence in children over the age of 6.

- *Presentation*: The presentation of retropharyngeal abscess is completely variable. The age of the child, as well as abscess size and location, determines the presentation. The disease is usually preceded by a URI and therefore symptoms of fever, cough, congestion, rhinorrhea, and sore throat are common.[3] Antibiotics may have been prescribed without improvement (or even worsening of symptoms). Older children may complain of pain with swallowing whereas children too young to verbalize complaints may simply have poor oral intake. More suggestive of the diagnosis is neck stiffness or torticollis. Trismus, neck swelling, or adenopathy may also be present. In the case of severe disease, symptoms of airway obstruction, such as respiratory distress or stridor, may be present. Children may also present with sepsis.

- *Diagnosis*: Physical examination findings of nuchal rigidity or neck stiffness in a child with the aforementioned presentation should prompt further investigation. Leukocytosis and elevated inflammatory markers such as sedimentation rate and/or CRP may also raise clinical suspicion.

Lateral neck radiographs are a reasonable screening test but may appear normal as often as 12 percent of the time.[2,4] Prevertebral edema is suggested when the distance from the anterior surface of the vertebrae to the posterior border of the airway exceeds 7 mm at the level of C2 or 14 mm at the level of C6 in a child.

When there is a high degree of suspicion, a contrast-enhanced CT of the soft tissue of the neck is the diagnostic study of choice. Sedation may be needed to obtain a contrast-enhanced CT scan. MRI is probably superior for the evaluation of soft-tissue infection but availability and the necessity for sedation limit its utility in the ED. Since these children may have airway compromise, sedation should be done for CT scanning cautiously. Prudence may warrant ENT consultation with examination under anesthesia in the OR for particularly ill children.

- *Treatment*: The mainstay of treatment is antibiotic therapy. Clindamycin or ampicillin–sulbactam are considered first-line treatment options. They will not, however, provide the ideal and perfect coverage for Gram-positive organisms. Therefore, vancomycin or linezolid may be added to combat MRSA or group A streptococci.

  Several recent studies have demonstrated that many children do well without surgical intervention.[5–9] A rational protocol for surgical intervention was suggested by Hoffman *et al.*, which suggests drainage only for abscesses greater than 20 mm in diameter or in the case of sepsis, airway obstruction, or vascular compromise.[5] If not responding to antibiotics within 24–48 hours, repeat imaging and consideration of surgery or CT-guided needle aspiration may be warranted.[5–9]

- *Disposition*: Children with retropharyngeal abscess should be admitted to the hospital for IV antibiotics. ENT consultation for management decisions is appropriate.

Historical clues	Physical findings	Ancillary studies
• Fever	• Fever	• Elevated WBC
• Recent URI	• Torticollis	• Negative LP (reducing likelihood of meningitis)
• Worsening on antibiotics		• Neck X-ray with widened prevertebral space
• Neck stiffness		• CT with abscess

Follow-Up

This patient was found to have a small retropharyngeal abscess on CT scan of the neck at a community hospital ED. The case was discussed with a pediatrician at a nearby tertiary care facility and the patient was transferred by ambulance and admitted to the pediatric floor. The following day she was evaluated by ENT who decided against draining the abscess due to the small size and positive response to IV antibiotics. She had an uneventful hospital course. She was noted to have some improvement in rotating her head on hospital day 3. On hospital day 4 she had resolution of her fever and was able to tolerate food by mouth. She was subsequently discharged on hospital day 4 with instructions to finish a 10-day course of oral clindamycin.

References

1. Woods CR, Cash AM, Smith MJ, et al. Retropharyngeal and parapharyngeal abscesses among children and adolescents in the United States: Epidemiology and management trends, 2003–2012. *J Pediatr Infect Dis Soc* 2016; 5: 259–68.

2. Coulthard M, Isaacs D. Retropharyngeal abscess. *Arch Dis Child* 1991; 66: 1227–30.

3. Stoner MJ, Dulaurier M. Pediatric ENT emergencies. *Emerg Med Clin N Am* 2013; 31: 795–808.

4. Craig FW, Schunk JE. Retropharyngeal abscess in children: Clinical presentation, utility of imaging, and current management. *Pediatrics* 2003; 111: 1394–8.

5. Hoffman C, Pierrot S, Contencin P, et al. Retropharyngeal infections in children. Treatment strategies and outcomes. *Int J Pediatr Otorhinolaryngol* 2011; 75: 1099–103.

6. Georget E, Gauthier A, Brugel L, et al. Acute cervical lymphadenitis and infections of the retropharyngeal and parapharyngeal spaces in children. *BMC Ear Nose Throat Disord* 2014; 14: 8.

7. Martin CA, Gabrillargues J, Louvrier C, et al. Contribution of CT scan and CT-guided aspiration in the management of retropharyngeal abscess in children based on a series of 18 cases. *Eur Ann Otorhinolaryngol Head Neck Dis* 2014; 131: 277–82.

8. Grisaru-Soen G, Komisar O, Aizenstein O, et al. Retropharyngeal and parapharyngeal abscess in children: Clinical presentation, utility of imaging, and current management. *Int J Pediatr Otorhinolaryngol* 2010; 74: 1016–20.

9. Cramer JD, Purkey MR, Smith SS, et al. The impact of delayed surgical drainage of deep neck abscesses in adult and pediatric populations. *Laryngoscope* 2016; 126: 1753–60.

Extremity Complaints

Chapter 6

Case 1

Contributing Author: Rebecca Jeanmonod

History

An 18-month-old girl presents to the ED with mom complaining of arm pain. Mom states the child was playing unsupervised with a 4-year-old sibling in their shared bedroom when she heard crying. When she went in the room, the 18-month old indicated she had pain in her right arm. The 4-year-old was unable to tell mom what happened. Mom did not see any signs of trauma to the child, so she did not bring her in immediately. However, after 3 hours, the child was still not using her arm, so mom brought her in for further evaluation. The child has been consolable since the event, but periodically cries when she attempts to move the arm. She has not had confusion, vomiting, difficulty breathing, or any other complaints.

Past Medical History

- The child was a term neonate born by NSVD. She has had all her immunizations and has not had any other health problems.

Medications

- None.

Allergies

- NKDA.

Physical Examination and Ancillary Studies

- *Vital signs*: T 98.6 °F, HR 110, RR 25, BP 90/40, O_2 sat 100% on room air.
- *General*: Awake, alert, interactive, with normal work of breathing, mental status, and perfusion. Child is not in distress.

- *HEENT*: No evidence of head trauma. Neck is supple.
- *Cardiovascular*: Normal heart rate, without murmur or arrhythmia. Normal capillary refill.
- *Lungs*: Clear and equal, with good air entry.
- *Abdomen*: Soft and non-tender, with no rebound, guarding, or masses.
- *Skin and extremities*: Radial and femoral pulses are 2+, and skin is warm and well-perfused. Child is holding her right arm semi-flexed and pronated. There is no swelling or deformity, no bruising or rashes.
- *Neurologic*: Normal sensation in affected limb, otherwise normal examination.

Questions for Thought

- Do you need to get a radiograph on this child's arm?
- What is the best way to reduce this injury?
- What are the items on the differential diagnosis that are important to not miss?

Diagnosis

- Radial head subluxation, or nursemaid's elbow.

Discussion

- *Epidemiology*: Nursemaid's elbow is a common injury of childhood. Most cases occur in children under the age of 5, with the majority under 2 years of age.[1,2] It is slightly more common in female children and more commonly involves the left arm.[1,2] It can recur in up to 25 percent of susceptible individuals.[1,2] It is rarely bilateral, and seldom occurs in adults.
- *Pathophysiology*: Nursemaid's elbow occurs when the annular ligament that attaches the proximal end of the radius to the ulna becomes displaced

and entrapped at the radiocapitellar joint. This is generally precipitated by tractional force applied to the pronated arm, although it has also been reported with falls and even with rolling over.[1,2] The force required to cause the injury is minor, and the elbow typically shows no evidence of swelling, ecchymosis, or deformity.

- *Presentation*: The patient usually presents with the history of tractional force applied to the arm, although the event may have been unwitnessed or unclear. The child will not use the arm, and often holds it semi-flexed and pronated, while supporting it with the unaffected arm.

- *Diagnosis*: It is important to consider the possibility of occult supracondylar fracture or child abuse in children with elbow pain. Arthritis, whether infectious (for example, Lyme disease or *Staphylococcus aureus*) or immune-mediated, may also present with elbow pain. One of the important distinguishing factors is that children with nursemaid's elbow have a normal examination, without systemic findings, skin findings, or musculoskeletal abnormalities. Their radiographs, if performed, are also typically normal.[3]

  The critical evaluation of a child with nursemaid's elbow is a thorough history and a careful examination. There is no role for radiography in the diagnosis of nursemaid's elbow, although imaging may rule out other pathologic entities. Certainly, in the child with a typical history, nursemaid's elbow can be treated presumptively. There is some evidence that, in children without the typical history but presenting with a benign examination and holding their arms in the typical position, reduction may be attempted without prior radiography. If reduction is not able to be performed empirically, radiography should be considered to rule out occult fracture.

- *Treatment*: Treatment of nursemaid's elbow involves manipulation of the elbow to reduce the interposed annular ligament. There are two commonly employed reduction techniques. In the first, the child is held firmly on the caregiver's lap and the affected arm is completely supinated and then fully flexed while pressure is placed on the child's radial head with the operator's thumb. In the second method, the child is held in the same

manner, but the affected arm is fully pronated and straightened while pressure is applied to the radial head. Both methods are similar in ease of performance as well as in terms of pain for the child, but the hyperpronation technique has a higher first-attempt success rate, and should be attempted first.[4,5]

- *Disposition*: Most children with a reduced nursemaid's elbow will move their arm within minutes after reduction. Some may be delayed for hours, however. If a child continues not to use the arm, the provider can consider performing a radiograph to rule out occult fracture or may attempt repeat reduction. With negative films and ongoing pain, the child can be placed in a splint and reassessed at 24 hours. Parents should be educated as to the etiology of this disease process, and may be taught reduction techniques to apply at home prior to deciding whether they need to visit the ED.

Historical clues	Physical findings
• Child in appropriate age group • Isolated elbow pain	• No musculoskeletal abnormality • Held in "nursemaid's position"

Follow-Up

The baby's elbow was reduced with hyperpronation and extension and she was pain free and using the arm prior to discharge.

References

1. Vitello S, Dvorkin R, Sattler S, et al. Epidemiology of nursemaid's elbow. *West J Emerg Med* 2014; 14: 554–7.

2. Irie T, Sono T, Hayama Y, et al. Investigation on 2331 cases of pulled elbow over the last 10 years. *Pediatr Rep* 2014; 6: 5090.

3. Guzel M, Salt O, Demir MT, et al. Comparison of hyperpronation and supination–flexion techniques in children presented to emergency department with painful pronation. *Niger J Clin Pract* 2014; 17: 201–4.

4. Eismann EA, Cosco ED, Wall EJ. Absence of radiographic abnormalities in nursemaid's elbows. *J Pediatr Orthop* 2014; 34: 426–31.

5. Gunaydin YK, Katirci Y, Duymaz H, et al. Comparison of success and pain levels of supination–flexion and hyperpronation maneuvers in childhood nursemaid's elbow cases. *Am J Emerg Med* 2013; 31: 1078–81.

Case 2

Contributing Author: Lauren Snyder

History

The patient is a 17-year-old male who presents to the ED following an ankle injury at school. The patient reports that he was playing catch and tripped as he was running for the football. The patient states he "rolled" his ankle, motioning to demonstrate ankle inversion. There was a hole in the grass that caught his right foot, which twisted his ankle. After the injury, he began to have pain and difficulty walking, prompting the school nursing staff to send him to the ED for evaluation. He reports right lateral ankle pain and swelling, but denies numbness or tingling. The patient notes he still has difficulty walking in the ED.

Past Medical History

- The patient denies any previous medical history and is UTD on his vaccinations. He lives with both parents and attends high school.

Medications

- None.

Allergies

- NKDA.

Physical Examination and Ancillary Studies

- *Vital signs*: T 97.9 °F, HR 62, RR 16, BP 129/70, O_2 sat 100% on room air.
- *General*: The patient is alert and with occasional facial grimaces secondary to ankle pain.
- *HEENT*: PERRL, intact extraocular movements. Oropharynx is clear.
- *Neck*: Supple, with no midline tenderness or step-offs.
- *Cardiovascular*: Regular rate and rhythm, no M/R/G, normal peripheral perfusion.
- *Lungs*: CTA bilaterally, respirations are non-labored, breath sounds are equal.
- *Abdomen*: The abdomen is soft and non-tender to palpation, non-distended, and with normal active bowel sounds.
- *Skin and extremities*: The right ankle has limited active and passive range of motion secondary to pain. There is no tenderness to palpation of the right medial malleolus, heel, mid foot, or right lower leg. There is mild swelling of the lateral right ankle without ecchymosis, with mild pain on palpation of the area anterior and inferior to the lateral malleolus, but non-tender over the bony malleolus itself. He has pain with talar tilt testing with varus stress. The patient has intact sensation and is able to move all toes of the right foot. Peripheral pulses are intact with 2+ dorsalis pedis pulse palpable on examination bilaterally. The patient is able to bear weight and take four steps with a slight limp while in the ED. The skin is warm and well-perfused.
- *Neurologic*: The patient is alert and is able to state his name, current location, and the date. No focal neurologic deficits are observed during examination.
- *Pertinent imaging*: Radiographic series of the right ankle is negative for fracture or dislocation, but does identify mild soft-tissue swelling surrounding the lateral ankle.

Questions for Thought

- What is the utility of obtaining X-rays in this patient?
- Which patients need X-rays with the complaint of ankle pain?
- Which ligaments are involved in the injury? How do you examine for these ligaments?
- How is the mechanism of injury helpful in determining the structures involved in the injury?

Diagnosis

- Grade I sprain of right anterior talofibular ligament.

Discussion

- *Epidemiology*: Ankle sprains, defined as a stretching, partial tear, or complete tear of at least one ligament, are one of the most common complaints in EDs. According to the CDC, in 2011 the USA had 1.6 million ED visits for injuries of the lower leg and ankle, with ankle sprains accounting for an estimated 85 percent of all ankle injuries.[1]
- *Pathophysiology*: The pathophysiology of all sprains is related to injury to ligaments, in

distinction from strains, which are related to injuries of tendon–muscle complexes. Any joint can be strained or sprained depending on the individual ligaments or tendons involved. As a general principle, joints with a greater degree of mobility (such as the shoulder) undergo strain more frequently, and those with less mobility (such as the knee) undergo sprain more frequently. Any joint that is completely disrupted by sprain or strain warrants urgent orthopedic consultation. Fortunately, it is relatively uncommon for a patient to have complete disruption of any joint, and most patients present with some combination of pain, swelling, and dysfunction that can be managed with immobilization, symptom management, and outpatient referral to sports medicine or orthopedics.

Ankles are the most common joint to suffer sprain injury.[1-4] The pathophysiology of ankle sprains is related to the mechanism of injury and the ligaments involved. The lateral ankle ligaments are most frequently injured, with medial ankle ligaments and ligaments between the tibia and fibula (including the IO membrane) less commonly involved.[2]

A grading system is traditionally used to classify ankle sprains, with grades I, II, and III describing the severity of ligamentous tear that occurred (Table 6.1). Based on the physical examination findings, clinicians can use the grading system to classify the degree of ankle sprain.[2-4]

Lateral ankle sprains are the result of foot inversion, often with the foot in plantar flexion. This mechanism causes damage to the lateral ankle ligaments in a predictable fashion as the forces of the injury increase. The lateral ankle ligaments include the anterior talofibular ligament, the calcaneofibular ligament, and the posterior talofibular ligament. Generally, the ligaments are injured in that order as the forces of the injury increase. In the majority of all ankle injuries, the anterior talofibular ligament is the only ligament that is injured.[2-4]

The ligament of the medial ankle, the deltoid ligament, is infrequently injured, as the mechanism of injury is forced eversion of the foot. This requires a larger amount of force due to the

Table 6.1 Grading of ankle sprains

	Ligamentous injury	Physical signs and symptoms	Ambulation
Grade I	Ligament stretched beyond normal range of motion resulting in microscopic tears	Mild swelling and tenderness	Minimal pain with weight-bearing and ambulation
Grade II	Incomplete ligament tear	Moderate pain, swelling, ecchymosis, and tenderness. May have joint instability and restricted range of motion	Weight-bearing and ambulating are painful
Grade III	Complete ligament tear	Severe pain, swelling, tenderness, and ecchymosis. Significant joint instability with loss of function and motion	Unable to bear weight or ambulate

strength of the deltoid ligament and thus is uncommon.[2-4]

A syndesmotic sprain, sometimes referred to as a "high ankle sprain," involves injuries to the ligaments connecting the tibia and fibula, which are also essential for ankle stability. Dorsiflexion and/or eversion of the ankle can cause injury to the anterior tibiofibular, posterior tibiofibular, transverse tibiofibular ligaments, or the IO membrane. A syndesmotic ankle sprain is more likely to occur in an individual with recurrent ankle sprains and chronic ankle instability.

- *Presentation*: In the majority of cases, patients will be able to identify the exact time of onset of their pain, as ankle sprains are an acute injury that most often result from stress to the ankle joint due to a traumatic event. Patients' major complaints will include pain, swelling, tenderness, and difficulty with ambulation and movement. Depending on the grade of the ankle sprain, the patient will have varying degrees of pain, swelling, ecchymosis, and inability to bear weight or ambulate. In patients who suffer major trauma, other injuries take priority and ankle sprains may go undiagnosed.

- *Diagnosis*: The diagnosis of ankle sprain is made clinically, based on the history and mechanism of the injury along with findings on physical examination.[2-4] Radiographs are not helpful in identifying sprains, although they are often obtained to identify associated fractures that may have resulted from the injury.[5] In pediatric patients, ankle injuries may also cause fractures through the growth plate (Salter–Harris fractures). The growth plate is a relatively weak structure and can fracture even without severe ligamentous injury. It is often difficult to distinguish Salter–Harris type I fractures from sprains, and so traditionally these injuries are treated as fractures with splinting of the ankle. There is some debate regarding how much immobilization should occur with possible Salter–Harris type I fractures of the distal fibula.[5,6]

  When evaluating a patient with ankle trauma, it is important to gather the following pieces of information:

  - the mechanism of injury;
  - the patient's ability to bear weight or ambulate following the injury;
  - prior injury to the ankle.

- A thorough physical examination in addition to the history and mechanism of injury will aid in forming the diagnosis of ankle sprain. In addition to examining the ankle itself, the fibula, distal tibia, foot, knee, and Achilles tendon should also be assessed for tenderness or injury, and a complete neurovascular examination should be performed.[2-4] Clinicians should assess the ankle's passive range of motion, checking for pain with gentle eversion and inversion, which can assist in localizing the area of injury. The clinician should also test for ligamentous instability with anterior drawer testing as well as talar tilt testing, comparing the affected to the unaffected side for firmness of endpoint and laxity.

- The Ottawa Ankle Rules were developed in an effort to reduce the number of plain films obtained in those acute ankle injuries in which fracture is less likely. The set of rules has been extensively tested and validated for ED adult patients with acute ankle injuries, and is very sensitive for excluding ankle fracture.[7,8] It should be noted

that while the Ottawa Ankle Rules have been tested and validated in adult patients, they can still be helpful when applied to pediatric patients.[7] If the following criteria are met, radiographs of the foot or ankle should be obtained:

Ankle series radiographs are indicated in patients with pain in the malleolar zone AND:

- bony tenderness at the posterior edge of distal 6 cm or tip of the lateral malleolus OR;
- bony tenderness at the posterior edge of the distal 6 cm or tip of medial malleolus OR;
- inability to bear weight both immediately after the injury and for four steps in the ED.

Foot series radiographs are indicated in patients with pain in the midfoot zone AND:

- bony tenderness at the base of the fifth metatarsal OR;
- bony tenderness at the navicular OR;
- inability to bear weight both immediately after the injury and for four steps in the ED.

- *Treatment*: For ankle sprains, initial treatment is conservative irrespective of the grade of the sprain. RICE (rest, ice, compression, elevation) is the treatment of choice for initial management, encouraging the patient to limit weight-bearing with use of crutches until their normal gait returns, applying ice or cold-water immersion every few hours initially, compression with soft elastic bandage to minimize swelling, and elevation above the level of the heart whenever possible, to minimize swelling. Additionally, NSAID medications can be used for pain control as needed.

  Once the pain and swelling abate, patients should be encouraged to gently exercise the ankle joint with gradual increase in range of motion. Ankle splints or braces can assist in limiting the extremes of joint motion and allow weight-bearing while protecting against re-injury.

  Grade 1 ankle sprains do not require immobilization, and a soft elastic bandage for swelling can be applied for a few days following the injury. Grade II and III sprains will require additional support, including an aircast or similar splint in addition to the elastic bandage, for up to a few weeks following the injury.[2-4]

- *Disposition*: Most patients with ankle sprain injury will be able to return home for the duration of their recovery without requiring a hospital stay. However, in a few cases that have additional injuries, complications, or other reasons for admission, the patient may require inpatient status. For cases involving fracture, dislocation or subluxation, syndemosis injury ("high ankle sprain"), tendon rupture, penetrating wound involving the joint, or a patient with neurovascular compromise (decreased sensation or circulation distal to the injury), prompt evaluation and possible orthopedic consultation should be completed. All ankle injuries should be re-evaluated in the outpatient setting, so the patient should be made aware of this and set up an appointment with their PCP, sports medicine, or orthopedic office for continued management and clearance to return to sports and activities.

Historical clues	Physical findings	Ancillary studies
• Inversion injury • Pain with ambulation	• Swelling to lateral aspect of ankle • Pain with talar tilt stress on anterior talofibular ligament	• Negative X-ray

Follow-Up

Although the child did not meet criteria for imaging as per Ottawa Ankle Rules, he received an X-ray, which was ordered from triage and was negative. He was given an elastic wrap for his ankle and discharged to follow up with sports medicine.

References

1. Centers for Disease Control and Prevention. National hospital ambulatory medical care survey: 2010 Emergency department summary tables. See www.cdc.gov/nchs/data/ahcd/nhamcs_emergency/2010_ed_web_tables.pdf (accessed January 2017).

2. Hanlon DP. Leg, ankle, and foot injuries. *Emerg Med Clin N Am* 2010; 28: 885–905.

3. Wedmore IS, Charette J. Emergency department evaluation and treatment of ankle and foot injuries. *Emerg Med Clin N Am* 2000; 18: 85–113

4. Tiemstra JD. Update on acute ankle sprains. *Am Fam Phys* 2012; 85: 1170–6.

5. Boutis K, Plint A, Stimec J, et al. Radiograph-negative lateral ankle injuries in children: Occult growth plate fracture or sprain? *JAMA Pediatr* 2016; 170: e154114.

6. Boutis K. Common pediatric fractures treated with minimal intervention. *Pediatr Emerg Care* 2010; 26: 152–7.

7. Plint AC, Bulloch B, Osmond MH, et al. Validation of the Ottawa Ankle Rules in children with ankle injuries. *Acad Emerg Med* 1999; 6: 1005–9.

8. Stiell IG, McKnight RD, Greenberg GH, et al. Implementation of the Ottawa ankle rules. *JAMA* 1994; 271: 827–32.

Case 3

Contributing Author: Melanie K. Prusakowski

History

The patient is a 9-year-old boy who presents with an inability to bear weight on his left leg. Five days ago he fell during a soccer game without any known resulting injury. He developed mild left knee pain the next day. For 3 days he has complained of increasing knee pain and developed a worsening limp. Yesterday he had less appetite and felt warm. His mother provided a weight-appropriate dose of ibuprofen and he seemed to improve. This morning he woke with a fever of 101.8 °F and cannot stand on his left leg. He reports no swelling of the knee. He denies numbness or tingling of the leg or foot, and has no back pain. The patient does not report dysuria but states that trying to stand makes his belly and knee hurt.

Past Medical History

- The patient had tympanostomy tubes placed when he was 3 years of age.
- Exercise-induced asthma.

Medications

- Ibuprofen, last dose yesterday.
- Albuterol metered-dose inhaler, last used 5 days ago.

Allergies

- NKDA.

Physical Examination and Ancillary Studies

- *Vital signs*: T 101.3 °F, HR 112, RR 18, BP 98/51, O₂ sat 98% on room air.
- *General*: The patient is a mildly anxious-appearing, well-developed boy, who appears somewhat uncomfortable.

- *HEENT*: PERRL. Oropharynx clear with no exudates. Mucous membranes moist.
- *Neck*: Supple and non-tender, with no adenopathy.
- *Cardiovascular*: Mild tachycardia, with no M/R/G.
- *Lungs*: Lungs are symmetric and clear, with no W/R/R.
- *Abdomen*: Soft, with active bowel sounds. Mild tenderness to palpation of the left lateral pelvis.
- *Extremities and skin*: There is full passive range of motion in the patient's left knee, but internal rotation of the left thigh results in pain. There are no knee joint effusions, no erythema of the knee or thigh, no calf tenderness, and no edema or clubbing bilaterally. His sensation and dorsalis pedis pulses are normal. There is no pallor or rash.
- *Pertinent laboratory values*: WBC 13,600, CRP 9.1 mg/dL.
- *Pertinent radiographs*: X-ray of the pelvis and left hip demonstrate no fractures, dislocation, or masses. No evidence of osteomyelitis. U/S of the left hip reveals a small intra-articular effusion.

Questions for Thought

- What other laboratory diagnostics could help make the diagnosis?
- What are the typical laboratory findings in this condition?
- What are some considerations to guide the use of radiographic diagnostic modalities?
- What treatment should be initiated in the ED?
- What is the definitive treatment of this condition?

Diagnosis
- Septic arthritis of the left hip.

Discussion
- *Epidemiology*: Septic arthritis is a joint-space and synovial-fluid infection, most commonly affecting large joints such as the hip (20 percent) or knee (40 percent). The incidence is about 10 cases in 100,000 children, with most cases occurring in children less than 3 years of age.[1] Boys are affected more commonly than girls.[1,2] At-risk populations include patients who are less than 3 years of age, immunocompromised hosts, or children lacking a functional spleen (i.e. splenectomy, sickle cell disease).[1,2]

- *Pathophysiology*: Most cases of pediatric septic arthritis are the result of hematogenous spread of bacterial infection, but direct inoculation can result from nearby bone and soft-tissue infection, penetrating injury, or iatrogenically.[1] Synovial tissue has no basement membrane, so blood-borne organisms can pass into the joint space and synovial fluid. The most common causative organism is *Staphylococcus aureus*, followed by group A streptococci and *Enterobacter*.[1] Children with sickle cell disease are also at risk for salmonella joint or bone infections. MRSA is an increasing consideration, especially in patients with a known prior history or current signs of MRSA soft-tissue infection. *Kingella kingae* has been increasingly implicated in osteoarticular infections of children less than 4 years old.[1,3] *Neisseria gonorrhoeae* is a consideration in sexually active adolescents and young adults. Once bacteria spread to the joint and initiate the inflammatory cascade, inflammatory mediators cause destruction to articular cartilage in as little as 8 hours.[1] Permanent damage to the cartilage and sub-chondral bone may occur within 3 days.[1]

- *Presentation*: Pediatric septic arthritis occurs in the lower limbs 80 percent of the time.[1] Patients often present with a limp or refusal to bear weight.[1,2] Classically, patients have pain with even very small passive movements of the affected joint. Fever is common, but absent in up to 20 percent of patients. For this reason, lack of fever cannot rule out septic arthritis. The classic signs of warmth, erythema, and edema are less often seen in septic arthritis of the hip, but may be more evident in smaller joints. Neonatal patients with septic arthritis can be difficult to diagnose, since they may lack classic signs of joint swelling or warmth and can present with only irritability or limited motion of a limb. It is not uncommon for the joint pain to be attributed to an incidental trauma that is unrelated.

- *Diagnosis*: A child presenting with an isolated limp or refusal to bear weight is a diagnostic challenge. The provider must determine if the abnormal gait is related to pain, weakness (as with neuromuscular disorders), or anatomic processes (for instance, dysplasia). Once the provider determines that the gait problem is secondary to pain, he or she must carefully consider other more common etiologies of pediatric joint pain, such as transient synovitis, trauma, and juvenile idiopathic arthritis, as well as other infectious etiologies, such as osteomyelitis, Lyme disease, cellulitis, and psoas muscle abscess.[2] History can help in narrowing down these possibilities. Pain that was acute in onset and is associated with an activity is more likely to be traumatic. Pain that is worse at night suggests malignancy. Pain that is better with activity suggests rheumatologic disease, while that which is worse with activity suggests an overuse injury. Pain with systemic symptoms is concerning for an infectious process, be it arthritis, osteomyelitis, or abscess, or potentially a malignancy.

Examination is also helpful to rule out other processes. It is important to examine the child thoroughly, assessing for rashes (that might suggest endocarditis or gonococcal infection or erythema migrans), abdominal pain (suggesting psoas abscess or acute abdomen with referred hip pain), strength and sensation (to assess for neuromuscular processes), and a thorough assessment of the limb itself, palpating for masses, effusion, tenderness, and deformity.

Radiographs can be helpful in the work-up of pediatric joint pain, as they are a reasonable initial screen for cancers, malformations, and abuse.[2] However, small effusions may be missed by plain film. MRI is sensitive and specific for detecting osteomyelitis or septic arthritis of the pediatric hip, but has not been tested in other joints.[2] U/S is a sensitive, non-invasive modality for hip effusion that can usually be performed without sedation in pediatric patients.[2] It can also aid arthrocentesis for diagnosis or treatment. However, an effusion seen on U/S cannot differentiate the more prevalent transient synovitis from bacterial septic arthritis, and it may not demonstrate an effusion in septic arthritis if it is performed very early in the course of illness.[4]

Elevated WBC, CRP, and ESR values suggest infection, but are non-specific for septic arthritis.[5-8] The Kocher criteria can be used as a clinical decision tool to differentiate septic arthritis from other painful hip etiologies. The four criteria are: refusal to bear weight on the affected side, an ESR > 40 mm/hr, WBC > 12,000, and presence of fever.[5] The presence of all four criteria has a 99 percent specificity for septic

arthritis in the study population; three of the criteria is 93 percent specific.[5] Similarly, having only one of the four criteria reduces the risk of a septic hip to only 3 percent.[5] Other studies have failed to reproduce this positive predictive value.[8]

Assessment of synovial fluid obtained by arthrocentesis is the standard diagnostic modality. Typically, the synovial fluid WBC will be > 50,000 in a septic joint.[9] Gram's stain is positive in only 30 percent of pediatric patients, but blood culture can identify the organism in some instances of hematogenous dissemination.[9] Molecular diagnostic studies, such as PCR, enhance discovery of infectious organisms such as *N. gonorrhoeae*, *Borrelia burgdorferi*, and *K. kingae*.[9] Although joint aspiration is the current gold standard for diagnosis, it is not perfectly reliable.[9]

- *Treatment*: Bacterial septic arthritis is a medical emergency. Treatment requires drainage and antibiotic therapy.[1,9] Drainage of the affected joint is traditionally done as an open procedure, but aspiration or serial aspirations can be part of the management of smaller joints, as well as part of the diagnosis.[9] Ideally, samples are obtained before beginning antimicrobial therapy unless patient acuity (i.e. sepsis) prohibits it. Because the causative pathogen in most pediatric septic arthritis is a Gram-positive microorganism, beta-lactam antibiotics are typical first-line treatment. Broader-spectrum antimicrobials are appropriate in children who present with signs of sepsis or underlying immune compromise. Gram's stain of the joint aspirate can direct treatment and coverage can be narrowed pending cultures.

The duration of IV antibiotic treatment for pediatric septic arthritis can be 1 to 7 weeks. Transition to oral antimicrobials is typically dictated by a combination of defervescence, return of joint mobility, and normalization of inflammatory markers like CRP.[10] A brief course of low-dose steroids may ameliorate some of the joint dysfunction after septic arthritis and may improve symptoms if started early in the disease course.[11]

Complications of late or inadequate treatment of pediatric septic arthritis include joint capsule damage, chronic arthritis, growth disturbances, osteomyelitis, joint subluxation, and sepsis.

- *Disposition*: Pediatric patients with septic arthritis should be admitted for joint drainage and IV antibiotics. Patients are at risk for sepsis and readmission for under-recognized associated osteomyelitis. Factors associated with poorer prognosis include delay in treatment (especially more than 4 days of symptoms), younger age, and *S. aureus* infection.

Historical clues	Physical findings	Ancillary studies
• Complaint of knee pain (hip often refers to knee) • Fever • Inability to bear weight	• Fever • Pain with internal rotation of left hip • Tenderness in left pelvis	• Elevated WBC • Elevated CRP • Negative X-ray • U/S with hip effusion

Follow-Up

The child received a left hip U/S-guided arthrocentesis. The joint aspirate had elevated WBC of 89,000. He was admitted for an operative joint drainage and 4 days of IV cefazolin. The child was intermittently febrile for the first 48 hours of admission. The joint aspirate culture grew *S. aureus* sensitive to cephalosporins. On the third day he had increased range of motion of the hip and was willing to bear weight. When he tolerated oral intake, the patient was discharged on 10 days of cephalexin.

References

1. Ceroni D, Kampouroglou G, Anderson della Llana R, et al. Osteoarticular infections in young children: What has changed over the last years? *Swiss Med Wkly* 2014; 144: w13971.

2. Naranje S, Kelly DM, Sawyer JR. A systematic approach to the evaluation of a limping child. *Am Fam Phys* 2015; 92: 908–18.

3. Yagupsky P, Porsch E, St Geme JW 3rd. *Kingella kingae*: An emerging pathogen in young children. *Pediatrics* 2011; 127: 557–65.

4. Gordon JE, Huang M, Dobbs M, et al. Causes of false-negative ultrasound scans in the diagnosis of septic arthritis of the hip in children. *J Pediatr Orthop* 2002; 22: 312–16.

5. Kocher MS, Zurakowski D, Kasser JR. Differentiating between septic arthritis and transient synovitis of the hip in children: An evidence-based clinical prediction algorithm. *J Bone Joint Surg Am* 1999; 81: 1662–70.

6. Caird MS, Flynn JM, Leung YL, et al. Factors distinguishing septic arthritis from transient synovitis of the hip in children. A prospective study. *J Bone Joint Surg Am* 2006; 88: 1251–7.

7. Levine MJ, McGuire KJ, McGowan KL, et al. Assessment of the test characteristics of C-reactive protein for septic arthritis in children. *J Pediatr Orthop* 2003; 23: 373–7.

8. Luhmann SJ, Jones A, Schootman M, et al. Differentiation between septic arthritis and transient synovitis of the hip in children with clinical prediction algorithms. *J Bone Joint Surg Am* 2004; 86-A: 956–62.

9. Kang SN, Sanghera T, Mangwani J, et al. The management of septic arthritis in children: Systematic review of the English language literature. *J Bone Joint Surg Br* 2009; 91: 1127–33.

10. Arnold JC, Cannavino CR, Ross MK, et al. Acute bacterial osteoarticular infections: Eight-year analysis of C-reactive protein for oral step-down therapy. *Pediatrics* 2012; 130: e821.

11. Odio CM, Ramirez T, Arias G, et al. Double blind, randomized, placebo-controlled study of dexamethasone therapy for hematogenous septic arthritis in children. *Pediatr Infect Dis J* 2003; 22: 883.

Case 4

Contributing Author: Dorka M. Jiménez Almonte

History

An 8-year-old boy presents with left knee pain and bleeding after he suffered an injury while running at the school gym just prior to arrival to the ED. The patient was playing at the gym when a friend accidentally pushed him. The patient fell and his left lower extremity slipped under a metal frame. The patient had immediate pain to his left knee area. He was able to stand and walk, but then noticed a cut on his knee. Moving the knee aggravates the pain, but the child denies any difficulty moving the knee otherwise. The patient denies any associated symptoms such as tingling or numbness. He also denies any other injuries. The patient's parents report his immunizations are current, he received the fifth dose of tetanus immunization at the age of 5.

Past Medical History

- Mild intermittent asthma.

Medications

- Albuterol as needed.

Allergies

- NKDA.

Physical Examination and Ancillary Studies

- *Vital signs*: T 98.9 °F, HR 105, RR 14, BP 105/65, O_2 sat 100% on room air.
- *General*: Well-appearing young male, in no acute distress.
- *HEENT*: There are no signs of head trauma. PERRL. Oropharynx clear, with moist mucous membranes.
- *Neck*: Supple, with no tenderness and normal range of motion.
- *Cardiovascular*: Regular rate and rhythm, with no M/R/G. Intact and equal distal pulses.
- *Lungs*: Normal work of breathing, with clear and equal breath sounds.
- *Abdomen*: Non-distended, soft and depressible, with no tenderness to palpation.
- *Musculoskeletal and skin*: There is a flap laceration measuring approximately 5 cm at the left anterior knee, just superior to the patella. There is no active bleeding. The subcutaneous adipose tissue is exposed, there are no visible tendons or deep structures. The range of motion is intact. The patient is able to extend the knee against gravity and against resistance without problems. Capillary refill < 2 seconds
- *Neurologic*: The left lower extremity strength is 5/5 and equal compared to the right lower extremity. The sensation to light touch is intact. Awake and alert.

Questions for Thought

- Is there any diagnostic testing (laboratory or imaging) indicated?
- Would you give a tetanus booster to this patient?
- Does this child require antibiotics?
- Would you close this wound primarily?
- Does the patient require referral to an orthopedic surgeon?

Diagnosis

- Knee laceration.

Discussion

- *Epidemiology*: Lacerations and other forms of wounds (such as abrasions) are an exceedingly common problem faced by the ED provider. One out of three injuries in children involve a laceration, with boys injured more commonly than girls. In younger children, the most common mechanism of injury is falling, whereas violent encounters are more likely in older children. Laceration repair accounts for approximately 50 percent of all the procedures performed in the ED.
- *Pathophysiology*: The skin is the largest organ of the body, and provides the critical service of a barrier to infection. Skin integrity is critical to this function. Breaks in integrity can occur from shear forces, tension, and compressive forces, with resulting lacerations, abrasions, avulsions, or pressure ulceration. Thermal injury can also disrupt skin integrity, and is discussed in Chapter 2, Case 5. The pathophysiology of wounds are dependent upon the type of wound, the location of the wound, the circumstances under which the wound was received, and the underlying comorbidities of the patient with the injury.[1-3] The skin is under constant tension due to high collagen content, and is increased in areas overlying dynamic structures such as tendons and muscles. Lacerations overlying joints or running perpendicular to skin tension lines are higher risk for poor cosmetic outcome. Dirty wounds (for example, those incurred in farming accidents or from bites), crush wounds (as opposed to wounds from a sharp object), wounds in areas of relatively decreased blood flow (for instance, the shin), and wounds in immunocompromised patients are higher risk for poor healing and infection.[1-3]

  The wound healing process begins with hemostasis via the coagulation cascade and platelet activation as well as an inflammatory response, which protects against infection.[4] Next, the proliferative phase is characterized by granulation, epithelialization, and contraction of the wound.[4] Wound edges should be slightly everted during wound closure in order for the skin to become flat after contraction occurs. Complete maturation and remodeling of the wound may continue for up to 2 years. Tensile strength is regained very slowly; with only 5 percent of the previous strength by 2 weeks, 30 percent at 2 months and 80 percent by 1 year. Scar formation ultimately results from the body's repair of injured tissue, as opposed to regenerative healing (for instance, with mild abrasions) that results in no scar.[4]

- *Presentation*: It is extremely important to obtain a detailed history of the time and mechanism of injury as it has a direct impact on management. Patients may present with an isolated soft-tissue injury, as in this patient, or may present with major trauma. A clear understanding of the mechanism of injury allows for thorough investigation of the possible magnitude of the injury such as an underlying fracture, violation of a joint space, or the possibility of a severe crush injury. Wounds caused by animal bites have a very high risk of infection, as do those caused by human bites, and patients may not readily admit that a hand injury was suffered as a consequence of punching another person in the mouth. The possibility of a retained foreign body in the wound also needs to be considered and explored, for instance from window glass in an auto accident or in a kitchen-related accident. Patients may present with loss of sensation or severe pain from underlying nerve injury, fracture, or compartment syndrome.[1-3] Preexisting or acute medical problems may impact presentation, such as a seizure or syncopal event that led to the injury.

- *Diagnosis*: The wound needs to be carefully examined, documenting the location, size, depth, presence of foreign matter, and any associated tissue injury.[1-3] Adequate illumination and hemostasis are imperative for an evaluation of the laceration. The vascular, neurologic, and tendon function need to be carefully assessed. A detailed vascular examination should include observation for the presence of pallor or cyanosis, capillary refill, and palpation of pulses distal to the wound, to assess tissue perfusion. A thorough motor examination should be performed, including flexor and extensor tendons near a wound. The sensation examination should include two-point discrimination when developmentally appropriate. If the laceration overlies a joint, the joint should be meticulously examined for signs of joint capsule penetration or damage to tendon structures. If the provider is unsure of joint involvement, methylene blue or saline may be injected into the joint to demonstrate joint integrity versus extravasation into the wound.

Clinical suspicion for a retained foreign body warrants imaging. Plain radiographs can detect radiopaque foreign bodies such as glass, stones, or metallic objects. U/S can locate radiolucent objects such as wood and plastic, and can be used real-time during wound exploration.[1-3] CT and MRI can be used, if necessary, to localize a foreign body if plain radiographs or U/S fail.[1-3] MRI should not be used for metal objects.

- *Treatment*: The "golden period" for wound closure was classically taught to be within 6 hours of injury; however, non-contaminated wounds can be closed successfully up to 12 hours after the injury, and in highly vascular areas like the face and scalp, 24 hours may be acceptable, as the risk of infection is lower.[1-3,5] There are no good data to establish any definitive time limit for wound closure.[5] In general, closure of animal and human bites is avoided and healing by secondary intention is preferred due to the high rate of infection, unless the wound is in a highly vascular area or is deforming.[1-3]

Abrasions require local care only, with irrigation and an occlusive dressing to optimize healing conditions.[2]

Pain management is a crucial aspect when providing care for the injured child. Whenever possible, the use of a topical anesthetic agent such as compounded lidocaine, epinephrine, tetracaine is preferred. Blanching of the site after application indicates effective anesthesia. A local anesthetic can also be applied using a small gauge needle to avoid pain associated to the injection, but this method usually causes significant anxiety in children. Benzodiazepines such as midazolam via an oral or intranasal route can help reduce patient anxiety. Procedural sedation and regional nerve blocks could be necessary for management of complicated wounds. Distraction techniques such as listening to music, watching a video, or listening to a story are also very effective in reducing anxiety, especially if a child life specialist is available.

Although traditional dogma would recommend sterile technique for wound repair, a large prospective randomized blinded trial found no difference in wound infection rate between wounds closed using clean technique (clean, non-sterile gloves) as compared to a sterile technique.[6] Wound irrigation with normal saline or tap water can significantly reduce the risk of infection by washing away foreign material and diluting bacterial concentration.[1,3] The fluid used for irrigation is less critical than the volume of irrigant used. Removal of hair around the wound is not recommended as it has been associated with increased rates of wound infection.[1]

Suturing with monofilament non-absorbable sutures of 4-0–5-0 thickness is commonly recommended for repair of lacerations located on the extremities or trunk. Monofilament of 6-0 is recommended for the face. Staples may be used on the scalp, and tissue adhesives provide equivalent repair to sutures in simple lacerations in low-tension, low-moisture areas.[2] Absorbable sutures are appropriate for oral mucosa.

Most wounds can be approximated effectively with simple interrupted sutures. The needle should pierce the skin at a 90-degree angle while pronating the wrist, causing the needle tip to penetrate deeply into the wound to attain adequate wound-edge eversion. Sutures should take equal bites from both wound edges to avoid margins from overlapping. Sutures should be placed close enough to approximate wound edges, but not excessively tight as to cause tissue necrosis, following the long-taught wisdom of "approximate, not strangulate." The knots are secured using an instrument tie and then pulled to one side of the wound, to decrease wound inflammation that may occur by a knot becoming incorporated into the wound. Oral antibiotic prophylaxis is only indicated for wounds with a higher risk of infection, and is most commonly used for cases of animal bites and open fractures.[1-3] Contaminated wounds also require antibiotics. Surgical consultation should be considered for deep wounds of the hand or foot, severe crush injuries, severely contaminated wounds, wounds that raise a concern for cosmetic outcome, and lacerations involving nerves, arteries, joints, or bones.[1,3]

Tetanus prophylaxis should be provided to children with no history of tetanus immunization and those with an incomplete series or who have not had a booster injection in 10 years.[2] Unimmunized children should also receive tetanus immunoglobulin if they have a deep puncture or contaminated wounds.[2]

- *Disposition*: Most patients are discharged home after wound management. Careful wound care instructions should be provided at discharge, as

wound aftercare is critical to cosmetic outcome. Wounds should be kept clean and dry. The child may shower after 24 hours, wash the wound with soap and water, and dry the wound gently. The patient should avoid soaking the wound in water (swimming, bathing) or scrubbing the wound. The patient's caregivers can administer oral pain medications such as acetaminophen or ibuprofen as needed. Topical antibiotics may be applied to the wound. Detailed instructions to monitor for signs of infection should be given (increased pain, swelling, redness, warmth, or drainage from the wound) as well as instructions to return if wound dehiscence occurs. Sutures in the face should be removed in 3–5 days, those in the scalp and arms can be removed in 7–10 days, those in the trunk, legs, hands, or feet can be removed in 10–14 days, and sutures on the palms and soles can be removed in 14–21 days.[3] Sunscreen may be applied to scars in areas exposed to sunlight to minimize wound hyperpigmentation for up to 1–2 years after injury.

Historical clues	Physical findings
• Fall injury • Sharp mechanism (metal frame) • Recent time interval • Able to bear weight • No numbness or tingling • No relevant medical or immunization history	• Flap laceration • Subcutaneous adipose with no foreign body and no visualized tendons • range of motion and tendon function intact • Palpable pulses, adequate perfusion

Follow-Up

Given there were no signs of tendon injury or violation of the joint space the laceration was repaired by the ED provider. A corner suture (half-buried mattress subcuticular suture) was used to approximate the triangular edge of the wound. Fifteen interrupted sutures were placed along the sides of the flap wound without complications. Lidocaine, epinephrine, and tetracaine was used for anesthesia with excellent results. The patient watched a movie during the procedure which provided distraction. Tetanus prophylaxis was not indicated given that the patient had received more than three doses of tetanus immunizations, with the last dose given 3 years ago (less than 5 years prior). Detailed wound care instructions were given upon discharge. The patient was instructed to visit his pediatrician in 10 days for suture removal.

References

1. DeBoard RH, Rondeau DF, Kang CS, et al. Principles of basic wound evaluation and management in the emergency department. *Emerg Med Clin N Am* 2007; 25: 23–39.

2. Worster B, Zawora MQ, Hsieh C. Common questions about wound care. *Am Fam Phys* 2015; 91(2): 86–92.

3. Forsch RT. Essentials of skin laceration repair. *Am Fam Phys* 2008; 78(8): 945–51.

4. Walmsley GG, Maan ZN, Wong VW, et al. Scarless wound healing: Chasing the holy grail. *Plast Reconstr Surg* 2015; 135: 907–17.

5. Zehtabchi S, Tan A, Yadav K, et al. The impact of wound age on the infection rate of simple lacerations repaired in the emergency department. *Injury* 2012; 43: 1793–8.

6. Perelman VS, Francis GJ, Rutledge T, et al. Sterile versus nonsterile gloves for repair of uncomplicated lacerations in the emergency department: A randomized controlled trial. *Ann Emerg Med* 2004; 43: 362–70.

Case 5

Contributing Author: Rachel A. Patterson

History

The patient is a 4-year old male who presents to the ED with his mother, complaining of left knee pain and swelling for 1 day. The patient's mother first noticed a limp the day prior to presentation while watching a parade outside. She noted continued worsening of his gait and swelling of the left knee over the next 24 hours to the point that the patient completely refused to stand or walk. He also complained of pain when the knee was touched or moved. The family does recall an erythematous rash on his arm during the summer but it resolved quickly so no further evaluation was performed at that time. The patient has otherwise been in his normal state of health and family denies any recent traumas, falls, or illnesses.

Past Medical History

The patient has a history of conductive hearing loss with developmental speech delay. He has had bilateral myringotomy tube placement and is UTD on his immunizations.

Medications

- None.

Allergies

- NKDA.

Physical Examination and Ancillary Studies

- *Vital signs*: T 98.8 °F, HR 108, RR 20, BP 108/60, O_2 sat 99% on room air.
- *General*: The patient is a well-developed child in no acute distress, playful and interactive until his knee is touched or he is stood up by his parents. He then begins to grimace and cry.
- *HEENT*: PERRL. No conjunctival injection or pallor. Oropharynx clear, with moist mucous membranes.
- *Neck*: Non-tender, with no adenopathy.
- *Cardiovascular*: Regular rate and rhythm. No M/R/G. Good capillary refill.
- *Lungs*: CTA bilaterally without W/R/R.
- *Abdomen*: The abdomen is soft, with bowel sounds present and no rebound or guarding.
- *Extremities and skin*: The patient's left knee is moderately swollen, mildly tender, and warm to palpation but without erythema or induration. He complains of pain when his knee is touched, extended, or flexed. He is otherwise able to move his bilateral hips, ankles, and arms without difficulty. There is no evidence of swelling to his extremities otherwise. He has no petechiae or rash.
- *Neurologic*: Appropriate for age, normal extremity strength and reflexes.
- *Pertinent laboratory values*: WBC 11,640, ESR 38, CRP 8.8.
- *Pertinent radiographs*: Knee X-ray and U/S with joint effusion.

Questions for Thought

- What are the important historical clues that should be obtained when evaluating this patient?
- What are the key physical examination findings?
- What is the typical diagnostic testing performed for this condition?
- What treatment should be initiated in the ED?

Diagnosis

- Lyme arthritis.

Discussion

- *Epidemiology*: Lyme disease was first identified in the 1970s in the Connecticut town of Lyme, when a cluster of children were being evaluated and treated for oligoarthritis.[1] Lyme disease is currently the most common vector-borne disease in the USA.[2] It is a tick-borne illness that is primarily caused by the spirochete *Borrelia burgdorferi* and according to the CDC, there are currently over 30,000 new cases of Lyme disease each year in the USA.[2]

- *Pathophysiology*: The spirochete of *B. burgdorferi* attaches to the skin and if not overwhelmed by host defenses it may cause the rash of erythema migrans. The spirochete can disseminate throughout the body with predilection for the skin, heart, joints, CNS, and eyes. Further discussion of this can be found in Chapter 10, Case 7.

- *Presentation*: Lyme disease can be divided into early localized, early disseminated, and late disease. Lyme arthritis is the most common late manifestation of the disease and occurs in approximately 50 to 60 percent of patients who go untreated for early Lyme disease.[3] Patients presenting with Lyme arthritis may have an antecedent history of erythema migrans, intermittent arthralgias, and myalgias; however, these are not necessary for the diagnosis.[4] The symptoms of arthritis generally occur within weeks to months of initial infection and tend to be characterized by either an acute onset of joint swelling that may persist, or recurrent episodes of self-resolving migratory monoarthritis of various large joints.[4–6] If untreated, approximately 10 percent of these patients will develop chronic monoarthritis.[5] Although it can be either mono- or oligoarticular, the knee is the most commonly affected joint and is involved in over 90 percent of patients presenting with Lyme arthritis.[5] Other commonly affected joints include the ankle, hip, and elbow.[5,6] On presentation, the affected joint is swollen and with limited range of motion to varying degrees. Although some patients are unable to bear weight, others are able to ambulate without significant difficulty. Fever, erythema, and warmth are variably present with Lyme arthritis but are much less common than with septic arthritis.[5,6]

- *Diagnosis*: The diagnosis of Lyme arthritis is initially based on clinical history and physical examination. This is especially true if the patient lives in an area or has traveled to an area that is endemic for Lyme disease and has the characteristic rash of erythema migrans. Most patients with Lyme arthritis have involvement of the knee or hip and also are less likely to have a fever or other systemic symptoms of illness at presentation.[5]

  When presenting with later stages of Lyme disease, additional testing in conjunction with a clinical examination and history is used to make the diagnosis. Unlike in early Lyme disease, patients with Lyme arthritis should have positive serologic antibodies to *B. burgdorferi*.[7] Serologic testing should be completed with a two-tier approach of ELISA followed by Western blot testing. It can take days, however, for these results to return, and a diagnosis often needs to be made urgently to differentiate Lyme arthritis from other septic and non-septic causes of monoarticular arthritis. Arthrocentesis of a joint for synovial fluid analysis should be performed. The synovial fluid can have varying WBC as high as 100,000, but often the WBC will be between 10,000 and 25,000 with polymorphonuclear leukocyte predominance.[8] Therefore, cell counts alone cannot be used to exclude or make a diagnosis of Lyme or septic arthritis, as there is considerable overlap between threshold values. A key laboratory criteria to differentiate Lyme from bacterial arthritis is a culture negative for a bacterial pathogen. Synovial-fluid PCR for *B. burgdorferi* DNA can also help make the diagnosis of Lyme arthritis.

  Laboratory evidence of inflammation includes elevated ESR levels, CRP levels, and peripheral WBC; however, these are not specific to Lyme arthritis and additional testing should be used to support the diagnosis. Markedly elevated peripheral WBC and ESR levels are more common in septic arthritis than Lyme arthritis, but lack sufficient specificity and sensitivity to be used to rule out the diagnosis.[9]

- *Treatment*: Successful treatment of Lyme arthritis can be achieved in over 90 percent of patients following a 28-day course of antibiotics. For pediatric patients who are less than 8 years old, amoxicillin is the initial recommended treatment regiment.[10] For children 8 years of age or older, doxycycline is first-line therapy.[10] Patients may have residual symptoms of mild joint swelling and pain after the initial course of antibiotics that continues to resolve slowly over weeks. Anti-inflammatories are key for adjunctive symptomatic control for these patients. Re-treatment with a 4-week course of oral antibiotics or IV antibiotics should also be considered in patients with only moderate or mild improvement of symptoms, respectively.[10]

- *Disposition*: When treated with antibiotics, Lyme arthritis has an excellent prognosis. If the patient has no systemic symptoms, can ambulate without difficulty, and has a physical examination/joint aspiration negative for septic arthritis, he or she can safely be discharged to home with initiation of oral antibiotics and follow-up with his or her PCP.

Historical clues	Physical findings	Ancillary studies
• Knee pain • Rash over the summer	• Joint pain and effusion • Absence of fever • Absence of warmth and erythema	• Negative X-ray (excluding occult trauma)

Follow-Up

The patient's clinical examination as well as history was concerning for Lyme arthritis. He had an U/S of his left knee that showed a moderately sized joint effusion, and an arthrocentesis was performed under U/S guidance, revealing cloudy, yellow joint fluid. The synovial fluid was sent for a Gram's stain, aerobic and anaerobic cultures as well as cell count, crystals, glucose, protein, and Lyme PCR. His synovial fluid was significant for over 60,000 WBC; however, the Gram's stain was negative. The joint fluid otherwise revealed normal glucose and protein and was negative for crystals. Because the patient was unable to ambulate, he was admitted to the hospital and started on anti-inflammatories for pain and oral antibiotics for presumptive Lyme disease while awaiting more definitive negative cultures. His Lyme titer was ultimately positive, as was his synovial fluid Lyme PCR. He was eventually discharged with an uneventful post-hospitalization course.

References

1. Steere AC, Malawista SE, Snydman DR, et al. Lyme arthritis: An epidemic of oligoarticular arthritis in children and adults in three Connecticut communities. *Arthritis Rheumatol* 1977; 20: 7–17.

2. Centers for Disease Control and Prevention. Lyme disease: Data and statistics. See www.cdc.gov/lyme/stats/index.html (accessed January 2017).

3. Warde N. Treating pediatric Lyme arthritis. *Nat Rev Rheumatol* 2010; 6: 312.

4. Rose CD, Fawcett PT, Eppes SC. Pediatric Lyme arthritis: Clinical spectrum and outcome. *J Pediatr Orthop* 1994; 14: 238–41.

5. Thompson A, Mannix R, Bachur R. Acute pediatric monoarticular arthritis: Distinguishing Lyme arthritis from other etiologies. *Pediatrics* 2009; 123: 959–65.

6. Wright WF, Riedel DJ, Talwani R, et al. Diagnosis and management of Lyme disease. *Am Fam Phys* 2012; 85: 1086–93.

7. Puius YA, Kalish RA. Lyme arthritis: Pathogenesis, clinical presentation, and management. *Infect Dis Clin North Am* 2008; 22: 289–300.

8. Deanehan JK, Nigrovic PA, Milewski MD. Synovial fluid findings in children with knee monoarthritis in Lyme disease endemic areas. *Pediatr Emerg Care* 2014; 30: 16–19.

9. Deanehan JK, Kimia AA, Tan Tanny SP, et al. Distinguishing Lyme from septic knee monoarthritis in Lyme disease-endemic areas. *Pediatrics* 2013; 131: e695–701.

10. Wormser GP, Dattwyler RJ, Shapiro ED, et al. The clinical assessment, treatment, and prevention of Lyme disease, human granulocytic anaplasmosis, and babesiosis: Clinical practice guidelines by the Infectious Diseases Society of America. *Clin Infect Dis* 2006; 43: 1089–134.

Case 6

Contributing Author: Benjamin Kitt

History

The patient is a 17-year-old male who presents to the ED for 2 weeks of steadily increasing left upper arm pain. The pain was initially mild and sporadic in nature. The pain is described as sharp and occurs both at rest and with movement. There is no known trauma or repetitive motion activity. The patient reports he was recently evaluated at another ED, where he was diagnosed with a muscle strain. Over the next 2 days, the pain increased substantially, which prompted this second ED visit. His pain has now increased to 10/10, which prevents him from sleeping at night. He also has developed numbness and throbbing in his forearm. He denies fever, rash, chest pain, shortness of breath, nausea, vomiting, abdominal pain, weakness, fatigue, or malaise. There hasn't been any recent travel or known sick contacts. The patient denies illicit drug use.

Past Medical History

- Mild intermittent asthma.
- UTD on immunizations.

Medications

- Albuterol inhaler as needed.

Allergies

- NKDA.

Physical Examination and Ancillary Studies

- *Vital signs*: T 99.7 °F, HR 88, RR 18, BP 109/61, O_2 sat 98% on room air.
- *General*: Lying in bed, clutching his arm, in moderate distress from pain.
- *HEENT*: PERRL. Mucous membranes are moist. No signs of trauma.
- *Neck*: Supple, with a midline trachea and no adenopathy.
- *Cardiovascular*: Regular rate and rhythm, with no M/R/G. Capillary refill < 2 seconds. No appreciable cyanosis.
- *Lungs*: CTA bilaterally with no W/R/R.
- *Abdomen*: Soft and non-tender to palpation, with normal bowel sounds.
- *Extremities and skin*: There is tenderness to palpation along the left shoulder laterally and the left upper arm. There are no palpable masses and there is no obvious deformity or edema. The left shoulder has limited range of motion secondary to pain but is without swelling. Muscular compartments are all soft. The right upper and both lower extremities are without swelling or tenderness. The skin is warm and dry with no erythema or rashes.
- *Neurologic*: Intact cranial nerves. Normal sensation, tone, and strength in the extremities.
- *Pertinent laboratory values*: WBC 13,500, Hb 11.6, ESR 91, CRP 25.

- *Pertinent radiographs*: Left humerus radiograph reveals a humeral midshaft lesion and a CT is recommended. CT demonstrates a 9-mm lucent lesion at the midshaft of the left humerus.

Questions for Thought

- What is the differential diagnosis of this lesion?
- Are there additional studies you would like to obtain?
- What are the next steps in the management of this patient?
- Who would you consult for further management?

Diagnosis

- Osteomyelitis of the humerus with abscess formation.

Discussion

- *Epidemiology*: Osteomyelitis is an infection of the bone resulting in inflammation of the surrounding tissues. It is a rare disease in pediatric populations, with an estimated annual incidence rate of 13 per 100,000 in patients under the age of 18.[1,2] The highest incidence occurs in children under the age of 3.[1-3] For unknown reasons, osteomyelitis tends to affect males more than females, in a ratio of 2:1. Osteomyelitis of hematogenous origin is more common in children than in adults.[2-4] Risk factors for osteomyelitis in infants less than 30 days of age include urinary tract anomalies, prematurity, CVC placement, complicated delivery, or overlying skin infection.[4] In older children, hematogenous risk factors for osteomyelitis include: sepsis, indwelling catheters, bacteremia secondary to trauma, sickle cell disease, and immunodeficiency disorders.[2-4] Osteomyelitis may be acute (less than 2 weeks of symptoms), subacute (symptoms for 2 weeks to 3 months), or chronic (symptoms for greater than 3 months).[2] Chronic osteomyelitis is rare in children.[3]
- *Pathophysiology*: There are various etiologies and sources of infection for osteomyelitis. One of the most common causes of pediatric osteomyelitis is via hematogenous seeding;[1-4] these are typically monomicrobial infections. Osteomyelitis can also occur secondary to a localized infection, such as a soft-tissue or joint infection, or through direct inoculation of infection to the bone from trauma

or surgery;[3] these are often polymicrobial infections. The development of osteomyelitis depends largely on the pathogen that infects the bone and the virulence of that organism. These factors can include the organism's ability to enter and adhere to the cells, as well as the immune status of the patient. For instance, patients with sickle cell disease lack functional spleens, which makes them more prone to bacteremia and therefore more likely to develop osteomyelitis.

As discussed above, hematogenous seeding is the most common cause of osteomyelitis in children, and the infection usually seeds to long-bone metaphysis. The exact mechanism for this process is unknown, but it is likely due to the large volume of blood that passes through the metaphysis as well as an increased permeability of the capillaries.[3] Once bacteria begin to proliferate within the area, they cause inflammation, with resulting destruction of trabecular bone and its vascular channels.[2] This destruction may make antibiotics ineffective, as they may not be able to reach the site of the infection due to the disrupted blood flow.[2]

The most common organisms isolated in osteomyelitis are Gram-positive bacteria and, in particular, MRSA. Other notable organisms include, but are not limited to: group A and B streptococci, *Streptococcus pneumoniae*, *Escherichia coli*, and *Kingella kingae*.[2] While less common than bacterial infections, fungal species have been known to cause osteomyelitis.[1]

- *Presentation*: Osteomyelitis often presents insidiously and can be missed on initial evaluation.[3] The symptoms are non-specific in nature and include decreased range of motion/weight-bearing on the affected bone, fever, malaise, pain, local swelling, tenderness, or warmth. Presentation also varies depending on the age of the child. Older children are often able to localize the pain and provide historical events of the progression of the pain. In young children who are unable to localize pain or communicate, the diagnosis can be even more difficult to make. The child may refuse to use the affected extremity, such as preferentially using the unaffected arm or, with lower extremity, refusing to weight-bear on the affected side. Infants may present by crying during diaper changing, crying when the affected extremity is touched, and refusing to crawl or sit.

- *Diagnosis*: The diagnosis of osteomyelitis is often difficult due to the non-specific presentation and nature of the disease. The provider must consider alternative possibilities, such as malignancy, septic arthritis, autoimmune disease, Lyme arthritis, occult or non-accidental trauma, and referred pain, and an evaluation must be undertaken to exclude these other diagnoses.

- In patients where osteomyelitis is suspected, a CBC with differential, CRP, ESR, and two blood cultures are generally recommended. Although not specific, elevations in acute phase reactants support the diagnosis. Radiographs are inexpensive and widely available, which make them a reasonable first choice for imaging. It is important to note that the sensitivity and specificity of plain films in the diagnosis of osteomyelitis is poor. The plain films can have suggestive features of osteomyelitis, such as soft-tissue swelling or cortical erosion. Although more difficult to obtain emergently, MRI is highly sensitive in detecting osteomyelitis.[1-3] It also has the added benefit of avoiding radiation in children. Although CT imaging is not as good as MRI in delineating osteomyelitis, it is a reasonable alternative.

- *Treatment*: The treatment of osteomyelitis is often an extended course of antibiotics. Due to this fact, it is important to obtain cultures with sensitivity testing to ensure the correct antibiotic is used as therapy.[1,2] Though blood cultures can be positive and aid in the diagnosis of the organism, a biopsy and culture of the lesion is ideal.[2] However, the condition of the patient must take priority, and if the patient is manifesting signs of serious infection, broad-spectrum antibiotics should be initiated. Consultation with orthopedics and infectious disease for assistance in starting appropriate therapy is recommended.

- *Disposition*: Patients with osteomyelitis require hospital admission for IV antibiotics and for surgical debridement and washout if they do not have a prompt clinical response.

Historical clues	Physical findings	Ancillary studies
• Gradually increasing pain • No improvement with conservative treatment • Pain with activity or rest	• Tenderness over humerus • No signs of trauma	• Elevated CRP • Elevated ESR • Abnormal X-ray and CT

Follow-Up

An MRI of the left humerus was obtained and demonstrated a 1-cm cortical lesion within the anterior cortex of the mid-humeral shaft suspicious for osteomyelitis. Orthopedics surgery and pediatric infectious disease services were consulted. The patient underwent biopsy and drainage of the bone abscess. He was initially started on IV vancomycin but did not achieve therapeutic levels, and was subsequently switched to daptomycin. Culture results from the abscess demonstrated MRSA. The patient then underwent another surgical drainage a week later due to persistent fevers, swelling of his arm, and drainage from wound. Vancomycin-impregnated beads were placed during the operation. The patient completed a 14-day course of daptomycin and was discharged on clindamycin for an anticipated 3-month course with orthopedic and infectious disease follow-up.

References

1. Riise, ØR, Kirkhus E, Handeland KS, et al. Childhood osteomyelitis: Incidence and differentiation from other acute onset musculoskeletal features in a population-based study. *BMC Pediatr* 2008; 8: 45.

2. Ceroni D, Kampouroglou G, Anderson della Llana R, et al. Osteoarticular infections in young children: What has changed over the last years? *Swiss Med Wkly* 2014; 144: w13971.

3. Hatzenbuehler J, Pulling TJ. Diagnosis and management of osteomyelitis. *Am Fam Phys* 2011; 84: 1027–33.

4. Dartnell J, Ramachandran M, Katchburian M. Haematogenous acute and subacute paediatric osteomyelitis: a systematic review of the literature. *J Bone Joint Surg Br* 2012; 94: 584–95.

Case 7

Contributing Author: M. Bryan Dalla Betta

History

A 3-year-old male presents by private vehicle to the ED complaining of right arm pain after a fall. According to the parents, the patient was playing basketball at the park when he tripped and fell forward onto both hands. There was no loss of consciousness and he cried immediately and clutched his right upper extremity. He has been in significant pain since the fall. The patient states that his pain is worst in his right elbow. The parents note elbow swelling and said that he doesn't want to move it. He has some pain in his hands but denies any numbness or tingling. He denies difficulty breathing, headache, pain in his chest or belly, and is acting normally according to his parents.

Past Medical History

- Prior tonsillectomy.
- UTD on immunizations.

Medications

- None.

Allergies

- NKDA.

Physical Examination and Ancillary Studies

- *Vital signs*: T 98.9 °F, HR 104, RR 22, BP 112/76, O_2 sat 99% on room air.
- *General*: Patient is tearful but awake and alert, looking around the room. He is well-nourished, appears mildly anxious, and has a normal body habitus for his age.
- *HEENT*: The head is atraumatic. There is no tenderness or swelling noted on palpation of the scalp. PERRL. Extraocular muscles intact.
- *Neck*: No midline tenderness, no step-offs.
- *Cardiovascular*: Regular tachycardia, with no M/R/G. Radial pulses are 2+ bilaterally and capillary refill is brisk in both hands.
- *Lungs*: The lung sounds are clear, with good air movement bilaterally.
- *Abdomen*: Soft and non-distended, with no signs of trauma. No tenderness or masses.
- *Extremities and skin*: The right arm is held in flexion with moderate swelling of the right elbow. The patient cries and withdraws at any attempt to manipulate the elbow. There is no deformity or tenderness to the right shoulder, clavicle, forearm, or wrist. There are superficial abrasions to the palms of both hands but otherwise the skin is intact, including at the right elbow.
- *Neurologic*: The grip strength of the right hand is decreased to 4/5 due to pain. When asked to make an "OK" sign, there is decreased flexion of the distal right index finger to a pincer-like configuration. Finger spread and wrist extension

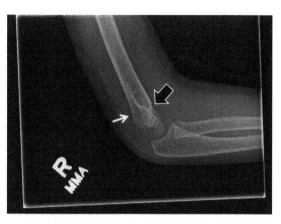

Figure 6.1 Lateral view of the right elbow shows a non-displaced supracondylar fracture (black arrow) with a posterior fat-pad sign (white arrow).

are intact with 5/5 strength. There is no sensory loss in the hand, forearm, or elbow.
- *Pertinent radiographs*: Elbow radiograph shown in Figure 6.1.

Questions for Thought

- What is the typical mechanism of injury for this condition?
- What vascular injury is associated with this condition?
- What radiographic views are best to evaluate for this kind of injury?
- What findings would mandate operative intervention in this injury?

Diagnosis

- Supracondylar fracture of the humerus.

Discussion

- *Epidemiology*: Supracondylar fractures occur in children primarily between the ages of 5 and 10 years old, but can be seen in the early or even late teenage years as well. Most are caused by a fall on an outstretched hand and they account for approximately 60 percent of pediatric elbow fractures.[1-3]
- *Pathophysiology*: In children, the humerus just proximal to the medial and lateral condyles is relatively weak. Falls on outstretched hands (or rarely, onto a flexed elbow) cause forces to be transmitted up the arm to this area of relative

weakness. Transverse fractures through this area of the distal humerus are termed supracondylar fractures.

The proximity of the brachial artery and median, ulnar, and radial nerves to the supracondylar fracture site adds to the clinical importance of the diagnosis.[2-5] Because of the proximity of these neurovascular structures, angulated or displaced supracondylar fractures can cause neurovascular compromise to the distal extremity.

- *Presentation*: The mechanism of supracondylar fractures can vary, but a history of a fall onto an outstretched hand or flexed elbow is most common. Some patients will have only elbow pain and mild swelling, while others can present with gross deformity, sensory deficit, or absent distal pulses. Patients will typically have considerable pain and significantly impaired range of motion at the elbow, and may cradle the extremity in flexion close to the body.
- *Diagnosis*: Diagnosing elbow fractures in general requires knowledge of appearance of growth plates, as growth centers can look like fractures. If you are unsure, you should obtain a radiograph of the other elbow for comparison. The capitellum is the first growth center to appear (at about age 1), followed by the radial head (at about age 3), the medial epicondyle (at about age 5), the trochlea (at about age 7), the olecranon (at about age 9), and the lateral epicondyle (at about age 11). The growth centers fuse and are no longer visible sometime around age 13.

The diagnosis of supracondylar fractures is made with anterior–posterior and lateral views of the elbow. The anterior humeral line, a line drawn down the anterior surface of the humerus, should pass through the middle third of the capitellum in a normal, true lateral film of the elbow, as it does in patients with non-displaced fractures like the one shown in Figure 6.1. An angulated fracture should be suspected if this line does not pass through the middle third of the capitellum (Figure 6.2). The presence of a posterior fat-pad sign or a sail sign (large anterior fat pad) should also raise suspicion for fracture. Radiographs of the forearm and proximal humerus may also be obtained due to the incidence of associated fractures in these areas.

Extension fractures are described using the Gartland classification system, where fracture

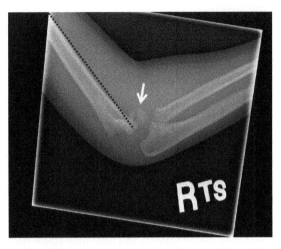

Figure 6.2 Radiograph demonstrating the anterior humeral line (black dotted line) that does not pass through the capitellum (white arrow), indicating a displaced fracture.

type ranges from I to III depending primarily on the amount of fracture angulation present. A supracondylar fracture without angulation or displacement is the least severe (type I), while fractures with angulation or displacement usually require surgical evaluation, reduction, and/or pinning (types II and III).[1,3,4] Type II fractures involve extension of the humerus with the posterior cortex still touching or even intact (angulated without complete translation), while type III involve a fully circumferential cortical break, with complete displacement of the distal fragment posteriorly.[1,3,4]

- *Treatment*: Treatment of supracondylar fractures begins on initial patient presentation with appropriate analgesia and temporary splinting for comfort. Any evidence of vascular compromise warrants immediate orthopedic consultation even if there is evidence of distal perfusion. The integrity of the brachial artery as well as the median, ulnar, and radial nerves should be assessed rapidly after initial presentation. A cold, pulseless, or pale distal extremity mandates emergent orthopedic involvement, and closed reduction should be attempted in the ED to restore distal perfusion and avoid ischemia.

  Supracondylar fractures without displacement, angulation, or other complicating factors can be managed with application of a long arm posterior splint in the ED. The splint should extend from the proximal humerus to the metacarpals, with the elbow in less than 90 degrees of flexion to prevent additional swelling.

  Displaced or angulated fractures, as well as any open fracture or fracture with neurovascular compromise or concern for compartment syndrome, require emergent orthopedic consultation in the ED. Displaced or considerably angulated fractures may require surgical pinning, open reduction, or exploration in the OR.[4]

- *Disposition*: Children with non-angulated and non-displaced fractures can be discharged home with long arm splint and sling. Consultation with orthopedics is recommended to determine a preferred time frame for follow-up, but generally this should occur within 2–3 days and no longer than 1 week. It is important to give parents good instructions regarding neurovascular compromise, and many physicians advocate either an observation admission or a return visit for an examination for neurovascular function at 24 hours.

  Any evidence of open fracture, compartment syndrome, neurovascular compromise, or any displaced or angulated fractures requires orthopedic consultation in the ED. These patients are often admitted to the hospital, and therefore decisions for these patients should be made in conjunction with the orthopedic surgeon.

Historical clues	Physical findings	Ancillary studies
• Fall on outstretched arm • Child 5–10 years • Elbow pain	• Elbow swelling/deformity • Restricted range of motion • Signs of neurovascular injury	• X-ray with fracture and posterior fat-pad and sail sign

Follow-Up

An orthopedic consultation was requested for this patient and after adequate pain control and re-examination it was determined that no reduction or operative intervention was emergently required. The patient was placed in a long arm splint with sling for immobilization and comfort, and arrangements were made for follow-up with the orthopedic department in the next several days. He was placed in a cast for 6 weeks but regained full function and range of motion of the affected arm.

References

1. Thornton MD, Della-Giustina K, Aronson PL. Emergency department evaluation and treatment of pediatric orthopedic injuries. *Emerg Med Clin N Am* 2015; 33: 423–49.

2. Lins RE, Simovitch RW, Waters PM. Pediatric elbow trauma. *Orthop Clin North Am* 1999; 30: 119–32.

3. Allen SR, Hang JR, Hau RC. Review article: Paediatric supracondylar humeral fractures: Emergency assessment and management. *Emerg Med Australas* 2010; 22: 418–26.

4. Abzug JM, Herman MJ. Management of supracondylar humerus fractures in children: Current concepts. *J Am Acad Orthop Surg* 2012; 20: 69–77.

5. Wu J, Perron AD, Miller MD, et al. Orthopedic pitfalls in the ED: Pediatric supracondylar fractures. *Am J Emerg Med* 2002; 20: 544–50.

Case 8

Contributing Author: Rebecca Jeanmonod

History

A 14-year-old girl presents to the ED with a chief complaint of left shoulder pain. The girl had been at rugby practice and was tackled from behind. She put her hands up to protect herself during the fall, and denies striking her head, but complains of left shoulder pain. Since the event, the child has been unable to move the shoulder. She denies neck pain, chest pain, or difficulty breathing. She has an area of tingling on the lateral aspect of her left shoulder, but otherwise denies numbness or sensory symptoms. She states she does not feel weak, but can't move the arm secondary to pain, which she localizes entirely to the shoulder. She denies elbow, wrist, or hand pain. She is right hand dominant. Her coach brought her to the ED, and her parents are on their way in to the ED, but have given verbal permission to treat the child by phone.

Past Medical History

- Prior open surgical repair of right-sided Colles fracture 1 year ago.
- Seasonal allergies.
- Immunizations UTD.

Medications

- Loratadine.

Allergies

- Peanuts and sulfa drugs.

Physical Examination and Ancillary Studies

- *Vital signs*: T 99.2 °F, HR 82, RR 15, BP 118/65, O_2 sat 100% on room air.
- *General*: Well-developed and well-nourished, sitting upright in stretcher with left arm held slightly abducted, internally rotated, with elbow flexed. She appears uncomfortable.
- *HEENT*: PERRL. No signs of trauma. No malocclusion. Oropharynx clear.
- *Neck*: No midline tenderness or step-offs. Trachea is midline. No adenopathy.
- *Cardiovascular*: Regular rate and rhythm. No M/R/G. 2+ radial pulses in both arms.
- *Lungs*: CTA bilaterally, with no W/R/R. No chest-wall tenderness or deformity.
- *Abdomen*: Soft, with no tenderness or masses. Pelvis stable.
- *Extremities and skin*: Extremities are warm and well-perfused. She has a small abrasion to her left palm. She has no edema and normal capillary refill. She has flattening beneath her left acromion, and her humeral head is palpable anterior to the glenoid. She has no arm or clavicular tenderness. She is unable to range the shoulder, but has intact range of motion of elbow, wrist, contralateral arm, and bilateral lower extremities.
- *Neurologic*: Her cranial nerves are intact. She has intact strength and sensation in her lower extremities. She has decreased sensation over her left lateral deltoid, but her radial, median, and ulnar nerves have intact function. She cannot participate in strength testing at the shoulder secondary to pain.

Questions for Thought

- What is the patient's diagnosis?
- Does the patient require imaging?
- What is the best way to treat this injury?
- What is the appropriate definitive treatment for this condition?

Diagnosis

- Anterior shoulder dislocation.

Discussion

- *Epidemiology*: Shoulders are the most commonly dislocated joint in the body, accounting for 50 percent of all dislocations.[1,2] Finger dislocations are also fairly common. Isolated patella and elbow dislocations occur less frequently, and hip dislocations typically only occur in the setting of high-energy trauma, such as dashboard injury in motor vehicle accidents. Ankle dislocations are rare in the absence of coincident fracture. The shoulder's high rate of dislocation is explained by its high degree of mobility. Although dislocations can occur at any age, the natural history of the disease differs by age. Younger patients have a much higher incidence of recurrence than older people, and age less than 20 at first dislocation confers a greater than $12\times$ risk of recurrence, with mean time to recurrence less than one year.[3]

- *Pathophysiology*: Shoulder dislocations are classified by location of the humeral head (anterior, posterior, or inferior) and by recurrence (acute traumatic versus recurrent). Ninety percent of shoulder dislocations are anterior, and are most commonly incurred by sporting injuries or direct shoulder trauma in teenagers.[2] The shoulder tends to dislocate anteriorly because of the relatively thinner joint capsule there. Inferior shoulder dislocations may be secondary to seizures or major trauma. Posterior dislocations are rare and are often missed on initial presentation, as the humeral head may be difficult to palpate in the posterior deltoid musculature and because the force necessary to cause a posterior dislocation often causes other more pressing and obvious injuries.

  When the shoulder dislocates, it can injure the anterior glenoid rim and avulse the labrum (Bankart lesion), leading to a predisposition to future anterior dislocations.[1-3] It can also cause rotator cuff tears or injure nerves in the brachial plexus. The most commonly injured nerve is the axillary nerve, which runs inferiorly to the shoulder joint capsule, and may be stretched or damaged during dislocation.[1] The axillary nerve is responsible for sensation over the lateral aspect of the deltoid. It is also responsible for arm abduction, which cannot be assessed until the shoulder is reduced.

- *Presentation*: Patients typically present immediately following trauma with shoulder pain and reduced range of motion after a mechanism of direct shoulder trauma or fall on outstretched hand. Rarely, patients will present in a delayed fashion, particularly if the dislocation occurred during intoxication or seizure. The patient with an inferior dislocation presents with an inability to adduct the arm, and it is easy to spot because the arm is extended over the head. The patient with a posterior dislocation presents with an internally rotated and adducted arm. He or she has shoulder pain and reduced range of motion, but it is often missed because radiographs may be misleading and the examination is subtle. Anterior dislocations may present acutely or in a recurrent fashion. Recurrent dislocations tend to occur while the patient is extending and externally rotating the shoulder during regular activities, such as hair brushing or bench pressing. These patients typically have a history of prior traumatic dislocation.

- *Diagnosis*: Diagnosis of dislocation is based on history and physical examination. A history of the mechanism of the injury and prior dislocations should be elicited, as well as a neurovascular review of systems. The patient with an anterior dislocation may have paresthesias or numbness in the distribution of the axillary nerve or in the entire arm from traction on the brachial plexus. The patient will typically have a sulcus just inferior to the acromion, which is easily palpable. Further palpation will often reveal the humeral head anteromedial to the glenoid. In posterior dislocations, palpation will reveal the humeral head in the posterior deltoid muscle.

  Radiographs are helpful in making the diagnosis of anterior shoulder dislocation, but are not necessary if the provider is clinically certain of the patient's pathology.[2] Particularly in the cases of dislocation at sporting events or ski slopes, if the provider has no immediate access to radiography, the better course of action is to reduce the injury, as delay to reduction prolongs patient discomfort and results in increasing difficulty in reduction over time. Although the presence of a fracture may have implications on long-term treatment and rehabilitation, it does not impact emergency management, and prompt reduction with referral for outpatient radiography is reasonable. The outpatient radiograph is important for assessment for occult physeal injury at the humeral head, which can have an impact on limb length in growing children. This child, who is 14, has likely reached her full growth potential.

When radiographs are obtained, the scapular Y view is the most important in determining humeral head location relative to the anatomic position. In this view, the X-ray beam passes through the axilla, projecting the appropriately placed humeral head at the center of a Y shape that is formed by the scapular body, the acromion, and the coracoid process. If the humeral head is anterior to this Y, the dislocation is anterior, and if it is posterior to this Y, it is a posterior dislocation.

- *Treatment*: The ED management of a shoulder dislocation is to reduce it. The first step is to provide adequate analgesia. For the calm and cooperative patient, several self-reduction methods are described.[4] Most patients require manual reduction by a healthcare provider. There are over 20 described reduction methods for shoulder dislocations, some of which rely on traction/countertraction, some of which rely on leverage, and some of which rely on manipulation.[4] Any one of these techniques is acceptable, and is largely a matter of provider preference.

Options for pain control range from oral anti-inflammatory medications to procedural sedation in intra-articular anesthesia. Intra-articular anesthesia with lidocaine or bupivacaine has been demonstrated to be as comfortable for patients as procedural sedation, with fewer complications and shorter ED stays, and is therefore a reasonable first-line choice for pain management.[5]

Once reduction is complete, the patient should be immobilized in a sling. There is no definitive evidence that external rotation immobilization provides better outcomes than a simple sling, and this is more difficult to apply.[6] Although many providers choose to obtain post-reduction radiographs, they do not add to the emergency management of these patients in most circumstances and are not strictly necessary.[7]

- *Disposition*: Once reduction is complete, most patients can be discharged home to follow up with orthopedic surgery. Since young patients are

extremely likely to have recurrent dislocations, surgical intervention is often indicated, and therefore referral to a surgeon is appropriate.[3,8]

Historical clues	Physical findings
- Fall on outstretched arm - Shoulder pain - Lateral shoulder tingling	- Sulcus beneath acromion - Humeral head palpable anteriorly - Decreased sensation over lateral deltoid (indicating axillary nerve traction)

Follow-Up

Radiology was delayed for this child due to a multiple trauma activation. The provider injected 20 cc of 1% lidocaine into her left shoulder joint via a posterior approach and let it dwell for 20 minutes. The child then underwent shoulder reduction with external rotation. She was placed in a sling and discharged home with her parents to follow up with orthopedic surgery.

References

1. Bonz J, Tinloy B. Emergency department evaluation and treatment of the shoulder and humerus. *Emerg Med Clin N Am* 2015; 33: 297–310.

2. Quillen DM, Wuchner M, Hatch RL. Acute shoulder injuries. *Am Fam Phys* 2004; 70: 1947–54.

3. Wasserstein DN, Sheth U, Colbenson K, et al. The true recurrence rate and factors predicting recurrent instability after nonsurgical management of traumatic primary anterior shoulder dislocation: A systematic review. *Arthroscopy* 2016; 32: 2616–25.

4. Alkaduhimi H, van der Linde JA, Flipsen M, et al. A systematic and technical guide on how to reduce a shoulder dislocation. *Turk J Emerg Med* 2016; 16: 155–68.

5. Kashani P, Zarchi FA, Hatamabadi HR, et al. Intra-articular lidocaine versus intravenous sedative and analgesic for reduction of anterior shoulder dislocation. *Turk J Emerg Med* 2016; 16: 60–4.

6. Whelan DB, Kletke SN, Schemitsch G, et al. Immobilization in external rotation versus internal rotation after primary anterior shoulder dislocation. *Am J Sports Med* 2015; 44: 521–32.

7. Hendey GW. Necessity of radiographs in the emergency department management of shoulder dislocations. *Ann Emerg Med* 2000; 36: 108–13.

8. Longo UG, Loppini M, Rizzello G, et al. Management of primary acute anterior shoulder dislocation: Systematic review and quantitative synthesis of the literature. *Arthroscopy* 2014; 30: 506–22.

Case 9

Contributing Author: Rebecca Jeanmonod

History

A 10-year-old boy presents to the ED with right ankle pain. The child was playing soccer in gym class when he tried to capture the ball from another player. His right foot became entrapped between the other player's feet. He lost his balance and fell to the ground, causing his foot to be twisted laterally. Since that time, he has been unable to walk on the ankle secondary to pain. He did not strike his head or lose consciousness. He denies neck pain, arm pain, chest pain, or abdominal pain. He denies numbness, tingling, or weakness in any of his extremities.

Past Medical History

- Transposition of the great vessels, which was corrected during infancy.
- Immunizations UTD.

Medications

- None.

Allergies

- None.

Physical Examination and Ancillary Studies

- *Vital signs*: 97.9 °F, HR 110, RR 19, BP 105/70, O_2 sat 99% on room air.
- *General*: Well-developed child, crying on the stretcher, holding onto his ankle.
- *HEENT*: PERRL. Oropharynx with moist mucous membranes and no lesions. Head is atraumatic.
- *Neck*: No midline tenderness, no step-offs or adenopathy.
- *Cardiovascular*: Regular rate and rhythm. No M/R/G. Brisk capillary refill.
- *Lungs*: CTA bilaterally, with no W/R/R. No chest-wall tenderness.
- *Abdomen*: Soft, no tenderness, no signs of trauma.
- *Extremities and skin*: Child with swelling and tenderness to right medial malleolus, with no obvious deformity. He has intact dorsalis pedis and posterior tibial pulses and a normal sensory examination of the foot. He has no tenderness at

the fibular head and has a normal range of motion at the hip and knee bilaterally. His lateral malleolus is not tender. His skin is warm and well-perfused. The remainder of his extremities are atraumatic and normal.

- *Neurologic*: Normal mental status. Intact sensation to the foot. Has minimal dorsi- and plantar flexion of the right ankle secondary to pain.
- *Pertinent radiographs*: X-ray demonstrating Salter–Harris II fracture of right distal tibia.

Questions for Thought

- How do children's fractures differ from adult fractures?
- What is the prognostic value of the Salter–Harris classification system for fractures?
- What are principles of splinting for fractures?

Diagnosis

- Salter–Harris II fracture of the distal tibia.

Discussion

- *Epidemiology*: Fractures are common in children, occurring with an annual incidence of 180 per 10,000 children younger than age 16.[1] Upper extremities are injured far more commonly than lower extremities, with the clavicle and distal radius being the most commonly fractured bones.[1,2]

  Ankle fractures account for about 5 percent of all pediatric fractures, and account for about 20 percent of pediatric physeal injuries.[3] They typically occur related to sporting injuries or motor vehicle accidents, and are more common in children with an elevated BMI.[1]
- *Pathophysiology*: Children's bones are more pliable and porous than adult bones, with a thicker and stronger periosteum and an increased ability to remodel.[2] These properties are largely responsible for the way in which children's bones fracture. These properties are also responsible for why children's fractures are less likely to displace, less likely to suffer non-union, and more likely to heal quickly.

  Because of the relative strength and flexibility of the periosteum, children may have *plastic deformity*, in which a force is applied to a bone

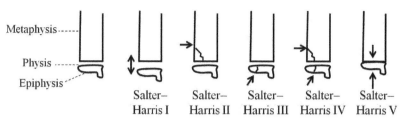

Figure 6.3 Salter–Harris fracture classification system for physeal injuries. Arrows indicate fracture location.

Metaphysis
Physis
Epiphysis

Salter–Harris I   Salter–Harris II   Salter–Harris III   Salter–Harris IV   Salter–Harris V

that is great enough to deform the bone without being so great as to break the periosteum.[2] Further force may break one side of the bone's periosteum, but may not extend completely through, causing an incomplete or a *greenstick fracture*.[2] A compressive force may cause a *buckle* or *torus fracture* which is identified by a loss of smoothness to the cortex on radiography. Finally, children have physes, or growth plates, that are made of cartilage and are a relatively weak area of pediatric bone. *Physeal fractures* are traditionally categorized by the Salter–Harris (S–H) classification system, which both describes the injury and is prognostically important. S–H I fractures are fractures through the physis only and may not be visible on radiography. These are diagnosed based on tenderness on examination, and have an excellent prognosis. S–H II fractures extend through the metaphysis into the physis, and are the most common S–H fracture. These are diagnosed by radiography, and also have an excellent prognosis. They often do not require surgery.[3,4] S–H III fractures extend from the physis through the epiphysis, and are therefore intra-articular fractures. These are higher risk for later arthritis or dysfunction, and require reduction, sometimes with open technique.[4] S–H IV fractures extend from the metaphysis, through the physis, and into the epiphysis. These injuries commonly require operative fixation, and have a high rate of later growth disturbance.[2,4] S–H V fractures are secondary to axial load and crush the physis. These are often missed on radiographs, and have a high rate of later growth failure and a poor prognosis.[2,5] Figure 6.3 demonstrates the S–H fracture classification system.

- *Presentation*: Children with a fracture typically present with pain and swelling at the affected site. Although most children present acutely after the index trauma, sometimes children present

remotely. It is not uncommon for a child to complain of wrist pain at the site of a torus fracture for a day or two before the caregiver brings the child in for medical care. Occasionally, the trauma history is unwitnessed or unknown. Particularly in non-verbal children, the chief complaint may be vague, such as "crying" or "fussiness." Children with lower-extremity fractures will generally refuse to bear weight or will limp. Those with upper-extremity fractures may refuse to use the affected limb, or may simply complain of discomfort. Children with clavicle fractures may have pain with head movement, or their caregivers may attribute their pain to an arm rather than a clavicle injury. The practitioner should always have a high index of suspicion for non-accidental trauma and injuries that are inconsistent with the stated mechanism.

- *Diagnosis*: Although most fractures are definitively diagnosed on radiography, the history and physical examination guides the provider to determine which areas to image. The medical provider should completely expose the patient and assess him or her just like any other trauma patient. Every bone should be palpated, every joint should be ranged. It is important to do a thorough neurovascular examination in all extremities. Some injuries, such as elbow fractures or dislocations, have exceedingly high rates of arterial and nerve injury (in this case, the brachial artery and the ulnar nerve in 5–10 percent of patients). Shoulder dislocations, humeral-shaft fractures, posterior clavicular dislocations, knee dislocations, and lower leg fractures all have well-described neurovascular complications, and any fracture has the potential to cause injury to surrounding structures.

Once the injured area has been identified, the provider should obtain appropriate radiographs to assess the injury. Classically, the radiograph should include imaging of the joint above and the joint below the injury to rule out associated injuries. Since pediatric growth centers can cause both false positive and false negative radiographs, if unsure, the provider should image the unaffected limb for comparison. If there is any doubt as to the presence of a fracture, the child should be splinted and referred to orthopedics.

- *Treatment*: Fractures that are minimally angulated and not rotated are generally treated with casting, although some debate exists as to the utility of casting for torus fractures.[6,7] Lower-extremity fractures should be made non-weight-bearing, typically for 6 weeks. S–H I and non-displaced S–H II fractures are usually treated with casting alone.[2-5] In the ED, it is appropriate to splint these children and call orthopedics to facilitate follow-up in the next 1–2 days for cast application after swelling has gone down. S–H III–V fractures, any fracture with rotational deformity, open fractures, fractures with neurovascular compromise, and fractures associated with compartment syndrome generally require emergency orthopedic consultation. The ED provider should attempt to reduce any fracture with neurovascular compromise rather than wait for a specialist, as ischemia time worsens prognosis.

  Splints should immobilize the joint above and below the injury, and should have one open side to allow for tissue swelling.

- *Disposition*: Non-displaced fractures in patients whose pain is adequately controlled may be discharged and orthopedic follow-up should be arranged. Family should be instructed regarding elevation, ice, and analgesia. Displaced, angulated, open, rotationally deformed, or complicated fractures require ED orthopedic consultation and often require admission for surgical reduction and fixation. Children with minor fractures in whom non-accidental trauma is suspected should also be admitted and CPS should be notified.

Historical clues	Physical findings	Ancillary studies
• Twisting injury to ankle • Inability to bear weight	• Tenderness and swelling over medial malleolus • Intact neurovascular examination	• X-ray with S–H II fracture of distal tibia

Follow-Up

The child's fracture was determined to be non-displaced. He was placed in a long leg splint and provided with crutches and teaching in crutch use. He followed up with orthopedics 2 days later and was casted. He had an excellent functional recovery.

References

1. Randsborg PH, Gulbrandsen P, Saltyté Benth J, et al. Fractures in children: Epidemiology and activity-specific fracture rates. *J Bone Joint Surg Am* 2013; 95: e42.

2. Thornton MD, Della-Giustina K, Aronson, PL. Emergency department evaluation and treatment of pediatric orthopedic injuries. *Emerg Med Clin N Am* 2015; 33: 423–49.

3. Su AW, Larson AN. Pediatric ankle fractures: Concepts and treatment principles. *Foot Ankle Clin* 2015; 20: 705–19.

4. Larsen MC, Bohm KC, Rizkala AR, et al. Outcomes of nonoperative treatment of Salter–Harris II distal radius fractures: A systematic review. *Hand (NY)* 2016; 11: 29–35.

5. Arora R, Fichadia U, Hartwig E, Kannikeswaran N. Pediatric upper-extremity fractures. *Pediatr Ann* 2014; 43: 196–204.

6. Firmin F, Crouch R. Splinting versus casting of "torus" fractures to the distal radius in the paediatric patient presenting at the ED: A literature review. *Int Emerg Nurs* 2009; 17: 173–8.

7. Yeung DE, Jia X, Miller CA, et al. Interventions for treating ankle fractures in children. *Cochrane Database Syst Rev* 2016; 4: CD010836.

Case 1

Contributing Author: Rebecca Jeanmonod

History

A 9-month-old boy is brought in by his mother for vomiting. The child has been having vomiting chronically on and off since birth, and mom has had him evaluated by pediatric gastroenterology, who diagnosed him with gastroparesis. The child has been receiving metoclopramide for this, but still has occasional paroxysms of vomiting. Mom told the triage nurse that the child has been having difficulty keeping anything down for the last 48 hours. He was seen by his pediatrician, who told her the child had gastroenteritis and prescribed a bland diet and ondansetron. Last night, the child was able to take 6 ounces of formula, but vomited during the night and then vomited again this morning. Mom states that the child has not had diarrhea, and his bowel movements have been normal. She has not noted fever or rashes. He has not had blood in his diaper. During the triage assessment, the child becomes unresponsive and has generalized seizure. The nurse rushes him back to an available room, where he continues to seize.

Past Medical History

- Induced at 37 weeks for intrauterine growth retardation, birth weight 5 pounds. The child had a brief NICU stay for hypoglycemia and hypothermia, and had feeding difficulty, resulting in him having a 10-day course in the neonatal nursery.
- The child has been consistently below the 5th percentile for body weight. He has lagged in his milestones and cannot sit unsupported yet.
- He is UTD on immunizations.

Medications

- Metoclopramide.
- Ondansetron.

Allergies

- None.

Physical Examination and Ancillary Studies

- *Vital signs*: T 99 °F, HR 180, RR UTO, BP UTO, O_2 sat UTO.
- *General*: The child is actively seizing.
- *Primary survey*: The child is drooling/foaming at the mouth. He is cyanotic. He has pulses. You do not have an IV line.

> #### Questions for Thought
>
> - Before moving on with your examination, what test must you have?
> - What interventions should you perform?
> - What medications should you give?

Physical Examination and Ancillary Studies

- *Bedside testing*: The child has a fingerstick glucose of 32. You recognize that the nurse has been unable to obtain peripheral access ×2, and place an IO line in the child's right tibia and give the child 2 cc/kg of 25% dextrose solution through the line. You place the patient on 100% oxygen by facemask and place the child on the monitor. The child stops seizing.
- *Vital signs*: T 99 °F, HR 150, RR 45, BP 95/60, O_2 sat 100% on room air.
- *General*: The child is lethargic and post-ictal.

- *HEENT*: There are no signs of head trauma. PERRL. The child has no oral lesions. His mucous membranes are somewhat dry.
- *Neck*: His neck seems supple, and you do not appreciate any adenopathy or masses.
- *Cardiovascular*: Regular tachycardia, with no M/R/G. > 3 second capillary refill.
- *Lungs*: CTA bilaterally, with good air movement.
- *Abdomen*: Soft, with normal bowel sounds. No masses. No hepatomegaly.
- *Extremities and skin*: Pale skin with no rashes or vesicles. No signs of trauma.
- *Neurologic*: The child is lethargic and has poor tone. He is becoming more responsive, moves all four extremities spontaneously, and is intermittently crying.
- *Pertinent laboratory values*: WBC 19,000, Hb normal. Na 141, K 5, Cl 105, bicarbonate 11, BUN 11, Cr 0.3. Urine dip + ketones. LP with low glucose, no cells.
- *Pertinent radiographs*: CXR and head CT negative.

Questions for Thought

- When faced with the seizing hypoglycemic infant, what laboratory tests should you draw to help with later diagnosis?
- If the child continues to be hypoglycemic, how would you manage him?
- If the child wakes up sufficiently and seems hungry, what should you feed him?

Diagnosis

- Inborn error of metabolism.

Discussion

- *Epidemiology*: Inborn errors of metabolism are a heterogeneous group of inherited disorders that involve problems of protein and carbohydrate metabolism and storage. Although each known syndrome is rare, all errors combined occur in about 1 in 2,500 births, making them a significant source of pediatric morbidity and mortality.[1,2] Although neonatal screening detects many disorders, it misses others. Furthermore, inborn errors of metabolism can present in any age group, with only half presenting in the neonatal period.[3] Therefore, it is important to consider this diagnosis in the appropriate clinical scenario.

- *Pathophysiology*: Inborn errors may disrupt carbohydrate metabolism, protein metabolism, fatty acid oxidation, or glycogen storage. When we eat, our bodies break down food into glucose and other metabolic products that are ultimately excreted. Excess glucose is stored as glycogen in the liver and muscle for use in times of fasting. When liver glycogen stores are depleted and the plasma glucose has been used, the body will make new glucose from amino acids (gluconeogenesis) and then, finally, will use fatty acid oxidation to create substrate for the Krebs cycle.[3] To broadly simplify, diseases that result in errors in breaking down foodstuffs will often cause hypoglycemia, ones that interfere with excretion of metabolites will cause intoxication (most commonly with ammonia), and ones that interfere with fatty acid oxidation can cause hypoglycemia and acidosis. Disorders of glycogen storage do not usually present acutely and will not be further addressed here.

- *Presentation:* Children with profound errors in carbohydrate metabolism present catastrophically in the neonatal period, and may be indistinguishable clinically from septic neonates. Because these are heterogeneous diseases, though, they can present in a variety of ways. Diseases that result in intoxication will typically progress over time with lethargy and altered mental status, diseases causing acidosis will present with vomiting and tachypnea, and diseases causing hypoglycemia will present with altered mental status and seizure. However, there is much overlap in different syndromes, and children can present with a mixed presentation or with episodic, seemingly non-progressive symptoms. The most common presentations for inborn errors of metabolism are neurologic (poor tone, poor suck, developmental delay or loss of milestones, seizure) or related to the GI tract (vomiting, food intolerance, hepatomegaly, diarrhea, dehydration).[3,4] Patients may also present with psychosis, behavioral, or learning disabilities, or autonomic instability.[3,4]

  Symptoms may be precipitated by an intercurrent illness that increases catabolism (i.e. febrile condition), fasting (whether because of progressive spacing of feeding during infancy or during GI illness that causes vomiting), dietary changes, or other stressor.[3-5] Often, a precipitant will not be identified, but a review of the child's history may reveal recurrent feeding issues, failure to thrive, or behavioral and developmental concerns.

- *Diagnosis*: Definitive diagnosis of a specific inborn error of metabolism is not a reasonable goal in the ED. That said, it is important not to miss these children, as delay to diagnosis can lead to morbidity and mortality. The first step to diagnosis is considering inborn errors of metabolism in the differential for the child with hypoglycemia, neurologic abnormalities, or GI complaints, or in any ill-appearing neonate. Although the specific diagnosis may require specialized testing that isn't usually performed in the ED, such as serum and urine amino and organic acids, most if not all symptomatic children with inborn errors of metabolism will have elevated lactate levels, hypoglycemia, hyperammonemia, or acidosis on blood testing, or ketonuria or elevated urine reducing substances on urine testing.[3-5] Therefore, a reasonable approach to the child with a possible inborn error of metabolism in the ED is to use serum pH, lactate, ammonia, electrolytes, and glucose testing, together with urine testing, as a screen for this group of diseases. Should the testing be concerning for inborn errors of metabolism, further more specific testing should be ordered in consultation with a metabolic specialist.

It is important to draw all blood for diagnostic testing at the time of the patient's presentation. Laboratory abnormalities in some inborn errors of metabolism may be transient and only present when the child is symptomatic. Therefore, the only opportunity for diagnosis may be on presentation, and diagnosis may be elusive after treatment is begun.[3-5] Because of this, even though the specific diagnostic tests are not typical "ED" tests, the blood should be drawn in the ED.

- *Treatment*: Ill children should be resuscitated, with careful attention to the ABC algorithm. Seizing children with hypoglycemia should receive dextrose. If seizures continue, benzodiazepines should be given. The treatment of a metabolic crisis in the child with inborn error of metabolism is dependent upon what is discovered during evaluation. All patients, however, should be made NPO. The reason for

this is that the provider has no way of knowing which dietary item is responsible for the child's symptoms, and therefore it is imperative to prevent ongoing metabolism.[3,5] Additionally, since the provider will have no way to know if the process involves gluconeogenesis or fatty acid oxidation, the provider must provide enough substrate (glucose) to the patient to prevent them from becoming catabolic and potentially worsening their status. Therefore, these children should be provided with 10% dextrose solution in 1/4 normal saline at 1 1/2 maintenance.[3,5] If the child develops hyperglycemia, insulin (0.2 IU/kg per hour) should be given. Nitrogen scavengers (sodium phenylacetate or sodium benzoate) can be used for patients with elevated ammonia, but toxic children and those with ammonia > 600 should be treated with dialysis.[3,5]

- *Disposition*: A child with a clinical and laboratory picture for inborn errors of metabolism should be admitted to a pediatric center with access to a metabolic specialist. Most children require ICU admission. Prognosis varies widely depending on the specific inborn error and the degree of enzymatic dysfunction.

Historical clues	Physical findings	Ancillary studies
• Failure to thrive • Developmental delay • Frequent vomiting • Prior episodes of hypoglycemia and hypothermia	• Seizure • Vomiting • Dehydration • Tachypnea (signaling acidosis)	• Hypoglycemia • Acidosis (elevated anion gap) • Ketonuria

Follow-Up

The patient remained lethargic with poor tone in the ED. He was given broad-spectrum antibiotics and IV access was attempted, which failed, but blood was drawn. The patient's IO line became dislodged. The patient had a second seizure after 45 minutes in the ED, and repeat glucose was 23. He was given a second IO line in the other leg and another bolus of dextrose. D10 was started, and IV access was obtained. Over the course of about 90 minutes, the child returned to his baseline functioning and mental status. He was transferred to a PICU at a nearby facility where he underwent extensive testing, but his precise diagnosis still eludes the metabolic specialists, as the ED was unable to obtain all necessary blood work prior to treating the child. The child's mother carries a written order for specific blood tests to be sent should the child become ill and present to an ED again in the hopes of establishing a definitive diagnosis and, therefore, a tailored treatment plan. In the meantime, the child is on a strict elemental diet with frequent feeds and blood glucose testing at home. He is enrolled in early intervention.

References

1. Dionisi-Vici C, Rizzo C, Burlina AB, et al. Inborn errors of metabolism in the Italian pediatric population: A national retrospective survey. *J Pediatr* 2002; 140: 321–7.

2. Applegarth DA, Toone JR, Lowry RB. Incidence of inborn errors of metabolism in British Columbia, 1969–1996. *Pediatrics* 2000; 105: e10.

3. Fletcher JM. Metabolic emergencies and the emergency physician. *J Paediatr Child Health* 2016; 52: 227–30.

4. Calvo M, Artuch R, Macia E, et al. Diagnostic approach to inborn errors of metabolism in an emergency unit. *Pediatr Emerg Care* 2000; 16: 405–8.

5. Long D, Long B, Koyfman A. Inborn errors of metabolism: An emergency medicine approach. *Am J Emerg Med* 2016; 34: 317–18.

Case 2

Contributing Author: Erica Escarcega

History

The patient is a 2-year-old male, who has been brought to the ED by his mother for vomiting, which began after waking up this morning. He has had three episodes of vomiting since onset 4 hours ago. He has not been able to tolerate solid food or liquids and vomited several seconds after attempting to eat breakfast. According to his mother, he has been feeling unwell and having diarrhea for the past 2 days. She states that she has changed four to five diapers with watery stools each day. He had been eating and drinking normally until this morning. He last ate at 6:00 pm last night. She is unsure of when he last urinated due to the watery nature of his diarrhea. She does not believe the patient has had a fever, but did not take his temperature. The child states that his belly hurts, but is unable to clarify further. The patient attends daycare regularly.

Past Medical History

- Delivered full-term at 39 weeks' gestation with no complications, immunizations UTD.

Medications

- None.

Allergies

- NKDA.

Physical Examination and Ancillary Studies

- *Vital signs*: T 99.1 °F, HR 135, BP 90/43, RR 25, O_2 sat 100% on room air.
- *General*: The patient appears sleepy, but is easily aroused. He becomes fussy during examination and cries, but with minimal tear production.
- *HEENT*: PERRL. Mucous membranes are tacky and stick to the tongue depressor. Posterior pharynx is clear.
- *Neck*: Supple, with midline trachea, and no adenopathy.
- *Cardiovascular*: The patient is mildly tachycardic, without M/R/G. Central pulses and peripheral pulses normal. Capillary refill 3 seconds.
- *Lungs*: The patient's lungs are CTA bilaterally, without W/R/R.
- *Abdomen*: His abdomen is soft, non-tender, and non-distended, with active bowel sounds throughout. There are no palpable masses.
- *Skin and extremities*: There is no peripheral edema. His skin is warm to the touch and there is no tenting of the skin.
- *Neurologic*: Sleepy and fussy. The child has good tone and normal reflexes.

Questions for Thought

- When would labs be indicated in the management of this patient?
- Is it possible to objectively determine the hydration status in this child without an invasive work-up?
- Should you rehydrate this child using oral rehydration or IV?
- What treatments can be used if the patient continues vomiting in the ED during attempts at rehydration?
- Are antibiotics indicated in the treatment of this condition?

Diagnosis

- Acute gastroenteritis.

Discussion

- *Epidemiology*: Acute gastroenteritis is a common diarrheal illness affecting children worldwide. In the USA alone, more than 1.5 million outpatient visits and 200,000 hospitalizations can be attributed to acute gastroenteritis.[1] As many as 300 children die each year in the USA from dehydration due to this prevalent illness, with approximately 1.5 billion deaths per year worldwide.[1] This number has been declining, likely due to efforts surrounding the development of oral rehydration fluids. Acute gastroenteritis is commonly of viral origin, with bacterial illnesses being less common in the developed world. Rotavirus is the most common cause of viral gastroenteritis.

- *Pathophysiology*: Typically, acute gastroenteritis is an osmotic diarrhea occurring in conjunction with vomiting. Rotavirus creates an osmotic diarrhea by both acting directly on the intestinal villi as well as through the production of an enterotoxin, which results in malabsorption.[2] Children can experience fluid loses exceeding 200 mL/kg body weight per day secondary to diarrheal illness alone, making dehydration the most common cause of morbidity and mortality that is associated with acute gastroenteritis.

- *Presentation*: Patients with acute gastroenteritis typically present with three or more episodes of loose or watery stools per day and a variable history of vomiting.[2] Variations can occur, however, and in some children, vomiting may be the primary complaint. Symptoms are generally present for less than 2 weeks and high-grade fevers are uncommon.[2] If symptoms are present for more than 2 weeks, the practitioner should consider parasitic causes of diarrhea.[2] Patients may present with varying degrees of dehydration. Parents may describe the child as being more irritable than usual, sleepy, or difficult to arouse. Eyes may appear sunken and mucous membranes may be sticky or dry. The child may have decreased tear production. Heart rate and respiratory rates may be elevated and pulses may be diminished.[2] Capillary refill may be prolonged and urine output may be decreased. Decreases in blood pressure generally portend severe dehydration and shock.[2] Although there are many scoring systems to help the clinician identify dehydration clinically, the assessment of hydration status is overall an imprecise science.[2]

- *Diagnosis*: Acute gastroenteritis is usually a clinical diagnosis. Laboratory tests are not routinely indicated.[2] However, it is important to distinguish this from dysenteric forms of diarrheal illness, which typically will require more extensive work-up and treatment. Children who have blood or mucous in their stool should have stool cultures performed and may require antibiotics.[2] Children with a prolonged course of illness should have stool studies, and those with neurologic abnormalities should be tested for toxin-producing pathogens.[2] Patients with fever or underlying medical conditions which may result in a compromised immune system will also require more extensive work-up. More severe illness can typically be ruled out through the history and physical. In cases of severe dehydration, obtaining serum electrolytes, bicarbonate, BUN, Cr, and glucose should be considered.[2] Hypernatremia may occur in more severe cases.

- *Treatment*: Treatment for parasitic infection or bacterial infection may require specific antimicrobial treatment, but most gastroenteritis is viral. Therefore, the treatment for acute gastroenteritis is supportive and centered around rehydration and maintenance of the patient's fluid status. Cases with mild to moderate dehydration are usually able to be managed with oral rehydration.[1] The child should be given small amounts of rehydration solution, beginning with 5 mL at first and gradually increasing, as tolerated. More recently, ondansetron has been used in children with acute gastroenteritis. Patients receiving ondansetron have been shown to be less likely to require admission to the hospital for rehydration, and are less likely to require IV rehydration, with one in five children having complete cessation of vomiting in the ED.[3] There are concerns, however, that ondansetron may result in cardiac arrhythmias after the finding of prolonged QT with 32 mg IV administration.[4] Despite this, there have been no reports of arrhythmias from single oral doses of ondansetron, which are typically administered in the ED. Antimotility agents should be avoided due to limited efficacy and side effects, such as ileus, increased nausea, and drowsiness. More severe dehydration may require IV resuscitation. Please see Case 7 in Chapter 2 for further discussion on rehydration techniques.

- *Disposition*: The vast majority of patients with gastroenteritis may be discharged home. Admission is appropriate for those with altered mental status, evidence of shock, and those who require ongoing volume resuscitation.

Historical clues	Physical findings
• Nausea	• Tacky mucous membranes
• Vomiting	• Tachycardia
• Diarrhea	• Minimal tear production

Follow-Up

This child had another episode of vomiting in the ED when his mother attempted to give him a small amount of rehydration fluid. The patient was given 2 mg ondansetron, after which he was able to tolerate oral rehydration without further episodes of emesis. He was discharged home in the care of his mother, at which point he was able to resume his normal diet. The patient had an uneventful recovery and was able to return to daycare after 2 days.

References

1. King C, Glass R, Bresee J, et al. Managing acute gastroenteritis among children: Oral rehydration, maintenance, and nutritional therapy. *MMWR Recomm Rep* 2003; 52: 1–16.

2. Churgay CA, Aftab Z. Gastroenteritis in children: Part I. Diagnosis. *Am Fam Phys* 2012; 85: 1059–62.

3. DeCamp L, Byerly J, Doshi N, et al. Use of antiemetic agents in acute gastroenteritis: A systematic review and meta-analysis. *Arch Pediatr Adolesc Med* 2008; 162: 858–65.

4. Freedman S, Uleryk E, Rumantir M, et al. Ondansetron and the risk of cardiac arrhythmias: A systematic review and postmarketing analysis. *Ann Emerg Med* 2014; 64: 19–25.

Case 3

Contributing Author: Kinsey Leonard

History

A 3-year-old boy is brought to the ED by his tearful mother with a chief complaint of vomiting. Mom states

she was bathing her 1-month-old infant while her toddler napped on the floor in the next room. She heard him playing and went to check on him after removing the infant from the bath. She noticed he had pulled several items off her dresser including some coins, a screw, a bottle of prenatal vitamins, a bottle of ibuprofen, and a bottle of acetaminophen. The pill bottles were open, but the child told his mother he did not eat anything. The child seemed to be fine at first, but started vomiting about 30–45 minutes later. She has noted blood in the emesis. He is now holding his abdomen and saying his tummy hurts.

On review of systems, mom states that he is a healthy boy and denies recent illness. She denies fevers, chills, headaches, cough, rhinorrhea, sore throat, difficulty breathing, or urinary complaints. She denies known sick contacts. He does not attend daycare.

Past Medical History

- No significant medical problems. He is UTD on immunizations.

Medications

- Pediatric chewable multivitamins.

Allergies

- NKDA.

Physical Examination and Ancillary Studies

- *Vital signs*: T 98.2 °F, HR 165, BP 75/40, RR 42, O₂ sat 100% on room air.
- *General*: The patient is awake, but not very interactive. He is laying on the stretcher looking at his mom. He is average size for a 3-year-old.
- *HEENT*: PERRL. No signs of trauma. No oropharyngeal erythema or foreign body.
- *Neck*: Supple neck, with midline trachea.
- *Cardiovascular*: Tachycardic with regular rhythm. No M/R/G. Capillary refill < 3 seconds.
- *Lungs*: Clear bilaterally. No W/R/R.
- *Abdomen*: The child has positive bowel sounds. He grimaces when the abdomen is palpated diffusely. No guarding or rebound tenderness.
- *Extremities and skin*: Extremities have no deformity or signs of trauma. Skin is warm and dry without rashes.
- *Neurologic*: Listless, but has symmetric strength and intact reflexes.

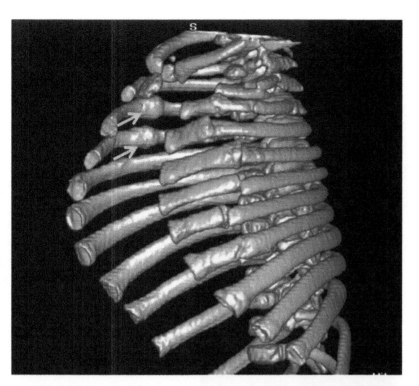

Figure 2.4 CT chest reconstruction: Lateral view showing multiple rib fractures.

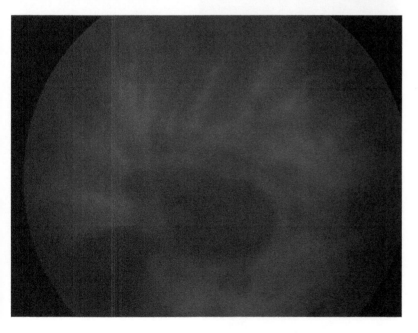

Figure 2.5 Retinal hemorrhages.

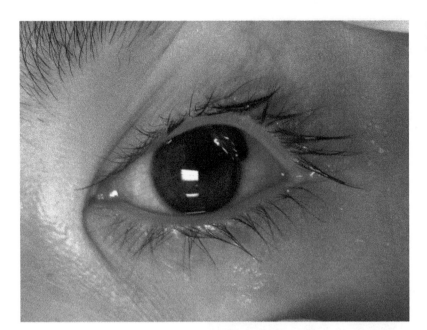

Figure 5.2 Photograph of patient's left eye, demonstrating an irregular pupil and extruded iris.

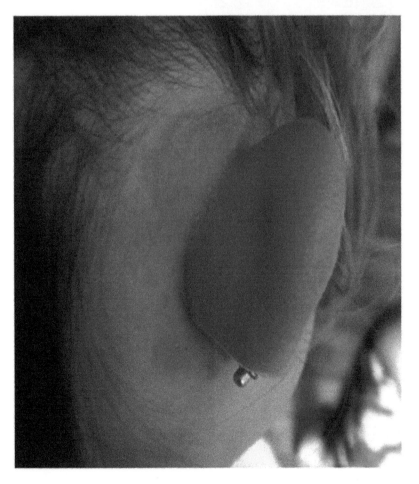

Figure 5.3 Erythema and swelling behind the pinna.

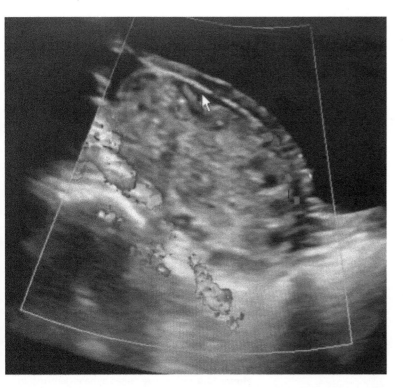

Figure 8.7 U/S of torsed ovary demonstrating decreased internal blood flow, but some evidence of peripheral flow. It is important to image both the affected and the unaffected side for comparison.

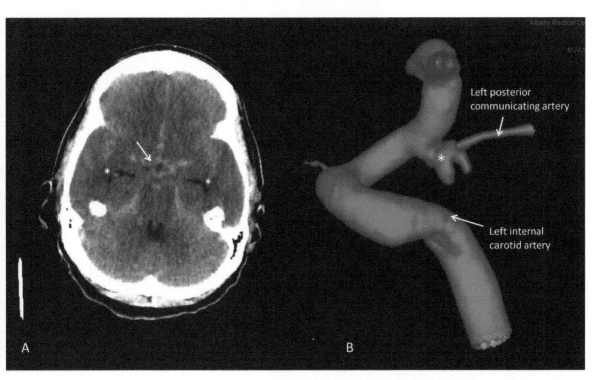

Left posterior communicating artery

Left internal carotid artery

A   B

Figure 10.5 (A) Non-contrast axial CT, demonstrating diffuse subarachnoid hemorrhage (arrow) as well as mild dilation of the temporal horns of the lateral ventricles (asterisk). (B) Three-dimensional angiography image of the left posterior carotid wall aneurysm (asterisk) associated with the left posterior communicating artery.

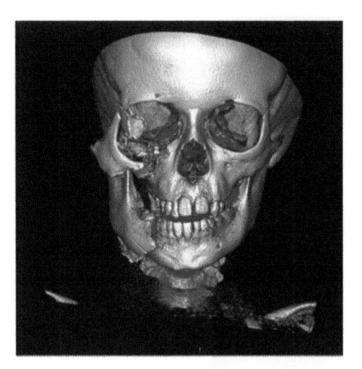

Figure 12.3 CT of head and face. There is no acute intracranial injury. There are numerous comminuted facial fractures, notably a comminuted orbital floor fracture, comminuted zygomaticomaxillary complex fracture, zygomatic arch fracture, fracture of the greater wing of the right sphenoid, and open comminuted mandible fracture–dislocation, with displacement of multiple primary teeth. The right orbit is also noted to be displaced inferiorly but without radiographic evidence of globe injury or optic nerve injury.

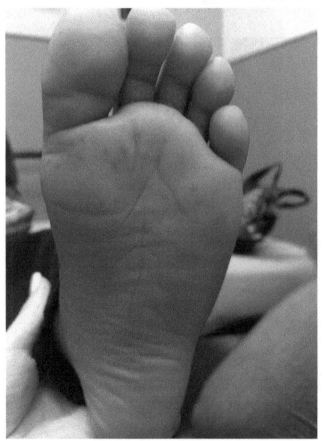

Figure 12.4 Rash on sole caused by hand–foot–mouth disease.

- *Pertinent laboratory values*: Na 144, K 4.7, Cl 103, bicarbonate 10, glucose 160, WBC 16,000, Hb 9.3, Plt 300,000.

Questions for Thought

- What imaging modalities would you use, if any, to make the diagnosis?
- What laboratories would you order and which would be abnormal?
- What treatments would you start in the ED?
- What determines the disposition of the patient?

Diagnosis

- Acute iron toxicity.

Discussion

- *Epidemiology*: In the USA, there are approximately 16,000 cases of iron ingestions reported annually in children under 6 years old.[1] Most ingestions are accidental, owing to the fact that iron pills and prenatal vitamins resemble candies, even coming in gummy formulations. Children with a sibling's birth in the prior 6 months and those age 3 and younger are at higher risk.[2] The risk of serious toxicity is greatest when the iron formulation is marketed for adults (e.g. adult pure iron pills or prenatal vitamins).[3] Children's chewable vitamins have not been found to cause serious harm.[3] Intentional overdoses typically occur in adolescent females.
- *Pathophysiology*: Iron is absorbed in the duodenum as ferrous iron and oxidized in mucosal cells to ferric iron. Once transferrin, the iron binding protein, and ferritin, the intracellular storage protein, are overwhelmed, ferric iron causes toxic effects by forming free radicals in multiple organ systems.[4]

  Free radicals cause mucosal cell damage in the GI tract with symptoms of abdominal pain, vomiting, diarrhea, and GI bleeding. Once free iron enters the bloodstream, systemic toxicity can be widespread. Effects include: uncoupling of the oxidative phosphorylation in the mitochondria, interference in the electron transport chain, and enzyme inhibition in the Krebs cycle. Acidosis results from hydroxyl free radicals and lipid peroxidation. Death usually results from shock or liver failure due to iron overload in the liver. Coagulation abnormalities may be seen due to the inhibition of an enzyme needed in thrombin formation. Shock results from hypotension and vasodilation. Iron deposits also accumulate in the myocardium, causing toxicity.

  Serum iron concentrations normally peak 6 hours after an overdose. Most studies agree that elemental iron ingestion of less than 20 mg/kg does not cause significant symptoms. Ingestion of greater than 60 mg/kg of elemental iron can cause serious morbidity and mortality.
- *Presentation*: Patient presentation depends on time since ingestion and is divided into five phases:
  - *GI irritation* (first few hours after ingestion): Symptoms resembling a GI illness, including abdominal pain, fatigue, nausea, vomiting, and diarrhea. There may be blood in the emesis or stool. Hypovolemic shock can result during this first stage.
  - *Latent phase* ($>$ 6 hours to 24 hours): GI symptoms resolve and the patient appears better clinically. Systemically, the child may become more hypovolemic and acidotic. Laboratory tests will differentiate worsening serious toxicity vs. recovery from mild toxicity. Vitals signs may also be abnormal, the patient may be tachycardic and/or hypotensive.
  - *Systemic toxicity* ($>$ 6 hours to 3 days): Patients who progress will develop lactic acidosis and hypovolemic shock during this phase. The child may also have worsening GI bleeding due to the disruption of the coagulation pathway. Organ failure may occur, including respiratory distress, cardiomyopathy (with subsequent cardiogenic shock), and renal failure.
  - *Hepatotoxicity* (48 hours to 5 days): Patients who continue to progress will develop elevated LFTs and may have liver failure secondary to lipid peroxidation.
  - *Gastric outlet obstruction* ($>$ 2 weeks after ingestion): This is a rarely seen late complication of iron toxicity, caused by scar formation from damage to the mucosa at the level of the gastric outlet.
- *Diagnosis*: History is key to making the diagnosis, as patients will typically present during the initial phase that resembles a GI infection.[3] Careful history taking from the parents should include if the patient was left unsupervised, had access to

any medications, and what medications are in the home. This should include the type of iron (ferrous sulfate pills vs. prenatal vitamins vs. multivitamins) and the suspected number of tablets ingested.

Once iron ingestion is suspected, laboratory tests should include a CBC, coagulation profile, LFTs, BUN/Cr, serum iron level, electrolytes, and glucose. If severe toxicity is suspected, a blood type and screen, ABG, and lactic acid level should also be ordered. If the child had access to other medications or drugs, acetaminophen and salicylate levels and urine toxicology may also be beneficial. An abdominal plain film may be ordered to see if any radiopaque tablets are visible. Chewable formulations are not usually seen on plain films.

Serum iron levels are helpful in confirming that iron was ingested, but less helpful in determining the degree of toxicity. Absorption time and peak levels vary depending on the iron formulation. The serum iron level reflects free iron, while intracellular iron is what causes toxic effects. Therefore, the iron level should not falsely reassure the clinician that the child will not have severe toxicity. The best time to draw serum iron levels is 4–6 hours after ingestion. Iron levels can also be trended over time during treatment, as treatment lowers the iron level. Generally, patients with levels < 300 mcg/dL have absent to mild symptoms, 300–500 mcg/dL usually have GI toxicity and possible systemic toxicity, > 500 mcg/dL have moderate to severe symptoms, and > 1,000 mcg/dL have significant morbidity and mortality.

- *Treatment*: The child's ABC should be addressed. Two IV sites should be established and the child should be given a bolus of crystalloid and placed on the monitor.

Charcoal is not recommended for iron toxicity since there is no evidence of benefit and it may be detrimental if the patient requires subsequent airway intervention or endoscopy. Orogastric lavage can be considered if the child presents within an hour of ingestion, but will not be beneficial in removing large pill fragments and has never shown a benefit in poisonings. Polyethylene glycol has been shown to be beneficial in cases where the child ingests several pills (dose is 250–500 mL/hr).

Children who present with severe systemic toxicity, shock, metabolic acidosis, or serum iron concentrations > 500 mcg/dL should be given deferoxamine, an iron chelating agent. It should be started at 5 mg/kg per hour because it can lead to hypotension. The rate can be slowly increased to 15 mg/kg per hour, as tolerated. The recommended dose in 24 hours is 36 mg/kg or 6 g. If treatment is being considered past 24 hours, dosing should be determined with the help of a toxicologist. Simultaneous fluid resuscitation should continue during treatment in the second IV site.

The decision to stop treatment is usually based on clinical recovery. Alternatively, serial urine samples can be used to determine therapy duration. Deferoxamine forms ferrioxamine when it chelates iron, which causes a characteristic orange to rusty color when it is excreted in urine ("vin rose"). As iron levels fall, the urine clears. This method is limited since the urine color change is not observed in all patients.

Deferoxamine treatment requires an ICU admission, given the side effects of the treatment, which include hypotension, renal failure, ARDS, mucormycosis, and sepsis.

If the patient has coagulation abnormalities, consider treatment with vitamin K or fresh frozen plasma. If the patient has GI bleeding and is anemic, transfusion should be performed.

Hemodialysis has been used in some cases after deferoxamine treatment in patients who have progressed to renal failure and cannot excrete the ferrioxamine.

- *Disposition*: If the patient is asymptomatic, has normal vitals, and ingested < 20 mg/kg, he or she can be observed in the ED for 6 hours. Mild symptoms, including abdominal pain and less than three episodes of emesis, can also be observed for 6 hours. Children with mild to moderate symptoms should be admitted for a longer observation period. If the child received deferoxamine, admission to the PICU is warranted.

Historical clues	Physical findings	Ancillary studies
• Child < 6 years	• Hypotension	• Anion gap
• Access to iron	• Tachypnea	acidosis
• Abdominal pain	• Tachycardia	• Non-specific
• GI symptoms	• Abdominal	leukocytosis
• Blood in emesis	tenderness	

Follow-Up

The child's serum iron level returned at 400 mcg/dL. He was given deferoxamine because of the severity of his symptoms and his acidosis. He improved over 24 hours and was ultimately discharged home with no sequelae.

References

1. Bronstein AC, Spyker DA, Cantilena LR Jr, et al. 2010 Annual report of the American Association of Poison Control Centers' National Poison Data System (NPDS): 28th Annual Report. *Clin Toxicol (Phila)* 2011; 49: 910–41.

2. Juurlink DN, Tenenbein M, Koren G, et al. Iron poisoning in young children: Association with the birth of a sibling. *CMAJ* 2003; 168: 1539–42.

3. McGregor T, Parkar M, Rau S. Evaluation and management of common childhood poisonings. *Am Fam Phys* 2009; 79: 397–403.

4. Tenenbein M. Toxicokinetics and toxicodynamics of iron poisoning. *Toxicol Lett* 1998; 102–103: 653–6.

Case 4

Contributing Authors: Angela Mastantuono and Melanie K. Prusakowski

History

The patient is a 4-month-old infant boy, born at term without complications, who presents to the ED with vomiting some of his feeds. He was acting normally last night but woke this morning unusually fussy. He remained fussy after his morning nap. While mom notes he has always been a gassy baby, today's fussiness is out of the ordinary. He is not interested in eating. He does not normally spit up, but today he seems to be choking and has spat up several times. He appears pale to his parents and has become less active.

Past Medical History

- Full-term born by spontaneous vaginal delivery, without complications in pregnancy or delivery.
- Recent allergy testing for "teal green" stool was negative. He was switched to an elemental formula, but parents have not noticed a difference in his gassiness or stools.
- He received his age-appropriate vaccines 5 days ago.

Medications

- None.

Allergies

- NKDA and recent allergy testing negative.

Physical Examination and Ancillary Studies

- *Vital signs*: T 98.3 °F, HR 140, RR 36, 103/43, O_2 sat 98% on room air.
- *General*: On initial evaluation the patient is limp in mom's arms and not responding to gentle stimuli of the examination.
- *HEENT*: Anterior fontanelle is soft and flat, mucous membranes are moist.
- *Neck*: Supple and non-tender.
- *Cardiovascular*: Regular rate and rhythm. No M/R/G.
- *Lungs*: Effort normal and breath sounds normal. No respiratory distress noted.
- *Abdomen*: Soft and mildly distended, patient awakes during palpation and begins crying.
- *Extremities and skin*: Pale, warm, dry. No signs of trauma.
- *Neurologic*: Tired and ill-appearing but can be stimulated, strong cry and normal tone after IV placement.
- *Pertinent laboratory values*: WBC 17,800, Plt 560,000, metabolic panel within normal limits.
- *Pertinent imaging*: U/S shows distended and fluid-filled stomach. There is a 5-cm tubular structure in the midline lower pelvis (Figure 7.1). Bowel and gastric gas prohibits full interrogation of the mesenteric vessels for malrotation.

> **Questions for Thought**
>
> - What diagnostic test can also treat the suspected condition?
> - Would any other laboratory tests be valuable?
> - Does this patient require inpatient admission?
> - Is this a typical presentation for this condition?
> - What vaccine was previously blamed for an increased incidence of this condition?

Diagnosis

- Intussusception (likely colocolic or colorectal).

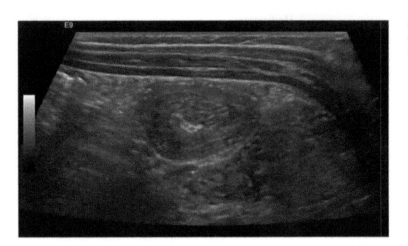

Figure 7.1 U/S demonstrating a cross-sectional image through a tubular structure in the pelvis.

Discussion

- *Epidemiology*: Intussusception is the most common cause of bowel obstruction in young children and the second most common pediatric surgical emergency.[1] It occurs when a portion of the bowel "telescopes" into another segment, potentially leading to bowel ischemia and necrosis. Intussusception is most common in children less than 5 years old (approximately 1 to 4 in 2,000 infants and children), with peak incidence less than 1 year of age.[1] A viral infection precedes intussusception in up to 20 percent of cases.

- *Pathophysiology*: The cause of intussusception is most often idiopathic. There is a correlation with viral infections and increased incidence of intussusception during viral seasons. Sometimes a mechanical lead point, such as a polyp, Meckel's diverticulum, lymph node, or tumor can be identified. Bowel is thought to telescope over such a structure. A malignant lead point is more typical in older children and adults.[2] Intussusception most commonly (75–95 percent of cases) occurs at the terminal ileum, but may occur anywhere along the bowel. This location is presumably due to the large amount of lymphoid tissue in the ileocolic region. A past formulation of the rotavirus vaccine was associated with an increased incidence of intussusception, but the newer formulation is not.[3] Intussusception can become a surgical emergency and, if left untreated, will lead to death.

- *Presentation*: Classic presentations of intussusception describe intermittent but severe abdominal pain. These children often vomit after the episodes of colicky pain. The pathognomonic "currant jelly stools" can be seen as a result of bowel-wall ischemia and venous engorgement, causing passage of mucous and blood that appears to look like red jelly, but this is a late finding.[1] A larger proportion of children will have hemoccult-positive stools.[1] Ideally, intussusception is diagnosed before the development of advanced ischemia, and so the classic triad of abdominal pain, vomiting, and bloody stools is present in only a small percentage of presentations. The abdominal examination can vary from soft and non-tender to acute. Some literature describes a palpable sausage-shaped mass in the right lower quadrant, but this may be difficult to appreciate in a squirming infant. Patients may be asymptomatic between episodes initially but, as the intussusception progresses, the infant or child can become lethargic. Lethargy may be the only presenting symptom in 10 percent of children, and small children may seem to have no pain at all.[1]

- *Diagnosis*: History and examination are important to diagnosis. Physician gestalt as to which patients do not have intussusception has a specificity of 85 percent and a negative predictive value of 94 percent.[1] Laboratory testing does not add much to the diagnosis, although it may support concern for ischemia (elevated lactate or WBC) or dehydration.

- Previously, the gold standard diagnostic and treatment modality for intussusception was an air- or water-soluble contrast enema. More recently, studies warn against moving directly to enema due to the risks of the procedure (bowel-wall perforation, infection) and exposure to radiation.[4,5] Plain radiographs can occasionally be useful, and may provide clues such as a paucity of gas in the right abdomen or findings consistent with bowel obstruction.[1] The use of screening U/S has decreased unnecessary enemas for clinically suspected intussusception, and has a sensitivity of 85 percent and a specificity of 97 percent.[1,4,5]

- *Treatment*: Initial management involves fluid resuscitation, pain control, and management of sepsis or shock, when present. Intussusception can become a surgical emergency and lead to death if untreated. Reduction of the intussusception occurs with air- or water-soluble contrast enema. If there are no signs of peritonitis (a contraindication to enema), enema may be attempted even with 24 hours of symptoms.[6] If the intussusception cannot be reduced with an enema, manual reduction with laparotomy is required. Resection of necrotic bowel may be necessary. Surgeons may also attempt to identify the "lead point" that caused the intussusception. Occasionally, complications of reduction, such as bowel-wall perforation, require surgical intervention.

- *Disposition*: There is a 5–10 percent recurrence rate in the first couple days after the reduction of an intussusception.[7] The decision to admit depends on the ease of the reduction, the clinical status at presentation, and practitioner practice. A period of observation in the ED following the reduction is considered safe practice.[7] Caregivers of patients who are discharged must be educated about signs and symptoms of recurrence, which generally is not associated with an unfavorable outcome.[7]

Historical clues	Physical findings	Ancillary studies
• Vomiting • Fussiness • Pallor	• Distended abdomen • Tender abdomen • Limp, lethargic child • Pallor	• Elevated WBC • Elevated Plt (acute phase reactant) • U/S with intussusception

Follow-Up

The baby underwent air-contrast enema reduction of the intussusception with no incident. He was admitted to the hospital for observation and was discharged home with no sequelae.

References

1. Smith J, Fox SM. Pediatric abdominal pain: An emergency medicine perspective. *Emerg Med Clin N Am* 2016; 34: 341–61.

2. Choi SH, Han JK, Kim SH, et al. Intussusception in adult patients: From stomach to rectum. *AJR Am J Roentgenol* 2004; 183: 691–8.

3. Tate JE, Yen C, Steiner CA, et al. Intussusception rates before and after the introduction of rotavirus vaccine. 2016; 138: e20161082.

4. Hentikson S, Blane CE, Koujok K, et al. The effect of screening sonography on the positive rate of enemas for intussusception. *Pediatr Radiol* 2003; 33: 190–3.

5. Bartocci M, Fabrizi G, Valente I, et al. Intussusception in childhood: Role of sonography on diagnosis and treatment. *J Ultrasound* 2015; 18: 205–11.

6. van den Ende ED, Allema JH, Hazebroek FWJ, et al. Success with hydrostatic reduction of intussusception in relation to duration of symptoms. *Arch Dis Child* 2005; 90: 1071–2.

7. Al-Jazaeri A, Yazbeck S, Filiatrault D, et al. Utility of hospital admission after successful enema reduction of ileocolic intussusception. *J Pediatr Surg* 2006; 41(5): 1010–13.

Case 5

Contributing Author: Rebecca Jeanmonod

History

A 38-month-old girl is brought into the ED by her distraught parents for vomiting. Her parents report that she was napping on the sofa when she woke suddenly and complained of not feeling well. She seemed pale and ill-appearing to them. She then began vomiting and lost consciousness, and has not woken up since. The parents attempted to revive her by putting cold water on her face and shaking her gently, but this was not successful. Her symptoms began about 10 minutes ago. Her parents, who live down the street from the hospital, brought her in immediately because "the ambulance takes too long." On arrival to triage, the parents are screaming "somebody help my baby." The child is brought to a resuscitation bay. As you initiate resuscitation, the parents report that the child has been otherwise healthy recently, with no fevers, weight loss, or difficulty breathing. They do recall that twice in the past 18 months, they had gotten up in the morning to get the child out of bed and noted that she had vomited in the bed, but they assumed this was likely secondary to reflux, as the child woke in good spirits and otherwise seemed well.

Past Medical History

- Born at 41 weeks, c-section for failure to progress, no complications. Child is UTD on immunizations and developmentally normal. She is potty-trained and attends preschool.

Medications

- None.

Allergies

- NKDA.

Physical Examination and Ancillary Studies

- *Vital signs*: T 100 °F, HR 90, RR 36, BP 90/60, O_2 sat 99% on room air.
- *General*: The child is pale and diaphoretic.
- *HEENT*: There are no signs of head trauma. The child has dilated pupils and tonic eye deviation to the right. She is drooling.
- *Neck*: Supple and non-tender, with no adenopathy.
- *Cardiovascular*: Regular bradycardia, with no M/R/G. >3 second capillary refill.
- *Lungs*: CTA bilaterally, with good air movement. There are transmitted upper-airway sounds.
- *Abdomen*: Soft with hyperactive bowel sounds. No masses. No hepatomegaly.
- *Extremities and skin*: Pale with no rashes or vesicles. No signs of trauma.
- *Neurologic*: The child is unresponsive, but breathing spontaneously. She occasionally vocalizes. She does not respond to voice but unreliably responds to pain.
- *Pertinent laboratory values*: Fingerstick glucose 75, CBC and chemistries normal, blood culture sent.

Questions for Thought

- What is the differential diagnosis for the vomiting child with an abnormal mental status?
- Are there any medications that you should begin prior to definitive diagnosis?
- What are your management priorities?

Diagnosis

- Panayiotopoulos syndrome (a common seizure disorder in children characterized by autonomic dysfunction).

Discussion

- *Epidemiology*: Panayiotopoulos syndrome was initially described in 1989, and is thought to affect greater than 10 percent of young children (age 3–6) with non-febrile seizures.[1] Seizure disorders in general affect children commonly: 2–4 percent of children will have at least one febrile seizure, 0.05–1 percent will have a seizure from a metabolic or neurologic process (most commonly in the first year of life), and about 0.1 percent will develop repetitive seizure episodes.[2]
- *Pathophysiology*: All seizures are a result of an abnormal discharge of electrical activity in the brain. This abnormal electrical activity may be present and evident on EEG all the time, or it may only be present during provocation or actual seizure. Seizures may be primary (genetically determined or idiopathic) or they may be secondary to trauma, structural lesions/masses, toxins, infections, or metabolic derangements. Depending upon the portion of the brain involved, seizures may present with focal or generalized motor activity, abnormalities in behavior, staring spells, syncope, thought disturbances, visual symptoms, or prominent autonomic symptoms. Autonomic symptoms such as ictal vomiting are common in temporal lobe seizures in infants and children as well as in Panayiotopoulos syndrome.[3]
- *Presentation*: Seizure patients may present in dramatic and obvious ways, such as those presenting in convulsive status epilepticus, or in more subtle ways, as in this case. The approach to treatment of convulsive status is addressed elsewhere in this book. It is critical that the EM provider remember that not all seizure patients move, and not all that move will do so convulsively. In myoclonic seizures, there may be a single jerking movement. In atonic seizures, the patient loses muscle tone and may fall to the ground. In tonic seizures, there may be generalized muscle stiffening. In complex partial seizures, the patient may seem confused and engage in automatic or restless behaviors, such as

lip smacking or repetitive movements. In absence seizures, the child may stare off into space. In small children, there may be no, or subtle, motor abnormalities and they often have prominent autonomic symptoms.[3,4] Because the clinician may not recognize this as a seizure, the child may be misdiagnosed and undergo invasive evaluation and treatment for the wrong condition.[5,6]

Children with Panayiotopoulos syndrome most commonly have seizures that occur during, or shortly after, sleeping. The seizures characteristically are long lasting, often greater than 30 minutes, and may have no motor findings, although some children will develop unilateral convulsions near the end of the seizure. To make the diagnosis of Panayiotopoulos syndrome, the child must meet five of the following criteria: infrequent seizures, prolonged seizures lasting greater than 5 minutes, ictal vomiting, eye deviation, autonomic manifestations, behavioral disturbances, and an altered level of consciousness.[5] Because of how long the seizures last, children may present with ongoing refractory vomiting, abnormal vital signs, incontinence, and confusion. As the seizures often occur at night or during naps, family may be unaware of the event and only note vomiting, or may bring the child in during the post-ictal period because of abnormal level of consciousness. Children typically recover completely within several hours and return to their normal level of consciousness.

- *Diagnosis*: The diagnosis of Panayiotopoulos syndrome or any seizure relies on clinical suspicion, a thorough history, a complete examination, and judicious ancillary testing. In any child with altered sensorium and abnormal vital signs, the provider should consider the dangerous differential diagnosis, *THE MISFITS* (*T*rauma, *H*ypovolemia/heart, *E*ndocrine, *M*etabolic, *I*ntestinal disasters, *S*eizures, *F*ormula misadventures, *I*nborn errors of metabolism, *T*oxicologic, and *S*epsis). Certainly in this case, this child is ill-appearing, and it is appropriate to pursue multiple differential items simultaneously while actively treating the child. A thorough head-to-toe examination may demonstrate clues to seizure like eye deviation, or autonomic symptoms such as drooling and mydriasis, but even once seizure is diagnosed, the underlying cause of the seizure must be considered. The

child's seizure could be from traumatic injury, CNS infection or masses, hypoglycemia, or toxins. Therefore, diagnostic evaluation should include laboratory chemistry studies (especially a fingerstick glucose!), toxicology screens, and neuroimaging.

The definitive diagnosis of seizure disorder relies on the clinical history, examination, and EEG. Not every patient with a seizure has an abnormal EEG, and EEG abnormalities can be transient or provoked. Furthermore, not every person with an abnormal EEG has a seizure disorder. Use of a video EEG may improve sensitivity and specificity. Although some advocate for use of prolactin levels to diagnose seizure, this is not a sensitive test and has not been studied in all subtypes of seizure disorder.[7]

- *Treatment*: Treatment of ongoing seizure activity in the ED is usually accomplished with benzodiazepines as a first-line agent, and any patient in status epilepticus should receive benzodiazepines. In the subset of patients with Panayiotopoulos syndrome, there is no evidence or even consensus regarding how to treat autonomic status epilepticus.[3] That said, a recent study suggests that there may be progressive cognitive dysfunction in children with Panayiotopoulos syndrome who present with status epilepticus, which suggests rescue treatment may still be indicated, and this is supported in several case reports as well.[5,6] It is unlikely that the EM provider will unilaterally make the diagnosis of this syndrome in the ED at the patient's first presentation. Therefore, if the child is recognized as actively seizing, the EM provider should treat the patient as any other seizing child.

In general, outpatient antiepileptic therapy is not prescribed to patients with Panayiotopoulos syndrome because their seizures are very infrequent and most patients will outgrow them in about 2 years. EM providers should not begin any seizing patient on prophylactic anti-seizure medications without consulting with a neurologist, as these medications may have deleterious effects and also may interfere with the child's future diagnostic testing.

- *Disposition*: A child with a first-time seizure who has returned to baseline, has a negative evaluation, and has reliable parents with good follow-up may be discharged from the ED with prescriptions and instructions for rescue medications. If any of these conditions are not met, the child should be admitted to the hospital for observation and to initiate neurology consultation, neuroimaging, and an EEG.

Historical clues	Physical findings
• Prior episodes of "isolated" vomiting • Onset during nap • Altered mental status	• Pallor • Eye deviaton • Autonomic findings (low-grade temperature, bradycardia, drooling, mydriasis, incontinence, diaphoresis)

Follow-Up

The patient was recognized to be having a seizure and was given a weight-based dose of IV lorazepam while being placed on the monitor. She was additionally given 20 cc/kg of normal saline and broad-spectrum antibiotics because of her ill appearance and poor perfusion. The child's eye deviation resolved and she was post-ictal, with lethargy for several hours. During that time, she underwent head CT, which was unremarkable, LP, which was normal, and was admitted to the PICU for ongoing monitoring. While inpatient, the child had a sleep EEG performed, which showed ictal occipital discharge spikes. The child was discharged home the next day with neurology follow-up. She had two more episodes over the following 2 years, and has since been seizure-free and developmentally normal.

References

1. Panayiotopoulos CP. Benign childhood epilepsy with occipital paroxysms: A 15-year prospective study. *Ann Neurol* 1989; 26: 51–6.

2. Hauser WA. The prevalence and incidence of convulsive disorders in children. *Epilepsia* 1994; 35 Suppl 2: S1–6.

3. Ferrie CD, Caraballo R, Covanis A, et al. Autonomic status epilepticus in Panayiotopoulos syndrome and other childhood and adult epilepsies: A consensus view. *Epilepsia* 2007; 48: 1165–72.

4. Aksoy A, Haliloglu G, Yalnizoglu D, et al. Childhood epilepsy with occipital paroxysm: Classification, atypical evolution and long-term prognosis in 35 patients. *Turk J Pediatr* 2015; 57: 439–52.

5. Zaki SA, Verma DK, Tayde P. Panayiotopoulos syndrome in a child masquerading as septic shock. *Indian J Crit Care Med* 2016; 20: 361–3.

6. Dirani M, Yamak W, Beydoun A. Panayiotopoulos syndrome presenting with respiratory arrest: A case
report and literature review. *Epilepsy Behav Case Rep* 2015; 3: 12–14.

7. Sundararajan T, Tesar GE, Jimenez XF. Biomarkers in the diagnosis and study of psychogenic nonepileptic seizures: A systematic review. *Seizure* 2016; 35: 11–22.

Case 6

Contributing Author: Jason Black

History

A 4-year-old male presents for evaluation of vomiting this morning upon awakening. Mom states that the child has had vomiting upon awakening two other times in the past week, but then had no further episodes during the day. Today he has continued to vomit. The patient's mother noticed some "twitching" in her son's right arm that lasted for a moment and stopped spontaneously 3 days ago. Mom also has thought that the child has been "less coordinated" the last couple days, bumping into things and less steady on his feet, which she believed was secondary to him napping less now that preschool has started. She does not recall any significant falls, although he does occasionally trip and fall when running. The patient has otherwise been in his normal state of health. His mother states he has had normal appetite and activity level and has not complained of any headache, fever, or abdominal pain. He has no history of seizure disorder; however, he does have intermittent breakouts of eczema that require application of a topical steroid cream. The patient was evaluated by his pediatrician 2 months ago for general well-child visit and is UTD with immunizations.

Past Medical History

- Eczema.

Medications

- Triamcinolone 0.1%.

Allergies

- Azithromycin.

Physical Examination and Ancillary Studies

- *Vital signs*: T 98.7 °F, HR 98, BP 94/52, RR 18, O$_2$ sat 100% on room air.
- *General*: The patient is awake, alert, and in no acute distress.

- *HEENT*: The patient's right pupil appears larger than the left and is sluggish to respond to light reflex or accommodation. There is slight blurring of the optic disk bilaterally. His cranial nerves are intact.
- *Neck*: His neck is supple, with a midline trachea.
- *Cardiovascular*: Heart is regular, with no M/R/G. Capillary refill < 2 seconds.
- *Lungs*: CTA bilaterally, with no W/R/R.
- *Abdomen*: Non-tender and soft, with normal bowel sounds. There is no rebound, rigidity, or guarding.
- *Extremities and skin*: Extremities are warm and well-perfused, with no rashes.
- *Neurologic*: The right upper extremity is weak, with decreased gross sensation compared to the left upper extremity; the lower extremities are equal in strength with no sensory deficits. The Babinski sign is negative when tested on both lower extremities. The child is mildly ataxic with a broad-based gait.
- *Pertinent laboratory values*: Fingerstick glucose 102.

Questions for Thought

- What further diagnostic modality could you use to evaluate this patient?
- What are the various neurologic findings in this condition?
- What are the typical causes?
- What treatments should be initiated in the ED?
- What is the definitive treatment for this condition?

Diagnosis

- Intracranial mass.

Discussion

- *Epidemiology*: Brain tumors are said to be either primary (originating from the brain tissue itself from an individual cell mutation) or secondary (metastatic from a distant primary site, with migration to the brain through the blood stream).[1] In the pediatric population, brain tumors are the second most common type of malignancy after leukemia, with an estimated 3.6 per 100,000 new cases annually.[2] Tumors of the posterior fossa are more common in pre-adolescence, after which supratentorial tumors tend to be more common. Between 54 and 70 percent of all childhood brain tumors are located in the posterior fossa.[2] Most brain tumors in children are primary, and most are gliomas.[2] Risk factors for developing a primary tumor include prior history of radiation or presence of congenital conditions, such as multiple endocrine neoplasia type 1, retinoblastoma, tuberous sclerosis, or neurofibromatosis.[2]
- *Pathophysiology*: Brain tumors cause symptoms by either their specific location disrupting brain function (causing seizures, weakness, sensory problems, or cerebellar findings) or secondary to increased intracranial pressure (vomiting, altered mental status). Symptoms depend on the location of the lesion, the rapidity of growth, obstruction of CSF drainage, and intracranial pressure.
- *Presentation*: Pediatric brain tumors, whether primary or secondary, will generally present with similar signs and symptoms. The onset of symptoms is usually subtle, with gradual progression, but can present acutely if there is tumor compressing the ventricular system and blocking flow of CSF in the brain.[3,4] This blockage could lead to more acute symptoms, such as vomiting, mental status change, and respiratory collapse.[4] The most commonly reported symptom is headache, occurring in about 40 percent of newly diagnosed pediatric brain tumors.[3,4] This headache is typically described as a non-specific tension type pattern with the location of the headache being non-specific to the actual location of the underlying tumor.[3] Although headache is a common first symptom of pediatric brain tumor, the average number of signs and symptoms at the time of diagnosis is six.[4] Specific signs and symptoms are related to the tumor size and location. Diplopia (double vision) or homonymous hemianopsia (loss of half of the field of view on the same side in both eyes) may indicate tumor compression on specific cranial nerves or visual field tracts.[4] Anosmia (loss of smell) is associated with frontal lobe tumors and ataxia is common in masses affecting the brainstem or cerebellum.[4] Other possible signs/symptoms include new-onset focal or generalized seizure activity, cranial nerve palsies, growth problems, head tilting, or changes in

behavior.[4] Papilledema (swelling of the optic disk) is a general sign of increased intracranial pressure, indicating possible swelling or edema, and is a serious sign that portends potential decompensation.

- *Diagnosis*: Blood chemistries may be helpful to establish baseline levels as pediatric brain masses can cause electrolyte disturbances, but these studies are usually normal in the setting of a primary intracranial mass. Diagnosis relies heavily upon good history taking to identify new red-flag symptoms and physical examination findings to identify evidence of new neurologic dysfunction. These findings should prompt further diagnostic imaging such as CT or MRI of the brain. Although an IV contrast CT provides better diagnostics than a non-contrasted CT, in the ED, non-contrasted CT is often performed initially. Imaging *should* be performed emergently in the ED if the provider is concerned that the patient may have increased intracranial pressure, in order to facilitate neurosurgical evaluation and possible decompressive surgery. In stable children in whom MRI can be performed on an urgent basis, it is reasonable to admit the child without ED imaging, to reduce the child's overall exposure to ionizing radiation, as most children with brain tumors or focal neurologic findings from other sources will require MRI. MRI is superior to CT in imaging the posterior fossa and does not expose the child to radiation, although many smaller children require procedural sedation to undergo MRI. In the ED, should a contrasted CT of the head be performed, primary tumors will generally appear as a single mass lesion, with secondary (or metastatic) disease appearing as multiple lesions. LP is generally not indicated for the detection of an intracranial mass, and in cases of obstructive hydrocephalus is actually contraindicated because of the increased risk of brainstem herniation.
- *Treatment*: The management of pediatric intracranial tumors is dependent upon the size, location, type, and acuity of the patient's condition. Children with rapidly progressive symptoms require resuscitation using the ABC algorithm. If elevated intracranial pressure is suspected, then osmotic agents such as mannitol may be necessary as a temporizing measure to prevent herniation until definitive decompressive

surgery can be achieved. In stable patients, the focus should be on symptom management and reducing the amount and progression of cerebral edema by use of corticosteroids, such as dexamethasone. Ultimate care may involve multiple specialties, including oncology, radiation therapy, neurology, and neurosurgery. Surgical options may include tumor removal or placement of a ventricular shunt and devices to measure intracranial pressure to guide medical management.

The prognosis for pediatric tumors is highly variable depending on the initial symptoms, tumor subtype, and management. Patients who survive their malignancy may have long-term deficits in memory and attention.[5] There is also concern of other sequelae in adolescence and adulthood, such as an increased risk of psychiatric illnesses, including depression and psychosis.[6]

- *Disposition*: Children with new diagnoses of brain tumors should be admitted to the hospital to facilitate coordination of care, and neurosurgery should be consulted. Patients with signs of increased intracranial pressure should be admitted to an ICU.

Historical clues	Physical findings	Ancillary studies
• Vomiting, particularly upon waking • Arm twitching • Balance problems • Fussiness • Pallor	• Abnormal pupils • Focal neurologic deficit • Ataxia • Papilledema	• Normal glucose

Follow-Up

The child was sent for contrast-enhanced CT of his head, which showed a single intracranial mass located in the posterior fossa, with moderate hydrocephalus. He was given 10 mg dexamethasone, with slight improvement in his pupillary response and vomiting. Neurosurgery was consulted and the patient was sent for a stat MRI-brain, with an anesthesiologist for sedation. The patient was admitted and subsequently underwent tumor resection and had a stable post-operative course. Repeat MRI testing showed resolution of the hydrocephalus and stable post-operative findings. The child was diagnosed with a pilocytic astrocytoma. He receives routine surveillance, but has had no recurrence of his tumor.

References

1. DeAngelis LM. Brain tumors. *N Engl J Med* 2001; 344: 114–23.

2. Johnson KJ, Cullen J, Barnholtz-Sloan JS, et al. Childhood brain tumor epidemiology: A brain tumor epidemiology consortium review. *Cancer Epidemiol Biomarkers Prev* 2014; 23: 2716–36.

3. Purdy RA, Kirby S. Headaches and brain tumors. *Neurol Clin* 2004; 22: 39–53.

4. Wilne S, Collier J, Kennedy C, et al. Progression from first symptom to diagnosis in childhood brain tumours. *Eur J Pediatr* 2012; 171: 87–93.

5. Tonning Olsson I, Perrin S, Lundgren J, Hjorth L, Johanson A. Long-term cognitive sequelae after pediatric brain tumor related to medical risk factors, age, and sex. *Pediatr Neurol* 2014; 51: 515–21.

6. Shah SS, Dellarole A, Peterson EC, et al. Long-term psychiatric outcomes in pediatric brain tumor survivors. *Childs Nerv Syst* 2015; 31: 653–63.

Case 7

Contributing Author: Kinsey Leonard

History

The patient is a healthy 16-year-old female who presents with vomiting episodes that have been occurring over the last 3–6 months, per her mother's report. The patient denies complaints. She states she vomits "now and again" when she's sick, but she isn't sick now. Mom also reports that the patient has seemed to have an increased appetite. She consumes larger than normal amounts of food at dinner, and mom has noted missing items from the pantry. Mom also states that the child eats very rapidly and asks to be excused from the table prior to the rest of the family.

On review of systems, the patient states that her last bowel movement was 3–4 days ago. She also reports mild generalized abdominal pain. She denies fevers, chills, headaches, cough, rhinorrhea, sore throat, difficulty breathing, or urinary complaints. She denies known sick contacts.

The patient states that she is sexually active with one partner in a monogamous relationship for over a year. She attends high school and denies any issues at school. She denies using drugs or alcohol.

Past Medical History

- No significant medical problems, UTD on immunizations.

Medications

- Oral contraceptive pills.

Allergies

- Penicillin.

Physical Examination and Ancillary Studies

- *Vital signs*: T 98.2 °F, HR 72, BP 120/69, RR 16, O$_2$ sat 100%.
- *General*: The patient is awake and alert. She is letting her mother answer most of the questions. She has a normal body habitus.
- *HEENT*: The patient has several filled caries. Mild erythema of the throat. Tonsils appear normal. The patient's parotid glands are enlarged bilaterally. Non-tender to palpation.
- *Neck*: Supple, with no adenopathy.
- *Cardiovascular*: Regular rate and rhythm, with no M/R/G.
- *Lungs*: CTA bilaterally, with no W/R/R.
- *Abdomen*: Soft, non-distended, positive bowel sounds. There is mild tenderness to palpation diffusely, with no guarding or rebound tenderness.
- *Extremities and skin*: Skin is warm and dry. Capillary refill < 3 seconds. No rash. Mild acne present on the patient's face. Calluses on patient's right hand over her metacarpophalangeal joints. Limbs are atraumatic.
- *Neurologic*: Alert and oriented, normal cranial nerves, strength, and sensation.
- *Pertinent laboratory values*: K 3.0, Cl 90, bicarbonate 32, amylase 130.

Questions for Thought

- How do you differentiate bulimia from anorexia?
- What are the criteria for making the diagnosis of bulimia or anorexia?
- What is the ED management of this condition?
- What are the worrisome physical complications of eating disorders that can result in immediate morbidity or mortality?

Diagnosis

- Bulimia nervosa.

Discussion

- *Epidemiology*: Bulimia and anorexia nervosa have a lifetime prevalence of 1 percent and under 1 percent, respectively, although there are conflicting data given the propensity to hide the disease.[1-3] Both are more common in women. The peak incidence of anorexia is in the 14–18-year-old age range, while the median age for bulimics is 18.

- *Pathophysiology*: The exact pathophysiology of both disorders is unknown. Eating disorders have been correlated with certain extracurricular activities (for example, cheerleading, dancing, or wrestling), having divorced parents, having underlying self-esteem issues, and having a perfectionistic personality.[2,3] Both conditions are associated with abnormalities in neurotransmitters, and both increase the patient's risk for depression, anxiety, and substance abuse.[2,4]

- *Presentation*: Both diseases are usually found in the teenage population. The adolescent may be apprehensive to present to the hospital or talk about eating habits. The teenager often has a long history of dieting and being preoccupied with weight and losing weight. Usually the teen continues to view herself as overweight, though she is either underweight (anorexia) or normal weight (bulimia). Parents may bring the adolescent to the ED with a medical complication of the disease as the chief complaint.[5]

  In anorectics, there are usually vague or no complaints.[2] Family members may bring the patient to the ED because of weight loss, weakness, fatigue, dizziness, or after a syncopal episode.[2,5] Other complications of starvation may be the presenting complaint, including low-impact fractures, amenorrhea, and poor growth. Patients may also present with abnormal vital signs, including hypothermia, hypotension, and bradycardia. Palpitations, chest pain, and cardiac dysrhythmias can lead to serious morbidity and mortality, including sudden cardiac death.[2,5] On examination, the patient will be very thin, with BMI < 19, with little muscle or subcutaneous fat. The patient may also have lanugo, fine soft hair, and appear dehydrated.

  Bulimics may be more difficult to discover since their body weight is usually normal. The patient may present with complications of repeated vomiting, such as Mallory–Weiss tears, GERD, dysphagia, sore throat, hoarseness, pancreatitis, or dehydration. They could also present with vague complaints similar to anorexia, including weakness, fatigue, dizziness, syncope, palpitations, or seizures. Generalized abdominal pain, constipation, or diarrhea might be the chief complaint. On examination, they may have dental caries, large parotid glands, and erythema on their palate and throat. They may also have Russell's sign, which are calluses over the metacarpophalangeal joints from inducing vomiting.

- *Diagnosis*: Both diseases are diagnosed on the basis of the Diagnostic and Statistical Manual 5 criteria. For *anorexia nervosa*, these are:[6]

  - Restriction of caloric intake relative to expenditure, leading to low body weight for age, sex, and development.
  - Intense fear of gaining weight or of becoming fat or persistent prevention of weight gain.
  - Disturbance in perception of body weight or acknowledgement of the seriousness of the low body weight.

  For bulimia nervosa, the criteria are:[6]

  - Recurrent binge eating – eating larger amounts of food than normal in a given period of time, where the patient feels out of control of eating.
  - Recurrent compensatory behavior to prevent weight gain.
  - Binging and compensatory behavior are at least once a week for 3 months.
  - Body shape and weight overly influence self worth.
  - Binging and compensatory behavior are not solely during anorexia.

  Work-up should include electrolytes, divalents, glucose, BUN/Cr, LFTs, CBC, and EKG. If the patient has abnormal vitals, TSH and T4 should be obtained. A U/A should also be performed to look for ketosis. A urine pregnancy test should also be performed.

- *Treatment*: Life-threatening arrhythmias and electrolyte abnormalities should be treated.[5] Rehydration may be needed in both anorexia and bulimia nervosa, and anorectic children may need to be admitted for refeeding.[2,5] Overaggressive rehydration and refeeding may lead to cardiopulmonary failure, and should not be undertaken in the ED. Psychiatric consultation or referral is warranted. Anorexia is usually treated with psychotherapy. Bulimia is generally treated with cognitive behavioral therapy. Antidepressants and selective serotonin reuptake inhibitors are also approved for treatment of bulimia nervosa.

- *Disposition*: Most patients with bulimia and anorexia are stable and safe to be discharged home with close follow-up with pediatrics and psychiatry. The Society for Adolescent Medicine compiled a list of admission criteria for children with eating disorders including: unstable vital signs, severe malnutrition, requiring aggressive rehydration, significant electrolyte abnormalities, dysrhythmia, refusal to eat, uncontrollable binging and purging, suicidal ideation, or the presence of other psychiatric diagnoses that make it unsafe for the patient to go home.[7]

Historical clues	Physical findings	Ancillary studies
• Repeated vomiting • Binge eating	• Russell's sign • Dental caries/poor dentition • Enlarged parotid glands • Throat erythema	• Hypokalemia • Hypochloremia • Metabolic alkalosis • Elevated amylase

Follow-Up

The patient's potassium was replaced. She was referred to psychiatry and ultimately spent 3 weeks in an inpatient eating disorder unit. She was begun on a selective serotonin reuptake inhibitor and is still undergoing cognitive behavioral therapy. She has shown improvement in her behaviors.

References

1. Hudson JI, Hiripi E, Pope HG Jr, et al. The prevalence and correlates of eating disorders in the National Comorbidity Survey Replication. *Biol Psychiatry* 2007; 61: 348–58.

2. Williams PM, Goodie J, Motsinger CD. Treating eating disorders in primary care. *Am Fam Phys* 2008; 77: 187–95.

3. Kessler RC, Berglund PA, Chiu WT, et al. The prevalence and correlates of binge eating disorder in the World Health Organization World Mental Health Surveys. *Biol Psychiatry* 2013; 73: 904–14.

4. Philipou A, Rossell SL, Castle DJ. The neurobiology of anorexia nervosa: A systematic review. *Aust N Z J Psychiatry* 2014; 48: 128–52.

5. Mascolo M, Trent S, Colwell C, et al. What the emergency department needs to know when caring for your patients with eating disorders. *Int J Eat Disord* 2012; 45: 977–81.

6. American Psychiatric Association. *Diagnostic and Statistical Manual of Mental Disorders*, 5th edition. Washington (DC): American Psychiatric Association, 2013.

7. Golden NH, Katzman DK, Kreipe RE, et al. Eating disorder in adolescents: Position paper of the Society for Adolescent Medicine. *J Adolesc Health* 2003; 33: 496–503.

Case 8

Contributing Author: Sarah Hudgins

History

A 4-week-old male with trisomy 21 (Down's syndrome) is brought to the ED by his parents for a 3-hour history of vomiting and irritability. The patient had a sudden onset of green-tinged, non-bloody emesis with multiple episodes of vomiting just prior to arrival. He has also had a decreased appetite accompanied by excessive and inconsolable crying. Both parents noted abdominal swelling. The mother gave the child acetaminophen, which was immediately followed by vomiting. The patient is described as healthy at baseline and was born full-term without any birth complications. He has had no trauma/injuries, respiratory symptoms, diarrhea, blood in his stool or vomit, and has remained afebrile. The child is bottle-fed with commercial formula that is mixed correctly, and he has had no history of feeding issues. He is an only child and lives with his mother and father. He does not attend daycare and has had no recent travel or sick contacts.

Past Medical History

- Trisomy 21
- Has not received 8-week vaccinations yet, but did receive vaccines at birth.
- Child has been circumcized.

Medications

- Acetaminophen prior to arrival.

Allergies

- NKDA.

Physical Examination and Ancillary Studies

- *Vital signs*: T 97 °F, HR 210, RR 50, BP 80/55, O_2 sat 99% on room air.
- *General*: The patient is crying during the examination, appears to be in moderate distress, parents and staff are unable to console the child. Child has flat facial features.
- *HEENT*: The head is normocephalic and atraumatic, with flat fontanelles. PERRL, with intact red reflex and upward slant to the eyes. The child is crying, with tears noted. No nasal congestion or rhinorrhea. Small, abnormally shaped ears. Tympanic membranes are intact, with a good cone of light and no erythema or effusion. Mucous membranes are moist, no pharyngeal erythema, no tonsillar edema/exudates. The tongue appears enlarged and is partially sticking out of the mouth.
- *Neck*: No cervical or occipital lymphadenopathy palpated. Neck is short and supple.
- *Cardiovascular*: Heart rate is tachycardic, with no audible M/R/G. Brachial and femoral pulses 2+ bilaterally. Capillary refill < 3 seconds.
- *Lungs*: Limited auscultation secondary to patient crying during examination; however, lungs appeared to be clear, without W/R/R.
- *Abdomen*: Soft, distended, abdomen which, with palpation, causes increased distress in the child. No audible bowel sounds auscultated. No umbilical hernia. No palpable masses.
- *Extremities and skin*: Child moving all extremities during examination, no external signs of trauma. Single deep crease seen in the center of the palm bilaterally. No peripheral edema. Skin is warm without any rashes. Extra space seen between first and second toes.
- *Neurologic*: Intact Moro and sucking reflex. Hypotonia (described as baseline).

Questions for Thought

- What is your differential diagnosis for this child?
- What tests would help guide you to this child's diagnosis?

- If you were a provider in a rural hospital without a pediatric surgeon, when would you obtain imaging and when would you consider transfer?
- What factors increase the child's likelihood of having a surgical disease?
- The child does not have a fever. Would you give antibiotics?

Diagnosis

- Intestinal malrotation with volvulus.

Discussion

- *Epidemiology*: Malrotation occurs at a rate of 1 in 500 live births with a male predominance of 2:1.[1] Children born with Down's syndrome, heterotaxy syndrome, or duodenal atresia have an increased risk of malrotation. Malrotation is asymptomatic but with volvulus it becomes a surgical emergency. In patients with malrotation, 90 percent will develop volvulus within the first year, with 75 percent of those having developed it within the first 4 weeks of life.[1,2] Although most cases occur in infancy, there have been reported cases in young children, adolescents, and even adults.[1,3–5] The mortality rate for volvulus ranges from 3 to 15 percent depending on the timing of the presentation and the extent of injury, and has improved dramatically over time.[1]
- *Pathophysiology*: Starting in the fifth week of embryologic development the fetal intestine, which begins as a straight tube, protrudes into the umbilical cord. As the GI tract returns into the abdomen, the intestines make a 270° counterclockwise turn, using the superior mesenteric artery as an axis. With normal development, the intestine, after rotation, will be fixed in place by peritoneal bands (called Ladd's bands). These bands adhere the cecum in the right lower quadrant and the duodenojejunal loop to the left of the midline. Malrotation occurs when there is any variation in either the fixation or rotation during this embryologic process. Without adequate adherence, the cecum and duodenum are left suspended by their vascular attachments, which contain the superior mesenteric artery. This mesentery, which hangs loosely as a short stalk within the abdomen, can easily twist on itself causing a compression of the

superior mesenteric artery. This compression can lead to bowel ischemia and necrosis/gangrene within as little as 1–2 hours. This obstruction of the bowel will clinically present as bilious emesis, with the underlying bowel necrosis manifesting as signs of shock.

- *Presentation*: A neonate with a sudden onset of abdominal pain with distension and bilious vomiting, who appears ill and/or in shock, is displaying the typical presentation of a patient suffering from malrotation with volvulus. The patient's presentation can vary greatly based on whether the condition is acute or chronic. With chronic volvulus, the intestines will twist and untwist, leading to intermixing symptoms of abdominal pain and vomiting with periods that are asymptomatic. The patient's presentation will greatly depend on the time between when they present to the hospital and the initiation of events. Children who present shortly after onset can appear well at the time of the examination, exhibiting only abdominal pain with non-bilious vomiting. Contrastingly, those receiving treatment later in the course will display signs of peritonitis with shock and can have GI hemorrhage, manifesting as bloody stools.

  Though this condition is typically a disease of infancy it can present at any age. Features most commonly associated with malrotation outside of infancy include: colicky abdominal pain, intermittent vomiting, and failure to thrive. GERD, pyloric stenosis, necrotizing enterocolitis, intussusception, and sepsis are other conditions that can have overlapping symptoms, complicating a timely diagnosis.

- *Diagnosis*: Any child with vomiting warrants consideration for the dangerous differential for the unwell infant, discussed further in Chapter 3, Case 7: *Trauma, Hypovolemia/heart, Endocrine, Metabolic, Intestinal disasters, Seizures, Formula misadventures, Inborn errors of metabolism, Toxicologic,* and *Sepsis (THE MISFITS)* can all present with vomiting. If the process is believed to be intra-abdominal, the provider should consider evaluation for appendicitis, intussusception, necrotizing enterocolitis, pyloric stenosis, volvulus, as well as medical pathologies such as pancreatitis. Especially in bilious vomiting, the child should be presumed to have an emergency surgical condition.

The test of choice in diagnosing malrotation with volvulus is the upper GI series with small-bowel follow-through. It has a 93–100 percent sensitivity for ruling out malrotation with a 100 percent specificity in diagnosing volvulus.[1,2,6,7] It is limited by its poor sensitivity (54–79 percent) for ruling out volvulus when the classic corkscrew appearance of the small bowel is not seen. This test is able to diagnose malrotation by identifying an abnormal position of the duodenal C-loop as well as a failure of the duodenojejunal junction to cross the midline.

The "double-bubble sign," in which one pocket of air is visualized from the dilated stomach and an additional pocket of air is visualized at the level of the obstructed proximal duodenum, is the hallmark abdominal X-ray finding. This test has been found to be neither sensitive nor specific in the diagnosis of malrotation as the double-bubble sign is also present in other conditions, such as pyloric stenosis and duodenal atresia.[1,2,6,7]

U/S is still a controversial yet increasingly popular method when evaluating children for malrotation. It has appeal as a low-radiation, non-invasive option that has been found to be accurate in studies with expertly trained ultrasonographers.[1,2,6,7] Malrotation can be evidenced via U/S by noting the abnormal position of the third portion of the duodenum outside of its normal retroperitoneal location. The U/S diagnosis of volvulus consists of a "whirlpool sign" in which the spiraled mesentery creates a distinct echogenic twisting pattern. U/S is very useful for diagnosing or excluding other pathologies, including appendicitis, pyloric stenosis, and intussusception. Laboratory studies are not helpful in diagnosing malrotation or volvulus but can be useful in determining the severity of the patient's condition.

- *Treatment*: A child that presents with symptoms that suggest possible volvulus should be treated as a surgical emergency. Emergent diagnosis and surgical intervention is necessary as intestinal necrosis and gangrene can occur in as little as 1–2 hours. A pediatric surgeon needs to be consulted even before imaging results are obtained. U/S imaging and/or upper GI series should be obtained to diagnose the condition. While in the ED the patient will need a baseline laboratory panel that includes: fingerstick glucose, CBC, electrolytes, LFTs, and a type and screen. IV access should be initiated and a 20 cc/kg bolus as well as maintenance fluids should be administered. Cultures including urine and blood should be obtained and antibiotics initiated. Recommended antibiotics for this condition are: ampicillin with gentamycin and clindamycin or metronidazole. In order to decompress the stomach a nasogastric tube should also be placed.

- *Disposition*: Ultimately, the child will need surgical intervention. Stable patients in rural facilities should be transferred to a facility with a pediatric surgeon. Unstable patients will require immediate surgical intervention and should not be transferred if a surgeon is present. Surgical intervention will consist of a Ladd's procedure in which the obstructing bands are removed and the intestines are carefully untwisted and then adhered to their proper anatomic location. If ischemic bowel is found it is resected and, if needed, a diverting ileostomy or colostomy is made. An appendectomy is also performed as the new position of the child's appendix will make future diagnosis of appendicitis difficult.

Historical clues	Physical findings
• Sudden-onset symptoms	• Ill-appearing
• Abdominal distension	• Abnormal vital signs
• Bilious vomiting	• Abdominal distension
• Irritability	• Abdominal tenderness
• Decreased appetite	• No bowel sounds
• Trisomy 21	

Follow-Up

Upon presentation to the ED, the patient received an IV fluid bolus and maintenance fluids. These initial measures resulted in the stabilization of the child's condition as well as an improvement in his vital signs. As this facility had no pediatric surgeons, a telephone consultation was placed while diagnostic imaging was being obtained. The upper GI series revealed an abnormally positioned C-loop with the classic corkscrew appearance that indicated a volvulus. Being that the child was hemodynamically stable at the time of diagnosis, he was immediately transferred to a nearby pediatric center where an emergent Ladd's procedure and appendectomy were performed. The child had no surgical complications. After an uneventful

recovery, he was discharged home from the hospital on day 13.

References
1. Ford EG, Senac Jr MO, Srikanth MS, et al. Malrotation of the intestine in children. *Ann Surg* 1992; 215: 172–8.
2. Smith J, Fox SM. Pediatric abdominal pain: An emergency medicine perspective. *Emerg Med Clin N Am* 2016; 34: 341–61.
3. Emanuwa OF, Ayantunde AA, Davies TW. Midgut malrotation first presenting as acute bowel obstruction in adulthood: A case report and literature review. *World J Emerg Surg* 2011; 6: 22.
4. Yanez R, Spitz L. Intestinal malrotation presenting outside the neonatal period. *Arch Dis Child* 1986; 61: 682–5.
5. Sipahi M, Caglayan K, Arslan E, et al. Intestinal malrotation: A rare cause of small intestinal obstruction. *Case Rep Surg* 2014; 2014: 453128.
6. Hamidi H, Obaidy Y, Maroof S. Intestinal malrotation and midgut volvulus. *Radiol Case Rep* 2016; 11: 271–4.
7. Khatami A, Mahdavi K, Karimi MA. Ultrasound as a feasible method for the assessment of malrotation. *Pol J Radiol* 2014; 79: 112–16.

Case 9

Contributing Author: Erica Escarcega

History

The patient is a 9-year-old female who has been brought to the ED for evaluation by her parents for vomiting this morning. The child had non-bloody, non-bilious vomiting after attempting to eat her breakfast this morning. The patient has not had any recent coughing or congestion. She denies diarrhea. She reports a sore throat that has been worsening over the past day. It is a burning pain that is made worse by swallowing both solids and liquids. She awoke this morning with a fever and had a maximum temperature of 101.3 °F taken orally just prior to arrival. The patient lives at home with her parents. She is in fourth grade and enjoys school. She states that two of her classmates have been absent from school, but she is unsure why.

Past Medical History

- Asthma, mild–intermittent, well controlled.

Medications

- Albuterol inhaler 90 mcg, two puffs every 4 hours as needed, last used 2 weeks ago.

Allergies

- NKDA.

Physical Examination and Ancillary Studies

- *Vital signs*: T 100.6 °F, HR 98, BP 100/60, RR 18, O_2 sat 100% on room air.
- *General*: The patient is alert and appears mildly distressed due to her throat pain. She is cooperative with the examination.
- *HEENT*: PERRL. Mucous membranes are moist. Posterior pharynx is erythematous. Tonsils are 2+, erythematous. White exudate is present on tonsils bilaterally. No trismus.
- *Neck*: Bilateral anterior cervical lymphadenopathy. Neck is supple and trachea is midline.
- *Cardiovascular*: Regular rate and rhythm, with no M/R/G. Peripheral pulses are normal. Capillary refill < 3 seconds.
- *Lungs*: CTA, with no W/R/R.
- *Abdomen*: The patient's abdomen is soft, non-tender, and non-distended, with normoactive bowel sounds throughout. There are no palpable masses.
- *Extremities and skin*: There is no peripheral edema. Her skin is warm to the touch and there are no rashes noted on examination.
- *Neurologic*: Alert. Age appropriate. No focal deficits.

Questions for Thought

- What items within the patient's history and physical can help lead you to the diagnosis?
- What tests would you run on this patient?
- Are antibiotics indicated?
- What complications may occur if you fail to treat this condition?

Diagnosis

- Streptococcal pharyngitis.

Discussion

- *Epidemiology*: Streptococcal pharyngitis is caused by group A streptococci and is most common in children ages 5–10. Atypical presentations are more likely in children under 5 and are often misdiagnosed as URIs. Complications of disease include peritonsillar abscess, retropharyngeal abscesses, suppurative cervical lymphadenitis, bacteremia, otitis media, sinusitis, mastoiditis, meningitis, pneumonia, and rheumatic fever.[1,2] Rheumatic fever is an exceedingly rare complication of strep throat with an annual incidence of less than one case per million population. This presents with fever, carditis, subcutaneous nodules, chorea, and migratory polyarthritis occurring 1–5 weeks after resolution of strep throat. The asymptomatic carrier rate of group A streptococci is 5–21 percent in children aged 3–5 and is lower in younger and older age groups.[2,3]
- *Pathophysiology*: Strep throat is caused by an inflammatory response to group A beta-hemolytic streptococci. Interleukins 1 and 6, tissue necrosis factor, and prostaglandins result in fever. Prostaglandins and bradykinin result in severe throat pain. Erythema and swelling of the tonsils, uvula, and soft palate result from the effect of prostaglandins and nitric oxide release. Tissue damage from lysosomal enzymes and oxygen free radicals generates a creamy exudate seen on the tonsillar pillars.
- *Presentation*: Classic symptoms only occur in approximately half of patients and are usually described as severe sore throat of sudden onset, with difficulty swallowing. Patients will often have a moderate fever, which rarely is accompanied by chills or rigors. Malaise, headache, mild neck stiffness, anorexia, nausea, vomiting, and abdominal pain are also commonly seen in cases of streptococcal pharyngitis.[1] GI symptoms are more common in younger patients.[1] On physical examination, patients will often have erythema and edema of the posterior pharynx and uvula, petechiae over the soft palate, and tonsillar hypertrophy often with a visible gray–white membrane or exudate over the tonsils. Frequently, acutely tender anterior cervical lymphadenopathy is present, which may be more pronounced at the angle of the jaw. Occasionally, patients may present with a scarlatiniform rash, which is characteristic of scarlet fever. This rash appears as fine erythematous "sandpapery" papules, which are initially present over the trunk and then

spread to the extremities, sparing the palms and soles.

- *Diagnosis*: Multiple clinical prediction rules have been developed to aid in diagnosis. The Centor score is most widely used. It was developed for adults but has been validated in children. Using the modified Centor criteria, patients are given a point for fever, anterior cervical adenopathy, tonsillar exudate, and lack of cough.[1,4,5] An additional point is given for patients age 3–14, and a point is subtracted for adults above 45 years old.[1] Patients with four or more points may be empirically treated for streptococcal pharyngitis, although the positive predictive value is only a little over 50 percent.[1] Newer rapid antigen testing, which boasts a sensitivity of 85 percent and specificity of 93 percent, can be used in patients with a low or intermediate likelihood of strep throat and should be confirmed with throat culture.

- *Treatment*: Untreated streptococcal pharyngitis lasts approximately 8–10 days, with an infectious period extending 1 week after resolution of the acute symptoms.[5] Antibiotic treatment reduces the symptom duration by a day.[5] Antibiotics have very little net benefit in protecting patients against suppurative and non-suppurative complications in developed societies where rheumatic fever is essentially non-existent, which has led some providers to forgo treatment of presumed strep throat in low-risk populations.[6]

  If antibiotics are given, first-line treatment consists of penicillin given either IM (benzathine penicillin G) or orally (either penicillin V or amoxicillin). Cephalosporins (such as cephalexin) are recommended in patients who have an allergy to penicillins without anaphylaxis. Even in those with anaphylaxis, there is only a 10 percent risk of cross-allergy to cephalosporins. Patients with a severe penicillin allergy may be treated with oral clindamycin or with macrolides.

  Steroids and anti-inflammatory medications have been shown to decrease pain and shorten disease course in adults when combined with antibiotics, but have not been adequately studied in the pediatric population.[7]

- *Disposition*: Patients with uncomplicated streptococcal pharyngitis may be discharged home to follow up with their pediatricians.

Historical clues	Physical findings
• Vomiting	• Erythema of posterior pharynx
• Sore throat	• Tonsillar hypertrophy
• Fever	• Exudates
• Abdominal pain	• Anterior cervical adenopathy
• Lack of cough	
• Age group	

Follow-Up

The patient was started on amoxicillin and discharged home with her parents. She was able to return to school 24 hours after starting antibiotics and had a full recovery after 4 days.

References

1. Choby BA. Diagnosis and treatment of streptococcal pharyngitis. *Am Fam Phys* 2009; 79: 383–90.
2. Hersh AL, Jackson MA, Hicks LA. Principles of judicious antibiotic prescribing for upper respiratory infections in pediatrics. *Pediatrics* 2013; 132: 1146–54.
3. Nussinovitch M, Finkelstein Y, Amir J, et al. Group A beta-hemolytic streptococcal pharyngitis in preschool children aged 3 months to 5 years. *Clin Pediatr (Phila)* 1999; 38: 357–60.
4. Ebell MH, Smith MA, Barry HC, et al. The rational clinical examination. Does this patient have strep throat? *JAMA* 2000; 284: 2912–18.
5. Sarrell EM, Giveon SM. Streptococcal pharyngitis: A prospective study of compliance and complications. *ISRN Pediatr* 2012; 2012: 796389.
6. Del Mar CB, Glasziou PP, Spinks AB. Antibiotics for sore throat. *Cochrane Database Syst Rev* 2004; 2: CD000023.
7. Hayward G, Thompson MJ, Perera R, et al. Corticosteroids as standalone or add-on treatment for sore throat. *Cochrane Database Syst Rev* 2012; 10: CD008268.

Case 10

Contributing Author: Kinsey Leonard

History

A 2-month-old infant is brought into the ED by her mother for vomiting. Mom reports that the child has been vomiting within an hour of feeding, and that the child is vomiting with almost every feed. She states that the vomiting does not appear to be everything the child eats, and she estimates that it's about 1–2 ounces each time. There has been no blood or bile in the vomit. The child has not appeared to be in pain. She has been making a usual amount of wet and dirty diapers. She has been acting like herself. The child is formula-fed, and takes 6 ounces every 2–3 hours. Mom follows the manufacturer guidelines for formula preparation, and only uses sterilized water. The child has not had fevers, diarrhea, sweating, pallor, cyanosis, or limp spells. The child will receive her 2-month immunizations next week. She has met all developmental milestones. She does not attend daycare. She has no sick contacts. Her review of systems is otherwise negative.

Past Medical History

- No significant medical problems.
- Normal pregnancy with spontaneous vaginal delivery at 41 weeks.

Medications

- None.

Allergies

- NKDA.

Physical Examination and Ancillary Studies

- *Vital signs*: T 99.0 °F, HR 120, BP 90/60, RR 30, O_2 sat 100%, weight 7 kg.
- *General*: The patient is awake and alert. She is looking around the examination room. She has a social smile.
- *HEENT*: Normocephalic and atraumatic. Anterior fontanelle is soft and flat. PERRL. Red reflex bilaterally. Moist mucous membranes. No pharyngeal erythema.
- *Neck*: Supple, with a midline trachea.
- *Cardiovascular*: Regular rate and rhythm, with no M/R/G.
- *Lungs*: Normal work of breathing, clear and equal breath sounds, with no W/R/R.
- *Abdomen*: Soft, non-distended, no organomegaly, positive bowel sounds.
- *Extremities and skin*: Skin is warm and dry. Capillary refill is < 3 seconds. No rash. No signs of trauma.

- *Neurologic*: Appropriate for age, normal Moro, grasp, and suck, symmetric face and extremities.

Questions for Thought

- What are some worrisome causes of vomiting in this age group?
- How much should a typical baby be fed?
- What is the ED management of this condition?
- What complications can result?

Diagnosis

- Overfeeding.

Discussion

- *Epidemiology*: Obesity is a problem in most Western societies and has become more prevalent in infants and children in recent years. In 2012, the CDC reported that close to 20 percent of children aged 6 to 19 years are obese.[1] Up to 10 percent of infants and toddlers are overweight in the USA.[1]
- *Pathophysiology*: Contributing factors to infant obesity include feeding infants too much, introducing solid foods too early, and having solid foods make up a large proportion of daily calories. Formula feeding also puts the infant at increased risk of overfeeding since different formulations have different calorie densities. Occasionally, caretakers may incorrectly mix formula, causing an overly concentrated bottle that results in overfeeding. There are differences amongst varying cultures in how overweight infants are perceived, which has led to infants of certain cultures being larger.[2] There are also differences in the feeding of infants among socioeconomic classes, with more educated mothers tending to breastfeed exclusively and continue breastfeeding for a longer period of time. One study has explored whether overfeeding is a consequence of mothers being more distracted during feedings and missing satiety signs from the infants.[3]

  The problem is similar in toddlers and older children. Parents feed children too much food for their caloric expenditure, and many foods consumed by children offer little nutrients and are calorically dense, with high concentrations of processed sugar, fat, and sodium. This is compounded by the fact that modern children are more sedentary than prior generations and as a result require fewer calories. The differences in obesity rates as a function of socioeconomic class persists in these older children, with Hispanic and black children at the highest risk.[1] Having parents who did not complete high school is independently associated with an increased risk of childhood obesity.

Overfeeding has been linked to GERD in infants, likely because overdistending the stomach leads to increased intra-abdominal pressure, encouraging regurgitation of the stomach contents. Overfeeding at an early age puts infants and children at increased risk of becoming overweight or obese adults. It also puts them at risk for impaired glucose tolerance, diabetes, and other metabolic problems.

- *Presentation*: The infant will present with vomiting or spitting up after eating. The infant may have been treated for GERD in the past. The infant will most likely be larger than normal for age, falling above the 95th percentile for weight. The child will otherwise have an entirely benign examination, with no worrisome findings.
- *Diagnosis*: All cases of vomiting in infancy deserve a careful history and physical examination, with consideration of the dangerous causes of vomiting in this age group, including trauma, cardiac disease, endocrine disease, metabolic disorders, inborn errors of metabolism, seizures, formula errors, intestinal disasters (such as volvulus), toxins, and sepsis. Overfeeding is diagnosed with careful history taking regarding the feeding practices, including how often the infant is fed, how much per feeding, how many times per day, and what the infant is fed.
- *Treatment*: Parents should be carefully counseled regarding the nutritional needs of their infants,

toddlers, and children. The AAP recommends breastfeeding exclusively for the first 6 months and continued breastfeeding to 1 year of life after the introduction of solid foods. Infants should not drink more than 32 ounces of formula in a 24-hour period. Parents should be encouraged to feed their older children healthier foods and engage in more physical activity. They should also be counseled regarding the risk of childhood obesity and increased risk of type 2 diabetes.

- *Disposition*: The patient can be discharged home with follow-up and further discussion with the family's pediatrician.

Historical clues	Physical findings
• Repeated vomiting after eating • Emesis of milk and no bile • Feeding practices that are above the needed caloric requirements	• Overweight but otherwise well-appearing infant

Follow-Up

The child had improvement in vomiting with adjustment of volume of feeds, and had an uneventful recovery.

References

1. Centers for Disease Control and Prevention. Prevalence of childhood obesity in the United States, 2011–2014. See www.cdc.gov/obesity/data/childhood.html (accessed March 7, 2015).

2. Cartagena D, Ameringer SW, McGrath JM, et al. Factors contributing to infant overfeeding in low-income immigrant Latina mothers. *J Obstet Gynecol Neonatal Nurs* 2014; 43:139–59.

3. Golden RB, Ventura AK. Mindless feeding: Is maternal distraction during bottle-feeding associated with overfeeding? *Appetite* 2015; 91: 385–92.

Chapter 8

Abdominal and Chest Pain

Case 1

Contributing Authors: Jonathan Nogueira and Janet Young

History

The patient is an 8-year-old female presenting to the ED with 4 days of generalized abdominal pain, now worse in the right lower quadrant. She has had nausea, vomiting, fevers, chills, decreased appetite, and worsening severity of abdominal pain over time. The patient's mother also states that she now prefers to stay rather still, with increased pain while moving or walking, stating it hurts more with any movement. She denies ever having symptoms like this in the past. There has been no constipation, diarrhea, or bloody stool. She has no known sick contacts, no rash, joint swelling, diarrhea, sore throat, rhinorrhea, cough, or difficulty in breathing. The patient's mother brought her to the ED due to worries of worsening abdominal pain.

Past Medical History

- Lyme disease approximately 2 years ago.

Medications

- None.

Allergies

- NKDA.

Physical Examination and Ancillary Studies

- *Vital signs*: T 101.7 °F, HR 132, RR 20, BP 124/44, O$_2$ sat 97% on room air.
- *General*: Appears well-developed and well-nourished, in moderate distress secondary to pain. Lying still on stretcher.

- *HEENT*: Mucous membranes are moist. PERRL. Bilateral conjunctival injection.
- *Neck*: Supple, with no adenopathy. Midline trachea.
- *Cardiovascular*: Regular rhythm. Tachycardia present. No murmur.
- *Lungs*: Breath sounds normal. No stridor. Tachypnea noted at time of examination. No respiratory distress. No wheezes or retractions.
- *Abdomen*: No distension. Bowel sounds are increased. Generalized tenderness most prominent in the right lower quadrant. There is rigidity, rebound, and guarding. Heel tap elicits abdominal pain.
- *Extremities and skin*: Warm and dry, capillary refill < 3 seconds. No petechiae and no purpura noted. No diaphoresis. No cyanosis.
- *Neurologic*: Age appropriate, normal mental status, strength, sensation, and reflexes normal.
- *Pertinent laboratory values*: WBC 12,000. Remainder of laboratory studies unremarkable.
- *Pertinent imaging*: Bedside point-of-care U/S: linear, non-compressible structure in the right lower quadrant, with associated tenderness. Hyperechoic area at the distal tip of this structure with a diameter > 6 mm, worrisome for appendicitis. Small amount of complex free fluid in the pelvis; see Figures 8.1 and 8.2.

Questions for Thought

- What are the typical laboratory findings in this condition?
- What is the appropriate first-line imaging study?
- What are the typical U/S and CT findings?
- What treatments should be initiated in the ED?
- What is the definitive treatment of this pathology?

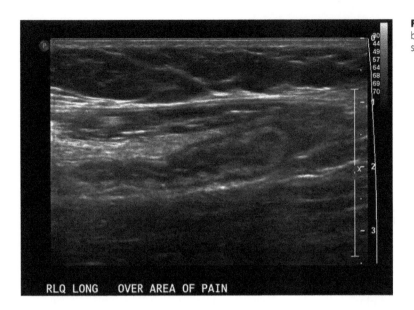

Figure 8.1 Long-axis view of the appendix by bedside point-of-care U/S in the ED, showing dilated distal appendix.

RLQ LONG   OVER AREA OF PAIN

Diagnosis

- Acute perforated appendicitis.

Discussion

- *Epidemiology*: It is estimated that the lifetime risk of developing appendicitis in the USA is about 9 percent for males and 7 percent for females, most commonly in patients aged 10–19 years old.[1,2] Appendicitis is a frequent cause of atraumatic abdominal pain in children greater than 1 year old as well as the most common non-obstetrical emergency in pregnancy. Appendicitis should be considered in any patient with acute atraumatic abdominal pain without prior appendectomy.

- *Pathophysiology*: Appendicitis is typically caused by luminal obstruction of the vermiform appendix by fecalith, lymphatic tissue, or, less commonly, tumor, foreign body, or parasitic infection. After obstruction occurs, continued secretion of the luminal mucosa results in increased intraluminal pressure, leading to inflammation, bacterial infection, and possibly necrosis or perforation due to increased intraluminal pressures. This leads to pain, initially visceral, then progressing to somatic, as the peritoneum becomes inflamed.

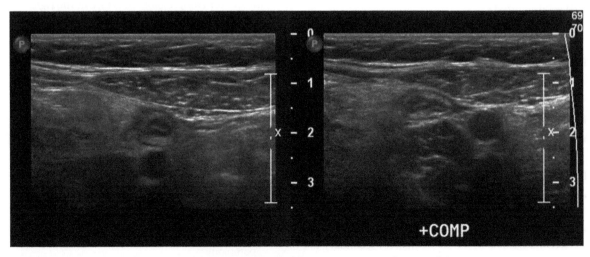

Figure 8.2 Short-axis view of the appendix showing non-compressible structure, suspicious for appendicitis.

Untreated appendicitis will lead to perforation and intra-abdominal sepsis or abscess and could cause death. Due to difficulties in obtaining history and ambiguity of examination, 80–100 percent of children less than 3 years old present with perforated appendicitis.[1] Perforation rates in older children are less, about 38 percent.[1]

- *Presentation*: Early appendicitis may begin with pain referred to the periumbilical area due to visceral innervation. Commonly associated symptoms include nausea and vomiting, anorexia, and pain migrating to the right lower quadrant at McBurney's point, one-third of the distance from the anterior superior iliac spine to the umbilicus. Other findings may include guarding, rebound tenderness, low-grade fever, obturator sign (pain with internal rotation of the leg with the hip and knee flexed), psoas sign (pain with extending the hip and the knee in full extension, or flexing the hip against resistance), and Rovsing's sign (pain in the right lower quadrant with palpation of the left lower quadrant). Once appendicitis has perforated, children may present with sepsis and with diffuse abdominal tenderness and guarding.
- *Diagnosis*: The critical evaluation of a child with appendicitis is a careful history and physical examination, looking for findings listed above.
  - Key diagnostic elements include right lower quadrant abdominal pain, anorexia, and fever. Many patients have an elevated peripheral WBC, but this is neither sensitive nor specific for appendicitis.[1,3]
  - May have elevated CRP and ESR.
  - U/S of the right lower quadrant with non-compressible tubular structure, appendiceal lumen greater than 6 mm, increased color flow indicative of inflammation and hyperemia, and periappendiceal inflammatory changes.[3–5]
  - If U/S is non-diagnostic, CT of the abdomen/pelvis showing periappendiceal fat stranding, appendiceal diameter greater than 6 mm, periappendiceal fluid, and possibly fecalith.[3–5]
- *Treatment*: Initially, patients should be made NPO due to the definitive need for surgical appendectomy. Fluid resuscitation as needed and maintenance fluids should be administered, as well as antiemetics and appropriate analgesia.

Perioperative antibiotics should be administered to cover common organisms such as Enterobacteriaceae (*Escherichia coli, Klebsiella* spp., *Proteus* spp.) and *Bacteroides*. Antibiotic choices for simple pediatric appendicitis may include ampicillin–sulbactam, cefoxitin, or metronidazole plus gentamycin. Antibiotic choices for complicated appendicitis, such as gangrenous, perforated, abscess, or phlegmon, may include imipenem–cilastatin, piperacillin–tazobactam, or metronidazole plus aztreonam.

- *Disposition*: When the diagnosis of appendicitis has been made, appendectomy is the definitive treatment of choice. Patients may be stable for discharge within 12–24 hours post appendectomy if they are tolerating oral intake and their pain is well managed. Patients with complicated appendicitis may need further monitoring and treatment as indicated.

Historical clues	Physical findings	Ancillary studies
• Right lower quadrant pain • Nausea and vomiting • Poor appetite	• Tender abdomen • Rebound and guarding • Positive heel tap (indicates peritoneal irritation)	• Elevated WBC • U/S with evidence of appendicitis

Follow-Up

The patient was made NPO and started on broad-spectrum antibiotics, as well as IV fluids, antiemetics, and analgesia. She was taken to the OR for urgent appendecomy and was found to have acute perforated appendicitis with periappendiceal abscess as well as diffuse peritonitis and adhesions to the anterior abdominal wall. There was turbid ascites in all four quadrants. Post-operatively, she was continued on IV antibiotics and slowly advanced to regular diet. She gradually recovered and was discharged home on hospital day 6.

References

1. Smith J, Fox SM. Pediatric abdominal pain: An emergency medicine perspective. *Emerg Med Clin N Am* 2016; 34: 341–61.
2. Addiss DG, Shaffer N, Fowler BS, et al. The epidemiology of appendicitis and appendectomy in the United States. *Am J Epidemiol* 1990; 132: 910–25.

3. Armstrong C. ACEP releases guidelines on evaluation of suspected acute appendicitis. *Am Fam Phys* 2010; 81: 1043–4.

4. Hansen LW, Dolgin SE. Trends in the diagnosis and management of pediatric appendicitis. *Pediatr Rev* 2016; 37: 52–7.

5. Kosloske AM, Love CL, Rohrer JE, et al. The diagnosis of appendicitis in children: Outcomes of a strategy based on ediatric surgical evaluation. *Pediatrics* 2004; 113: 29–34.

Case 2

Contributing Author: Michelle Clinton

History

The patient is a 14-year-old female who was referred to the ED by her PCP for evaluation of abdominal pain. She complains of lower abdominal pain and cramping over the past day, and has had decreased urine output over the last 2 days. The patient states that she was started on an oral contraceptive pill 16 days ago due to amenorrhea and her menstrual period started 2 days ago. She reports that she missed a few days of taking the pill. She states that she had a normal stool this morning and denies history of constipation, stating she generally has a bowel movement every 1–2 days. She states she was also started on metformin 16 days ago due to insulin resistance. Patient denies history of difficulty urinating prior to this episode. She also denies fever, chills, nausea, vomiting, hematuria, urinary frequency, and dysuria. She denies episodes of incontinence of urine or stool. She does have a history of hemorrhoids. The patient's mother states that she has to hold her urine for long periods of time because she recently started high school. On further questioning, the patient admits to having slightly less frequent, harder, smaller stools over the past several weeks.

Past Medical History

- Hyperinsulinemia.
- Hyperandrogenemia.
- Abnormal weight gain.

Medications

- Norgestimate/ethinyl estradiol 0.25 mg/35 mcg daily.
- Metformin 1,000 mg daily.

Allergies

- NKDA.

Physical Examination and Ancillary Studies

- *Vital signs*: T 99.1 °F, HR 70, BP 123/79, RR 18, O_2 sat 98% on room air, weight 129 kg.
- *General*: Awake, alert, appears uncomfortable. Obese.
- *HEENT*: PERRL. Mucous membranes moist.
- *Neck*: Supple, with no adenopathy.
- *Cardiovascular*: Heart has regular rate and rhythm. No M/R/G.
- *Lungs*: Clear bilaterally. No W/R/R.
- *Abdomen*: Obese and soft. Normal bowel sounds; suprapubic tenderness to palpation without guarding or rebound. Fullness is palpated in the suprapubic region. There is no costovertebral angle tenderness. Normal genitalia.
- *Extremities and skin*: No edema, no extremity tenderness; distal pulses are intact.
- *Neurologic*: Cranial nerves intact, normal strength and sensation. No saddle anesthesia.
- *Pertinent laboratory values*: U/A is negative for nitrite, leukocyte esterase, WBC, RBC, protein, glucose, and ketones. Specific gravity is 1.009. WBC 10,800, Hb 12.9, HCT 38.9, and basic metabolic panel is within normal limits.
- *Pertinent imaging*: Bedside U/S shown in Figure 8.3.

Questions for Thought

- What further diagnostic modalities could you use to evaluate this patient?
- What are the typical laboratory findings in this condition?
- What are the typical U/S findings?
- What treatments should be initiated in the ED?
- What underlying causes contribute to this condition?
- What is definitive treatment of this condition?

Diagnosis

- Bladder and bowel dysfunction with urinary retention and constipation.

Discussion

- *Epidemiology*: Constipation is generally defined as two or fewer bowel movements per week with an

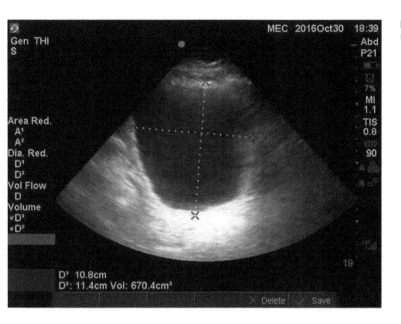

Figure 8.3 U/S demonstrating 664 mL of urine in the bladder.

episode of fecal incontinence, in the setting of a history of excessive stool retention, painful or hard bowel movements, presence of a large fecal mass in the rectum, and a history of stools that may stop up the toilet.

Constipation is a common condition affecting an estimated 5–10 percent of children and accounting for 3–5 percent of pediatrician visits.[1–3] ED visits for constipation are increasing steadily, with one study showing a 50.7 percent increase in constipation-related ED visits in children of ages 1 to 17 from 2006 to 2011.[4] Constipation affects all ages of children, but is most prevalent in the preschool years. Functional constipation is the cause of about 95 percent of pediatric constipation.[1–3,5] Organic causes of constipation in children should be considered when the presentation and physical examination are not consistent with a functional cause. Presenting factors that make an organic cause of a child's constipation more likely include neonatal constipation, history of constipation since birth, delayed passage of meconium, failure to thrive, vomiting, blood in the stool, abdominal distension, anal stenosis, and an empty rectum on physical examination.[3]

Neonatal constipation should raise concern for anatomic causes, Hirschsprung's disease, intestinal obstruction, or metabolic causes such as hypothyroidism or cystic fibrosis.[3] Children with neurologic disorders commonly suffer from constipation as a result of delayed colonic transit times, abnormal innervation, and poor muscle tone. Most constipation presenting after infancy is functional constipation and is often related to social factors.

Dysfunctional elimination syndrome or bladder-bowel dysfunction refers to the condition in which constipation is associated with bladder dysfunction. It is common for ano-rectal dysfunction to be associated with urinary symptoms; more than 50 percent of children evaluated with lower urinary tract symptoms meet the diagnostic criteria for functional constipation.[6,7] Bladder dysfunction associated with constipation can manifest as bladder under- or over-activity, urgency, or frequency.

- *Pathophysiology*: Painful defecation is often an underlying cause of functional constipation, which is in turn frequently related to social factors that lead to stool retention. Toilet training, inaccessible toileting facilities or unwillingness to use public toilets, dehydration, viral illness, and stress often contribute to stool-holding behavior in children. This leads to increased colonic water absorption from the feces and creates hard, large stools that are painful to pass, perpetuating the problem when not properly treated. Dietary factors such as lack of fiber or water intake also contribute. Infant dyschezia is rather common in

177

the first year of life and is caused by the incoordination of abdominal muscle contraction and anal relaxation necessary to produce a bowel movement, causing straining and grunting with attempted defecation. The large majority of constipation in children over 1 year of age is functional constipation; however, organic causes must always be sought, particularly in young children and infants.

Congenital aganglionic megacolon, or Hirschsprung's disease, is a rare condition caused by an absence of ganglion cells in the rectum and often presents at birth with delayed passage of meconium. The rectum is usually empty on digital examination in patients with this condition. Cerebral palsy and spina bifida are potential neurogenic causes of constipation. Abnormal findings in neurologic examination should raise concern for an underlying congenital neurologic problem or lesion involving the spinal cord, such as a neuroblastoma. Anatomic causes of constipation, such as imperforate anus, anterior displaced anus, fissures, or strictures, should be assessed for on physical examination.

Other potential contributing factors to constipation include medications, lead toxicity, endocrine disease, and metabolic conditions. Anticholinergics, opiates, iron supplements, and antidepressants are pharmacologic agents that can cause constipation. Endocrine conditions such as diabetes mellitus, hypothyroidism, or hyperparathyroidism may contribute to constipation. Electrolyte disturbances are a metabolic factor that often incites constipation, while cystic fibrosis, celiac disease, and milk protein intolerance are underlying conditions whose pathophysiology and effect on electrolytes both contribute to constipation.

- *Presentation*: Constipation in children may present with a wide variety of subjective complaints. Older children frequently present with symptoms of crampy, intermittent, central abdominal pain. Parents may be unaware that the child is constipated, but further questioning often reveals that symptoms improve after a large stool. Other symptoms that may be noted include abdominal distension, irritability, soiling, and decreased appetite. Parents of infants with constipation frequently describe straining, grunting, and the infant turning red in the face, as well as the passage of small, hard stools.

- *Diagnosis*: History should focus on identifying signs and symptoms that are associated with the increased likelihood of an organic cause of constipation, including melena, history of constipation since birth or delayed meconium passage, urinary retention, vomiting, fever, failure to thrive, severe abdominal distension, and neurologic deficits. The presence of any of these symptoms or physical examination findings should prompt more in-depth evaluation with focused laboratory tests, imaging, and consultation as deemed appropriate by the emergency physician.

The absence of any of the above alarm signs makes functional constipation the likely diagnosis in patients presenting with symptoms of constipation. The Rome IV criteria were established to aid in the diagnosis of functional constipation in children aged 4 or above and is defined as the presence of at least two of the following criteria occurring at least once weekly over a period of at least 1 month: less than three stools per week, at least one episode of stool incontinence weekly, stool mass palpated on rectal or abdominal examination, history of retentive posturing or stool withholding, history of painful, hard stools, and history of large-volume stools that may obstruct the toilet. Focused history and physical examination are generally sufficient for the diagnosis of functional constipation in children and further diagnostic studies are unwarranted.

The physical examination should include a global assessment of development, weight gain, hydration, and nutrition status. A detailed abdominal examination should be performed and the presence of bowel sounds, tenderness, distension, and stool mass should be assessed. The back and perianal area should be evaluated for evidence of a sacral dimple (which is associated with spina bifida), perianal strep infection, skin tags, anal fissure, and anal wink. A detailed neurologic examination should be performed and should include an assessment of tone, deep tendon reflexes, saddle anesthesia, and gait.

A digital rectal examination is invasive and uncomfortable and is generally not necessary in evaluating children presenting with constipation.

Digital rectal examination should be performed in infants and patients with history of constipation since early infancy to assess for anatomic abnormalities, and when alarm symptoms suggestive of an organic cause of constipation are present. It may also be considered when the degree of constipation is uncertain. A large amount of hard stool is generally present in the rectum of patients with functional constipation, while children with colonic neuropathy tend to have scant stool and a narrow ampulla.

Imaging does not generally play a role in the diagnosis of constipation. A recent study involving 3,685 pediatric patients evaluated in an ED who were diagnosed with constipation revealed that, unless an alternative diagnosis is being considered, abdominal X-rays are not helpful and can delay recognition of more serious diagnoses.[8] An abdominal radiograph was performed more frequently in children with misdiagnosis of constipation (75 percent vs. 45 percent).[8] These children more frequently had abdominal pain and tenderness on examination. Nevertheless, if plain films are done, the provider may see stool in the rectal vault as well as formed stool throughout the colon (Figure 8.4 in Case 4 below).

- *Treatment*: The treatment of pediatric constipation is multidisciplinary and close follow-up with the patient's PCP is important to assess response to treatment started in the ED, to reinforce parental education, and to establish a maintenance treatment plan. Oral, rectal, or a combination of treatments is usually effective; however, it should be considered that rectal treatments might exacerbate the psychologic components contributing to constipation. An aggressive oral disimpaction protocol is generally very effective in treating functional constipation. For children under the age of 5 it is recommended that a solution of eight capfuls of polyethylene glycol electrolyte lavage solution 3350 in 64 ounces of liquid be made. For children 5 years and older, 16 capfuls of polyethylene glycol is mixed in 64 ounces of liquid. Eight ounces may be administered every 15 minutes until finished. If results are unsatisfactory, this protocol may be reattempted the following day. Lower doses of polyethylene glycol or milk of magnesia may be used in less severe cases of constipation.

Rectally administered glycerin suppositories are safe in young infants and are often effective in treating infant dyschezia. Addition of carbohydrate-containing osmotic liquids such as prune juice, corn syrup, or malt syrup extract to breast milk or formula will help soften stools. Two to four ounces per day of fruit juice is the suggested dose for children 4 months or older. Polyethylene glycol may be given to infants 6 months and older with ongoing constipation after above treatments. Sodium phosphate or mineral oil enemas may be administered to children age 3 and above in whom oral treatment is resisted by the child or ineffective. An enema solution of 15–30 mL per year of age is the recommended dose. Maintenance treatment is recommended for at least 6 months after an acute episode of constipation and is generally accomplished with a lower dose of polyethylene glycol: one-half to one capful of polyethylene glycol in 8 ounces of liquid, one to two times daily.

Dietary changes should be discussed and the parents instructed to increase fiber by assuring the child gets at least five servings of fruits and vegetables per day. Fluid intake must also be increased. Positive reinforcement is encouraged and parents should be instructed to create protected time for children to have a bowel movement by placing the patient on the toilet for 5–10 minutes two to three times daily to encourage stooling.

- *Disposition*: Constipation may be treated as an outpatient, with close follow-up with the child's PCP.

Historical clues	Physical findings	Ancillary studies
• Change in stool habits • Abdominal pain • Difficulty urinating	• Suprapubic fullness • Essentially benign examination otherwise	• Bedside U/S with urinary retention

Follow-Up

This patient's diagnosis of bladder-bowel dysfunction was determined by a thorough history and the absence of physical examination or laboratory findings concerning for acute infectious or other obstructive intra-abdominal or genitourinary pathology. Bladder catheterization was performed and 700 mL of urine drained from the patient's bladder. She was observed and unable to urinate within 2 hours of initial catheterization. Repeat bladder U/S revealed 550 mL of urine in the bladder. Subsequently, the patient was able to urinate spontaneously and final bedside U/S revealed only 50 mL of urine in the bladder. The patient's mother expressed that the patient had to hold urine for long periods of time due to not being able to use the bathroom very often after recently starting high school. The patient was discharged home with instructions for timed voiding every 2 hours. She was also prescribed 17 g of polyethylene glycol in 8-ounce liquid twice daily for constipation because it was felt that her urinary retention was related to stool withholding.

Unfortunately, this outpatient treatment was initially unsuccessful and the patient returned to the ED 4 days later with persistent abdominal pain. Laboratory tests were unremarkable on repeat ED evaluation. CT imaging was performed to evaluate for appendicitis as the patient had right-lower-quadrant tenderness and her morbid obesity precluded appendicitis evaluation by U/S. The CT was negative for evidence of appendicitis or other acute intra-abdominal pathology. A very large stool burden was noted on CT and the patient was admitted to the inpatient pediatrics team and underwent fecal disimpaction with polyethylene glycol 3350 via a nasogastric tube. The patient passed a large amount of stool, progressing to clear diarrhea. The difficulty in urinating and abdominal pain resolved and the patient was discharged home with a continued daily regimen of oral polyethylene glycol.

References

1. van den Berg MM, Benninga MA, DiLorenzo C. Epidemiology of childhood constipation: A systematic review. *Am J Gastroenterol* 2006; 101: 2401–9.

2. Getto L, Zeserson E, Breyer M. Vomiting, diarrhea, constipation, and gastroenteritis. *Emerg Med Clin N Am* 2011; 29: 211–37.

3. Nurko S, Zimmerman LA. Evaluation and treatment of constipation in children and adolescents. *Am Fam Phys* 2014; 90: 82–90.

4. Sommers T, Corban C, Sengupta N, et al. Emergency department burden of constipation in the United States from 2006 to 2011. *Am J Gastroenterol* 2015; 110: 572–9.

5. Hyams JS, DiLorenzo C, Saps M, et al. Childhood functional gastrointestinal disorders: Child/adolescent. *Gastroenterology* 2016; 150: 1456–68.

6. Burgers RE, Mugie SM, Chase J, et al. Management of functional constipation in children with lower urinary tract symptoms: Report from the Standarization Committee of the International Children's Continence Society. *J Urol* 2013; 190: 29–36.

7. Burgers R, de Jong TP, Visser M, et al. Functional defecation disorders in children with lower urinary tract symptoms. *J Urol* 2013; 189: 1886–91.

8. Freedman SB, Thull-Freedman J, Manson D, et al. Pediatric abdominal radiograph use, constipation, and significant misdiagnoses. *J Pediatr* 2014; 164: 83–8.

Case 3

Contributing Authors: Alyssa Milano and Sadé McKenzie

History

The patient is a 16-year-old male who presents to the ED with nausea for the past several days. He complains of abdominal pain and several episodes of non-bloody, non-bilious vomiting earlier today. His abdominal pain is diffuse, constant, and described as crampy. He denies associated fevers and diarrhea. He also complains of a sore throat and sinus congestion. On further questioning, the patient reports recent weight loss and generalized fatigue. He denies having a headache, cough, chest pain, or shortness of breath. He denies experiencing similar episodes in the past, sick contacts, or recent travel.

Past Medical History

- Inguinal hernia repair.
- Seasonal allergies.
- UTD on immunizations.

Medications

- Cetirizine.

Allergies

- Amoxicillin–clavulanate.

Physical Examination and Ancillary Studies

- *Vital signs:* T 97.6 °F, HR 110, RR 25, BP 121/72, O_2 sat 97% on room air.
- *General:* The patient is awake and alert, appears to be in a moderate amount of distress.

- *HEENT*: PERRL. Mucous membranes are dry.
- *Neck*: Supple, with no adenopathy.
- *Cardiovascular*: Tachycardic, with no M/R/G.
- *Lungs*: CTA bilaterally, without W/R/R. Patient is tachypneic but not dyspneic.
- *Abdomen*: Soft, non-tender, non-distended, with normoactive bowel sounds. No guarding or rebound tenderness.
- *Extremities and skin*: No rashes. Skin is warm and dry. No peripheral edema. Pulses are intact in all extremities.
- *Neurologic*: Cranial nerves II–XII are intact. Motor strength and sensation are intact.
- *Pertinent laboratory values*: Serum glucose 666 mg/dL, Na 130, K 5.1, Cl 106, bicarbonate 6, serum acetone 1+, urine ketones positive.

Questions for Thought

- What laboratory tests would be diagnostic in this patient?
- What treatments would you initiate in this patient?
- How would you monitor the response to therapy in this patient?
- What complication is unique to the pediatric population?

Diagnosis

- Diabetic ketoacidosis in type 1 diabetes mellitus, new onset.

Discussion

- *Epidemiology*: Diabetes mellitus is a common endocrine disorder seen among pediatric and adult patients. There are two types of diabetes mellitus, type 1 and type 2. In general, type 1 occurs in a younger population secondary to insulin deficiency while type 2 occurs in the middle-aged to older population, due to insulin resistance. Type 1 diabetes mellitus is the most common pediatric endocrine disorder. Of children presenting in diabetic ketoacidosis (DKA), 27–40 percent of them will be diagnosed with new-onset type 1 diabetes mellitus.[1–4] Children less than 5 years old are more likely to present in DKA.[1–3] Children with a prior diagnosis of diabetes mellitus are less likely to have recurrent episodes of DKA, approximately 1–10 per 100 patients per year.[1,2] Risk factors for recurrent episodes of DKA include poor metabolic control, psychiatric diagnoses, difficult or unstable family, limited access to medical services, and coexisting infection. DKA is the leading cause of mortality in diabetic patients less than 24 years old.[4]

- *Pathophysiology*: DKA is caused by the absolute loss of insulin, which leads to upregulation of counterregulatory hormones, including glucagon, catecholamines, cortisol, and growth hormone. With the increase in these hormones, cells begin to undergo lipolysis, proteolysis, glycogenolysis, and decreased glucose utilization. After upregulation of these pathways, patients develop ketogenesis with ketone body production and hyperglycemia. The major ketoacid produced (and subsequently measured) is β-hydroxybutyrate. Elevated levels of β-hydroxybutyrate ultimately cause the metabolic acidosis associated with DKA. Hyperglycemia leads to glucosuria, osmotic diuresis, dehydration, and elevated serum osmolality.

- *Presentation*: Patients presenting in DKA can have a wide variety of complaints; however, most complain of vague abdominal pain, nausea, and vomiting.[3] Patients may complain of generalized malaise, getting progressively worse over the recent weeks. Further questioning may reveal a history of polyuria, polydipsia, and recent weight loss.

  On physical examination, patients will likely appear dehydrated; vital signs may reveal tachycardia and hypotension, depending on the severity of dehydration. The characteristic smell of acetone on the breath may be appreciated. Patients may also have Kussmaul breathing, the body's compensatory response to the overwhelming acidosis. The remainder of the physical examination may reveal findings associated with coexisting infection, as many patients with DKA have an infectious precipitant. The abdominal examination is usually benign, and if abdominal tenderness is appreciated, frequent re-evaluations must be done to monitor its resolution with DKA treatment. Neurologic examination may reveal an altered level of consciousness, ranging from lethargy to coma. Cerebral edema occurs in 1 percent of all patients with DKA, most commonly in children less than

5 years old.[1-6] Cerebral edema carries significant morbidity and mortality, accounting for 57–87 percent of all pediatric DKA-associated deaths.[1] If cerebral edema is present, patients may have cranial nerve palsies, abnormal motor or verbal responses, and posturing.

- *Diagnosis*: The diagnosis of DKA is based on laboratory values. DKA is defined by the presence of metabolic acidosis (pH less than 7.3 or bicarbonate less than 15), with concomitant hyperglycemia, ketonemia, glucosuria, and ketonuria.[1-4] The clinician should maintain a high index of suspicion for DKA in the vomiting child, particularly in the absence of diarrhea. When concern for DKA is present, the clinician should obtain serum glucose, VBG or ABG, U/A, and an electrolyte panel including potassium, sodium, calcium, and phosphate. Patients are usually found to have hyponatremia on initial testing, secondary to hyperglycemia and cellular fluid shift. The corrected sodium is obtained by the following formula: Na + [1.6 × (glucose – 100)]. Serum sodium levels should normalize with fluid and insulin therapy. Patients typically also have abnormalities in potassium levels. Overall, patients have a total body decrease in potassium secondary to osmotic diuresis; however, at presentation patients may appear hyperkalemic as a result of an extracellular potassium shift in response to acidosis. Potassium levels will begin to decrease with insulin treatment. Additional laboratory tests to consider include serum ketone levels, LFTs, serum osmolality, and magnesium.

  The diagnosis of cerebral edema is overwhelmingly a clinical one because CT scans are found to be normal in up to 40 percent of symptomatic children.[1,3,6] Symptoms of cerebral edema tend to occur 6–12 hours after therapy onset; however, cases have been reported at the time of presentation before therapy initiation.[1,3]

- *Treatment*: The goals of DKA treatment are to restore circulating volume, replace water deficits, and clear serum glucose and ketones. Treatment of DKA is started with an assessment of the dehydration status and peripheral perfusion. If the patient is hemodynamically unstable or reveals signs of poor peripheral perfusion and shock, a fluid bolus dosed 10–20 cc/kg of normal saline can be given.[1-4] A bolus can be repeated if shock persists. After the patient stabilizes, the remainder of the fluid should be administered as 0.45% saline over the next 48 hours. Potassium, dosed 30–40 mEq/L, should be added to the maintenance fluid to prevent and treat hypokalemia. Because of arrhythmia from very low potassium, the provider should not start insulin until the potassium level is known.[3] If the potassium is normal, potassium should be added (40 mEq/L) to fluids, and if it is low, it should be repleted concurrently with insulin initiation.[3] Once the patient is hemodynically stable, a continuous infusion of insulin at 0.1 unit/kg per hour is started. An insulin bolus is strongly advised against, due to the fear of developing cerebral edema, with a rapid drop in serum osmolality. Once serum glucose has decreased to 300, 5% glucose is added to the maintenance fluids with goal glucose levels of 150–300.[1-3] If the glucose cannot be maintained in that range, the insulin infusion can be decreased to 0.05 unit/kg per hour. Bicarbonate is contraindicated in children with DKA as it is associated with a fourfold increase in cerebral edema.

- *Disposition*: The vast majority of patients with DKA will require admission to the hospital. In patients with severe acidosis, admission to an ICU is warranted. Patients will require close monitoring with hourly glucose and vital-sign checks, along with a reassessment of electrolytes and acid–base status every 2 hours. A small subset of patients, who are clinically stable with resolving acidosis and close follow-up, may be discharged home.

Historical clues	Physical findings	Ancillary studies
• Abdominal pain	• Tachycardia	• Hyperglycemia
• Vomiting without diarrhea	• Tachypnea without increased work of breathing	• Elevated anion gap
• Recent viral illness	• Benign abdomen	• Ketonuria
• Weight loss		• Ketonemia

Follow-Up

The child was admitted to the step-down unit after appropriate resuscitation in the ED. He was placed on an insulin drip and his anion gap and serum glucose normalized. He required supplemental potassium during his hospital stay. While inpatient, he and his parents received diabetic education and had an endocrinology consultation. He was discharged on hospital day 3 on a home insulin regimen.

References

1. Rosenbloom AL. The management of diabetic ketoacidosis in children. *Diabetes Ther* 2010; 1: 103–20.

2. Wolfsdorf J, Glaser N, Sperling MA. Diabetic ketoacidosis in infants, children, and adolescents. *Diabetes Care* 2006; 29: 1150–9.

3. Olivieri L, Chasm R. Diabetic ketoacidosis in the pediatric emergency department. *Emerg Med Clin N Am* 2013; 31: 755–73.

4. Westerberg DP. Diabetic ketoacidosis: Evaluation and treatment. *Am Fam Phys* 2013; 87: 337–46.

5. Glaser NS, Wootton-Gorges SL, Marcin JP, et al. Mechanism of cerebral edema in children with diabetic ketoacidosis. 2004; 145: 164–71.

6. Levin DL. Cerebral edema in diabetic ketoacidosis. *Pediatr Crit Care Med* 2008; 9: 320–9.

Case 4

Contributing Authors: Holly Stankewicz and Rebecca Jeanmonod

History

The patient is a 10-year-old boy brought in for what his parents believe is abdominal pain. The child is non-verbal at baseline, related to trisomy 21 and "autism spectrum." The child knows a few signs and usually "makes himself understood." His parents state that, while walking, he periodically stops and crouches down and appears uncomfortable. He has been playing and running around less than usual. They have not noted fevers, and state that he is still eating well. He has had his normal appetite, frequently putting his hand up to his mouth to signify that he is hungry. There have been no episodes of vomiting. He has chronic constipation, but they do not believe that it is any worse than usual. The child is toilet trained, so they do not know when he last defecated, but they report they have not had to plunge the toilet in the last week or so. He has not had any incontinence. They are unaware of any trauma. The child attends school, and his aide at school says he has been reluctant to participate in gym for the last 2 weeks or so. The parents have not noted any coughing, runny nose, or sneezing. They have not noticed any rashes. They don't think he has lost any weight.

Past Medical History

- Trisomy 21.
- Autism spectrum disorder.
- Was seen in the ED 3 months ago and underwent CT scan under sedation, which was remarkable for constipation and no other abnormalities.
- UTD on immunizations.

Medications

- None.

Allergies

- NKDA.

Physical Examination and Ancillary Studies

- *Vital signs*: T 97 °F tympanic thermometer, HR 115, RR 24, BP 125/80, O_2 sat 98% on room air.
- *General*: Agitated and difficult to assess, attempts to strike anyone who gets near him. Refuses to get on the bed, is sitting in a chair, making the sign for "hungry" to his parents.
- *HEENT*: PERRL, atraumatic, normocephalic, mucous membranes are moist, tympanic membranes normal.
- *Neck*: Child moves neck all around with no pain. No adenopathy.
- *Cardiovascular*: Regular, without murmurs. Good peripheral pulses and normal capillary refill.
- *Lungs*: Clear and equal, with no W/R/R.
- *Abdomen*: Child is not compliant with examination. He kicks and claws when attempts are made to palpate the abdomen. Child seems to range the hip without difficulty. Testicles are descended bilaterally. No penile lesions. Cannot appreciate masses. Cannot adequately assess for tenderness, guarding, or rebound.
- *Extremities and skin*: Warm and well-perfused without rashes or deformity. Moves all four extremities spontaneously. Child can ambulate, but seems to be limping, favoring the right, and crouches down every 3–4 steps.
- *Neurologic*: Non-verbal, but interacts with parents. No focal abnormalities.
- *Pertinent laboratory values*: WBC 16,800, remainder of CBC and all chemistries normal.
- *Pertinent imaging*: Abdominal series with stool throughout colon (Figure 8.4).

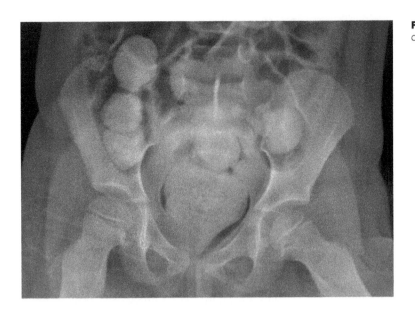

Figure 8.4 Abdominal series demonstrating constipation.

Questions for Thought

- What are possible sources of this child's symptoms that should be considered?
- Does this child warrant imaging? Does he warrant admission?
- Does the finding of constipation on radiograph adequately explain the patient's presentation?

Diagnosis

- Bowel perforation secondary to ingested foreign body.

Discussion

- *Epidemiology*: It is difficult to determine the exact incidence of pediatric foreign-body ingestions but it is a common pediatric ED complaint. Infants and young children explore objects by putting them in their mouths, and studies suggest that there are more than 125,000 presentations of foreign-body ingestions by children yearly.[1,2] The most commonly ingested foreign bodies are coins. However, magnets and batteries are increasing in frequency, due to increasing numbers of electronic toys and devices and small magnets used for play or to imitate piercings. Children 6 years old and younger are the most likely to ingest foreign bodies, and the frequency is higher in underdeveloped countries.[1-3] In young children, males and females are equally affected. In older children and adolescents, males are more likely to ingest foreign bodies than females.

- *Pathophysiology*: Once a foreign body is swallowed, the most common site of impaction is the thoracic inlet where skeletal muscle changes to smooth muscle in the esophagus. The majority of esophageal impactions occur at this point, followed by the mid esophagus and the lower esophageal sphincter. Children with previous esophageal abnormalities are likely to have a foreign body become lodged at the site of the abnormality. Sharp objects may become impaled anywhere in the esophagus, or indeed anywhere in the entire GI tract. If the foreign body reaches the stomach, it is less likely to cause complications. Exceptions include stomach ulceration from interaction of zinc (in coins) and stomach acid, pointed objects, toxic objects, objects unable to pass through the pyloric sphincter due to length over 6 cm or width greater than 2 cm, multiple magnet ingestion, or problems related to previous GI-tract abnormalities.[1-6] If a foreign body does become impacted it may cause local irritation, obstruction, bleeding, mucosal erosion, perforation, pain, or no symptoms at all. Erosions through the esophagus may cause mediastinitis or even aortoenteric fistulas.

  Objects that pass the pylorus, even straight pins, are likely to pass through the GI tract completely, without complication. However, occasionally, objects will cause obstruction at the ileocecal valve or cause perforation at any area within the bowel. These perforations can self-seal with granuloma formation, abscess formation, or cause intra-abdominal sepsis. These can present in a delayed fashion and with no apparent history of foreign-body ingestion.

- *Presentation*: Children may present with symptoms including (but not limited to) drooling, fussiness, stridor, pain including chest or abdominal pain, refusal to eat or drink, wheezing, fevers, respiratory distress, cough, vomiting, altered mental status, abdominal distension, hematemesis, or hematochezia. Children may also be asymptomatic but present due to caregiver suspicion of an ingested foreign body or after passing a foreign body in their stool.

- *Diagnosis*: A good history and physical will aid in the diagnosis in most cases, although not in this case. Chest and/or abdominal X-rays will show ingested foreign bodies that are radiopaque. If the object is identified below the diaphragm, a single frontal radiograph is usually sufficient. If the object is seen in the esophagus, frontal and lateral CXRs are indicated to assess location as well as to determine what the object is and to make sure it is one object and not two stuck together.[3,4] Additionally, the lateral CXR can aid in confirmation that a coin, for example, is in the esophagus and not the trachea, since coins in the esophagus typically appear in the coronal orientation as opposed to a coin in the trachea, which is typically seen in the sagittal orientation. If a radiolucent object is suspected, diagnosis may be aided by having the child drink a small amount of dilute contrast and repeating the study, or one can proceed directly to endoscopy. Similarly, if foreign-body ingestion is strongly suspected on clinical examination and history, direct visualization may be the most efficient method to both diagnose and remove the object. Another possible diagnostic strategy is to use a metal detector to identify the location of a metallic object such as a coin. CT imaging may be of benefit in the assessment of foreign-body ingestion where bowel perforation or obstruction is suspected. Further information on this can be found in Chapter 5, Case 1.

Although observation is a strategy for foreign body, it is predicated upon the diagnosis being made. Likewise, in cases of non-specific abdominal pain, observation and serial abdominal examinations represent a reasonable option. In this case, there was no diagnostic certainty, and there was no ability to follow serial examinations. The child had an X-ray that demonstrated constipation, but does that adequately explain the child's symptoms? It has been shown in a large study that there is no difference between the amount of stool seen on radiographs of children with serious pathology compared to those with a final diagnosis of simple constipation.[7] In those with pain and tenderness, constipation is a diagnosis of exclusion.[7]

When possible, it is preferable to avoid CT in children due to the radiation burden. However, this child illustrates an important point: serial examinations only work in children who can be examined. U/S is an option to evaluate for appendicitis or intussusception or even torsion, but is dependent upon the operator, and is best used to seek for a specific clinical entity. CT scanning gives a more comprehensive assessment of the bowel, liver, and retroperitoneum, and is a reasonable option when the clinician frankly is looking for something, but is not entirely sure what. The differential diagnosis in this child included surgical pathology such as appendicitis, psoas abscess, hip pathology, renal or testicular pathology, or infectious disease. This particular case has the added risks associated with sedation for imaging, and is a difficult judgment call.

- *Treatment*: If there is concern that the child is unable to protect their airway, intubation may be necessary. Most children who swallow a foreign body do not require any intervention at all. If the child is symptomatic (cough, stridor, drooling, pain, etc.) and there is a foreign body impacted in the esophagus, endoscopy is recommended. If the child is asymptomatic and there is a blunt foreign body in the esophagus, especially if located at the lower esophageal sphincter, these children may be observed for 12–24 hours with hope of spontaneous passage. If smooth objects have passed the duodenal sweep, they can be managed conservatively with stool inspection and possibly X-ray surveillance. If the object fails to pass through the GI tract or if the patient becomes symptomatic, endoscopic or surgical intervention may be needed. Alternatives to endoscopy for esophageal foreign bodies include the foley catheter method and the bougienage method to remove esophageal foreign bodies.[1-6] Blunt foreign bodies may be removed by passing an uninflated Foley catheter distal to the object in a patient who is positioned head-down on the table. The catheter is then inflated and gently withdrawn, potentially bringing the foreign body with it. The object may also be dislodged and passed into the stomach during this technique. This technique is often performed under fluoroscopy and should be carried out by experienced clinicians only. It should also only be done in cases where there was a witnessed ingestion of a blunt object less than 24 hours before the procedure, in a healthy child. The bougienage method involves passing a bougie down the esophagus in an attempt to dislodge and push the object into the stomach. It should be performed with the patient sitting upright. This technique should only be performed in a healthy child who had a witnessed foreign-body ingestion less than 24 hours prior to procedure. The bougienage method has been shown to be safe and highly effective as well as more time- and cost-efficient than other treatment options. Surgery may be indicated if there are suspected complications, such as bowel perforation or obstruction.

- Button batteries: Patients with button batteries lodged in the esophagus are at high risk for perforation due to the caustic nature of the battery. If there is concern that the foreign body lodged in the esophagus is a button battery, then endoscopy should be performed. If a button battery has passed into the stomach it does not need to be removed immediately, as it will likely pass through the lower GI tract without complication. Parents should be instructed to observe the stool for 2–3 days and if the battery has not passed, they must return for repeat X-rays. If the button battery remains in the stomach or is at a fixed spot in the intestines, it should be removed.
- Magnets: Patients with ingestion of one magnet do not carry any additional risk of bowel injury. In the setting of ingestion of multiple magnets, there is an increased risk of bowel injury due to magnetic attraction across the bowel wall and resulting pressure necrosis. Patients with

ingestion of multiple magnets should be observed carefully with a low threshold for endoscopic or surgical removal of the magnets.
- Children with perforation or abscesses may need laparotomy or interventional radiology drainage as well as IV antibiotics.

- *Disposition*: After uncomplicated removal of an esophageal foreign body, a healthy child may be safely discharged. Further evaluation for underlying esophageal problems should be done in a child with repeated foreign-body impaction or impaction at an unusual location. If the child has a foreign body in the stomach or lower GI tract without symptoms or obvious complications, he or she may be discharged with instructions to return if any symptoms develop, such as pain, vomiting, constipation, or fever. Children with GI-tract abnormalities, unusual foreign bodies, or frequent foreign-body ingestion may require additional evaluation and management. While most foreign bodies pass without complication, follow-up imaging should be performed for sharp foreign bodies or button batteries which did not require urgent retrieval from the esophagus.

Historical clues	Physical findings	Ancillary studies
• Abdominal pain • Crouching when walking	• Tachycardia • Difficult examination	• Plain film with constipation

Follow-Up

Although the child had had a prior CT with no significant diaognsis, the parents' concern and the provider's inability to assess the child led to the child undergoing procedural sedation and CT scanning (Figure 8.5). The child's CT demonstrated a needle-like foreign body that had perforated the child's intestine near the ileocecal valve. The child was admitted for IV antibiotics and underwent interventional radiologic drainage of the abscess and a prolonged course of antibiotics via a PICC line.

References

1. Hesham A-Kader H. Foreign body ingestion: Children like to put objects in their mouth. *World J Pediatr* 2010; 6: 301–10.
2. Kay M, Wyllie R. Pediatric foreign bodies and their management. *Curr Gastroenterol Rep* 2005; 7: 212–18.

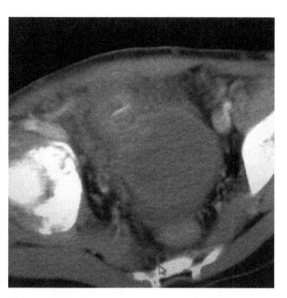

Figure 8.5 CT scan demonstrating needle-like foreign body in the right lower quadrant with a related abscess.

3. Uyemura MC. Foreign body ingestion in children. *Am Fam Phys* 2005; 72: 287–91.

4. Kramer RE, Lerner DG, Lin T, et al. Management of ingested foreign bodies in children: A clinical report of the NASPHAN Endoscopy Committee. *J Pediatr Gastroenterol Nutr* 2015; 60: 562–74.

5. Şahin A, Meteroğlu F, Erbey A, et al. Insidious threat of children: Esophageal foreign body ingestion. *JAEM* 2014; 13: 159–61.

6. Cevik M, Gökdemir MT, Boleken ME, et al. The characteristics and outcomes of foreign body ingestion and aspiration in children due to lodged foreign body in the aerodigestive tract. *Pediatr Emerg Care* 2013; 29: 53–7.

7. Freedma SB, Thull-Freedman J, Manson D, et al. Pediatric abdominal radiograph use, constipation, and significant misdiagnoses. *J Pediatr* 2014; 164: 83–8.

Case 5

Contributing Author: Sadé McKenzie

History

The patient is a 17-year-old healthy female who presents with bilateral lower quadrant abdominal pain. The pain started 5 days prior to presentation, with a severity of 7 out of 10. The pain is equally severe on either side. She cannot describe any alleviating or aggravating factors. Associated symptoms include nausea and feeling bloated. She denies vomiting, vaginal bleeding or abnormal discharge, changes in bowel habits, dysuria, fever, chills or diaphoresis, chest pain, shortness of breath, or any correlation with meals. She has a history of chronic constipation, with her last bowel movement the day prior to presentation; she denies the presence of blood in the stool. She does have unprotected sexual intercourse with one male partner, with no history of sexually transmitted infections (STIs).

Past Medical History
- Spontaneous abortion.

Medications
- Oral contraceptives.

Allergies
- Peanuts.

Physical Examination and Ancillary Studies
- *Vital signs*: 98.5 °F, HR 114, RR 20, BP 128/76, O$_2$ sat 100% on room air.
- *General*: Well-appearing young female; does not appear to be in acute distress.
- *HEENT*: PERRL, mucous membranes moist, no signs of trauma.
- *Neck*: Supple and non-tender, with no adenopathy and midline trachea.
- *Cardiovascular*: Regular tachycardia, with no M/R/G.
- *Lungs*: Normal work of breathing, with clear lungs.
- *Abdomen:* Soft and flat abdomen, normal bowel sounds, moderate tenderness at right lower quadrant and suprapubic area, no rebound or guarding.
- *Pelvic examination*: No lesions to external genitalia; age-appropriate development of external labia; vaginal mucosa pink, with no lesions; mucopurulent discharge within vaginal vault, no foul odor; mucopurulent discharge from cervical os with associated generalized erythema of cervix; no cervical motion tenderness, uterine fundal tenderness, no adnexal tenderness or masses.
- *Extremities and skin*: Warm and well-perfused, with normal capillary refill and no rashes.
- *Neurologic*: Alert, with no focal abnormalities.

- *Pertinent laboratory values*:
  - Urine pregnancy test: negative;
  - CBC: WBC 11,000, Hb 13.4, HCT 39.6, Plt 381,000;
  - U/A: 1+ leukocyte esterase, 2+ hemoglobin, WBC 5–10, RBC 5–10, slight epithelial cells, slight bacteria;
  - *Neisseria gonorrhoeae* and *Chlamydia trachomatis* probes sent. Wet mount with no clue cells, budding yeast, or trichomonads.
- *Pertinent imaging*: Pelvic U/S reveals a small amount of fluid in the pelvis, otherwise unremarkable.

Questions for Thought

- What genitourinary pathologies can present with abdominal pain?
- What are the complications of this diagnosis?
- What practices can be employed to better ensure gathering of a complete sexual history when treating adolescents and young adults?
- What treatments can be initiated in the ED?

Diagnosis

- Chlamydial infection.

Discussion

- *Epidemiology*: The prevalence of STIs is dependent upon age, gender, and race/ethnicity. In the USA, adolescents and young adults aged 15–24 years old account for almost 50 percent of all cases of STIs each year.[1] Females are generally infected at a higher rate than males, with females of African American, Native American/Alaska Native, and Hispanic ethnicities disproportionately affected.[1] Social factors, such as poverty, limited access to healthcare services, homelessness, and sexual abuse and violence, are additional factors that increase adolescents' susceptibility to contracting STIs.[1] Last year, there were over 1,500,000 STIs reported to the CDC.[1]
- *Pathophysiology*: *Chlamydia trachomatis* is an obligate intracellular bacterium responsible for chlamydial infections. Other organisms responsible for bacterial STIs include *Neisseria gonorrhoeae* and *Trichomonas vaginalis*. Although not considered STIs, women may present with co-infections due to *Candida albicans* (vulvovaginal/vaginal candidiasis) or *Gardnerella*

vaginalis (bacterial vaginosis). The former group of organisms cause inflammation of the cervix, uterus, and fallopian tubes. These may progress to frank peritonitis and abscess of the fallopian tubes. The latter group of organisms primarily cause irritation of the vagina and vulva and are discussed in detail in Chapter 11, Case 7.

- *Presentation*: Both men and women with STIs are commonly asymptomatic. *C. trachomatis* and *N. gonorrhoeae* can cause urethritis, epididymitis, orchitis, proctitis, or Reiter syndrome in men; in women, they cause urethritis, cervicitis, pelvic inflammatory disease, and infertility. Urethritis may present with urethral discharge, dysuria, or meatal pruritis in men. Epididymitis may present with unilateral scrotal swelling and tenderness.

  Pelvic inflammatory disease is defined as a spectrum of inflammatory disorders of the female upper genital tract, including endometritis, salpingitis, tubo-ovarian abscess, and pelvic peritonitis. It is the sequela of an untreated STI. Although pelvic inflammatory disease is predominantly caused by *N. gonorrhoeae* and *C. trachomatis*, it should be considered a multiorganism process. The presence of abnormal cervical or vaginal mucopurulent discharge, cervical motion tenderness, uterine tenderness, or adnexal tenderness should raise the suspicion of pelvic inflammatory disease.

  Vaginitis, by comparison, refers to the superficial infection of the vaginal mucosa; it is commonly associated with vaginal discharge and may involve the vulva. Vaginitis can coexist with STIs but is not itself classically considered an STI, and is discussed in more detail in Chapter 11, Case 7. Trichomoniasis classically presents with malodorous, yellow-green vaginal discharge, and may be associated with vulvar irritation. In men, urethritis may develop, but they are often asymptomatic.

  Patients may also present with comorbid disease related to unprotected sex, such as primary HIV infection, HSV infection, syphilis, or pregnancy-related complications.
- *Diagnosis*: Nucleic acid amplification tests allow for very sensitive and non-invasive testing for chlamydial and gonorrheal infections. Nucleic acid amplification tests are licensed for use with urine, urethral, vagina,[1] and cervical specimens. When collecting specimens, male first-void urine

and female vaginal or cervical specimens are considered optimal. Nucleic acid amplification tests work well in the diagnosis of oropharyngeal or rectal gonorrheal or chlamydial infections. The turn-around time on these tests can be longer than the time a patient typically remains in the ED, so high-risk patients should undergo empiric treatment.

- *Treatment*: When treating an STI empirically, both gonorrheal and chlamydial infections should be covered, as concomitant infections are common; treat with single-dose regimens when possible, to ensure compliance.
  - *C. trachomatis*: azithromycin 1 g orally, single dose, or doxycycline 100 mg orally, twice a day for 7 days.
    - Alternatives: erythromycin base 500 mg orally, four times a day for 7 days; oxofloxacin 300 mg orally, twice a day for 7 days; levofloxacin 500 mg orally, once a day for 7 days.
    - Pregnant patient: azithromycin 1 g orally, single dose; amoxicillin 500 mg orally, three times a day for 7 days; erythromycin base 500 mg orally, four times a day for 7 days.
  - *N. gonorrhoeae*: ceftriaxone 250 mg IM, single dose.
    - Alternatives: cefixime 400 mg orally, single dose; cefotaxime 500 mg IM, single dose.

- *Disposition*: Patients should be screened for other STIs (HIV, syphilis, other viral infections) and be provided counseling for STI/HIV prevention and contraception. The local health department should be notified per protocol. Patients should establish follow-up with a PCP or local clinic, and partner(s) should be advised to seek treatment. Patients should be advised to abstain from sexual activity for at least 7 days after treatment. If sexual abuse is suspected, the incident should be reported to CPS, and the collection of forensic evidence may be indicated. Prepubertal girls who are the victims of sexual assault should be tested for STIs, and adolescent victims of sexual assault should be treated prophylactically, regardless of whether STI testing occurs. Patients who are ill with pelvic inflammatory disease should be admitted for IV antibiotics and gynecology consultation.

Historical clues	Physical findings	Ancillary studies
• Abdominal pain • Indolent course • Sexually active adolescent	• Tachycardia • Abdominal tenderness • Erythema of cervix • Mucopurulent cervical discharge	• Negative pregnancy test • Negative wet mount

Follow-Up

The patient was treated empirically for cervicitis in the ED but failed to keep a follow-up appointment with the local health department clinic. She re-presented to the ED several months later with recurrent infection, which had now progressed to pelvic inflammatory disease with tubo-ovarian abscess, and was admitted for surgical management and parenteral antibiotics.

Reference

1. Centers for Disease Control and Prevention. Sexually transmitted diseases (STDs). https://www.cdc.gov/std/stats/ (accessed January 2017).

Case 6

Contributing Author: Brian Kelly

History

A 5-year-old male presents to the ED with his parents for abdominal pain. The onset of the pain was yesterday while the patient was at school. He was subsequently sent home due to concerns that he had the "stomach flu." His parents were concerned that his pain was not going away and that he developed a fever this afternoon of 100.7 °F. They brought him for evaluation because the mother remembers having similar symptoms when she had appendicitis as a child. He describes the pain as cramping in nature. When asked to point to where his pain is, he points to his umbilicus. The patient also admits to having a cough over the past 2 days that has been intermittently productive. He has some nausea but denies vomiting, diarrhea, or dysuria. He is able to tolerate fluids but has not had an appetite over the past day. Neither the patient nor his family have been out of the country recently and he has not had any sick contacts.

Past Medical History

- Seasonal allergies.

Medications

- Cetirizine 5 mg daily.

Allergies

- NKDA.

Physical Examination and Ancillary Studies

- *Vital signs*: T 101.2 °F, HR 94, BP 110/68, RR 30, O_2 sat 96% on room air.
- *General*: The patient is alert but appears to have slightly increased work of breathing. He is interactive and cooperative but appears listless.
- *HEENT*: PERRL. Moist mucous membranes. Posterior pharynx is erythematous. No exudate is noted on tonsils. Tympanic membranes normal bilaterally.
- *Neck*: There is no anterior or posterior cervical lymphadenopathy. Neck is supple and trachea is midline.
- *Cardiovascular*: The patient's heart rate is regular, with normal rhythm and no M/R/G. Peripheral pulses are normal. Capillary refill < 3 seconds.
- *Lungs*: Increased work of breathing. Rhonchi at the right lung base. Otherwise there are no wheezes or rales in other lung fields.
- *Abdomen*: The patient's abdomen is diffusely tender in all quadrants but is soft, without rebound or guarding. There is no splenomegaly or hepatomegaly.
- *Extremities and skin*: Skin is warm to the touch but there are no rashes or mottling.
- *Neurologic*: Grossly intact with no focal deficits.

Questions for Thought

- What diseases, common and life-threatening, should be on your differential diagnosis?
- What imaging studies should this patient undergo?
- What is the disposition for this patient?

Diagnosis

- Community-acquired pneumonia.

Discussion

- *Epidemiology*: Acute abdominal pain is one of the most common chief complaints in the ED. According to retrospective analyses, a large majority of patients presenting with acute abdominal pain are diagnosed with "acute non-specific abdominal pain," with acute appendicitis and UTI as the next two most common entities.[1] Approximately 2–5 percent of children with pneumonia present with abdominal pain; some with abdominal pain as the only presenting symptom.[1-3] Viral and bacterial pneumonia can both present as abdominal pain.
- *Pathophysiology*: Pneumonia results from infection of the lung parenchyma and consolidation of that part of the lung and a subsequent inflammatory cascade from the body's immune system. Basilar pneumonia may present with abdominal pain from diaphragmatic irritation or through referred pain via a shared dermatome. Additionally, patients with pneumonia may have inflamed abdominal lymph nodes, causing their pain.[2]
- *Presentation*: Given that pneumonia is an infection primarily affecting the respiratory system, the classic symptoms include cough, fever, dyspnea, tachypnea, generalized malaise, as well as a constellation of other symptoms. However, referred abdominal pain may be the only presenting symptom. It is important for clinicians to be cognizant that abdominal pain can commonly stem from extra-abdominal disease processes.[1] Abdominal pain without vomiting or diarrhea should prompt the clinician to evaluate the patient for pneumonia as well as other intra- and extra-abdominal causes, such as pneumonia, acidosis, or tonsillitis.[1] According to one retrospective study, fever was the most common symptom prevalent in cases of pneumonia presenting as abdominal pain, followed by cough and signs of upper-respiratory-tract infection.[3] Although rare, pneumonia and other extra-abdominal causes of abdominal pain can be life-threatening and should not be missed, as diagnostic delay worsens outcomes. These include, but are not limited to, diabetic ketoacidosis, meningitis, Henoch–Schönlein purpura, hemolytic uremic syndrome, leukemia, sickle cell crisis, and streptococcal pharyngitis.[1]
- *Diagnosis*: As with any presentation, a thorough physical examination can aid in avoiding misdiagnosis of pneumonia causing abdominal pain (i.e. rhonchi on lung auscultation). The gold standard for diagnosing pneumonia is chest

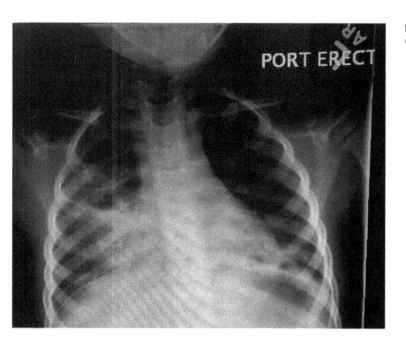

Figure 8.6 Typical pediatric radiograph demonstrating right lower lobe infiltrate.

radiography (Figure 8.6). Chest radiography does sometimes lag behind the clinical presentation and may miss diagnosing early pneumonia, and it is not unreasonable to treat a patient for pneumonia based on clinical presentation in the absence of radiographic findings. In children with viral syndromes, who are well-appearing, with non-focal examinations, CXR is not necessary or indicated. Generally, viral and bacterial pneumonias appear as interstitial infiltrates on CXR.[4] Alveolar pneumonia and especially lobar infiltrates tend to be indicative of a bacterial pathogen.[4] In terms of the presenting symptom of abdominal pain, some studies suggest that any child who also has a cough, fever, or dyspnea should receive a CXR before any abdominal imaging.[2] U/S is being studied as a potential diagnostic alternative to chest radiography for pneumonia, although currently its use is limited. CT has very high sensitivity and specificity but is generally only indicated when there are complications of pneumonia, such as concerns for empyema or abscess.

- *Treatment*: As with any patient, the first priority in treatment is appropriate respiratory and hemodynamic support, if necessary. Supplemental oxygen or IV fluid resuscitation may be required in severe cases of pneumonia. The variance of causative organisms for pneumonia depends partly on the patient's age, risk factors, geography, and clinical presentation. There does not appear to be an association with a specific organism in patients presenting primarily with abdominal pain. For newborns and young infants, empiric treatment is with ampicillin and cefotaxime or gentamycin.[5] Outpatient management for infants and toddlers is appropriate with beta-lactam antibiotics. School-aged children have a higher incidence of atypical pneumonia (i.e. *Mycoplasma pneumoniae*) and therefore macrolides are the agent of choice, as pneumococcus is susceptible as well.[5]

- *Disposition*: The majority of children, other than newborns and infants, can be managed on an outpatient basis, depending on the clinical scenario and patient comorbidities.

Historical clues	Physical findings
• Cough • Fever • Lack of vomiting/diarrhea	• Rhonchi • Lack of focal abdominal tenderness • Tachypnea

Follow-Up

Given the fever and the abdominal pain, U/S was ordered to evaluate for acute appendicitis. The appendix was not visualized, however, and the patient had undergone laboratory work, and a CT of the abdomen and pelvis with oral and IV contrast. This showed a normal appendix but also a right-lower-lobe infiltrate as the scan extended into the thorax. The patient was placed on antibiotics and discharged after being observed tolerating oral intake and followed up with his pediatrician as an outpatient.

References

1. Ttsalkidis A, Gardikis S, Cassimos D, et al. Acute abdomen in children due to extra-abdominal causes. *Pediatr Int* 2008; 50: 315–18.

2. Moustaki M, Zeis PM, Katsikari M, et al. Mesenteric lymphadenopathy as a cause of abdominal pain in children with lobar or segmental pneumonia. *Pediatr Pulmonol.* 2003; 35: 269–73.

3. Homier V, Bellavance C, Xhignesse M. Prevalence of pneumonia in children under 12 years of age who undergo abdominal radiography in the emergency department. *CJEM* 2007; 9: 347–51.

4. Virkki R, Juven T, Rikalainen H, et al. Differentiation of bacterial and viral pneumonia in children. *Thorax* 2002; 57: 438–41.

5. Bradley JS, Byington CL, Shah SS, et al. The management of community-acquired pneumonia in infants and children older than 3 months of age: Clinical practice guidelines by the Pediatric Infectious Diseases Society and the Infectious Diseases Society of America. *Clin Infect Dis* 2011; 53: 617–30.

Case 7

Contributing Authors: Cara V. Tillotson, Melanie K. Prusakowski, and Rebecca Jeanmonod

History

The patient is a 13-year-old male who presents to the ED with sudden-onset abdominal pain for the last hour. His mother states that he woke up this morning complaining of extreme pain and has not been able to get out of bed except to ride to the hospital. The pain is located in his lower abdomen bilaterally, but is worse on the left. He rates the pain 9 out of 10. He has vomited once since the onset of symptoms. The vomit was non-bilious and non-bloody. He denies any recent illness or injury. He has had no fever, diarrhea, dysuria, or hematuria. You interview the patient without the mother present and he reports that he has never been sexually active.

Past Medical History

- Attention deficit–hyperactivity disorder.

Medications

- Methylphenidate, extended release, daily.

Allergies

- NKDA.

Physical Examination and Ancillary Studies

- *Vital signs*: T 99.5 °F, HR 112, RR 12, BP 128/75, O_2 sat 98% on room air.
- *General*: Patient is alert, oriented, well-developed, and appears very uncomfortable. He is grimacing and holding his lower abdomen.
- *HEENT*: No signs of trauma. PERRL. Mucous membranes moist. Oropharynx clear.
- *Neck*: Supple, with midline trachea and no adenopathy.
- *Cardiovascular*: Tachycardic; regular rhythm, no M/R/G; bilateral radial pulses equal and 2+.
- *Lungs*: Clear, equal air entry bilaterally; no W/R/R.
- *Abdomen*: Normoactive bowel sounds; tender to palpation on bilateral lower quadrants, worse on the left, no masses, negative Rovsing's sign, negative obturator sign, negative psoas sign.
- *Genitourinary examination*: The left testicle is high-riding with some mild erythema and edema. The patient is unable to tolerate palpation of the testicle due to pain. There is no movement of the testicle upon stroking of the medial inner thigh. Inguinal canals are normal bilaterally. The right testicle is non-tender to palpation.
- *Extremities and skin*: No rashes, purpura, petechiae, or pallor. No signs of trauma.
- *Neurologic*: Alert and age-appropriate, with no focal deficits.
- *Pertinent laboratory values*: WBC 7,000, CRP < 3, U/A normal.
- *Pertinent imaging*: Pertinent radiologic studies: U/S with color Doppler: left testicle mildly enlarged with homogeneous echotexture; twisting of the spermatic cord, and absent blood flow to the left testis and epididymis.

Diagnosis

- Torsion of the left testicle.

Discussion

- *Epidemiology*: Testicular torsion is the twisting of the spermatic cord and has an annual incidence of about 1 in 4,000 males who are less than 25 years old.[1] It is the most common cause of testicle loss in the USA. The peak incidence occurs in ages 12–18 years and the neonatal period, although it can occur at any age. Adolescents and neonates are more likely to have torsion of the spermatic cord (true testicular torsion), while prepubertal boys are more likely to have torsion of the appendix testes or epididymis.[2,3] Neonatal torsion can occur prenatally (70 percent) or postnatally (30 percent).[2,3] Torsion more commonly occurs on the left side.

  Young females may also present with acute abdominal pain related to gonadal torsion. Gonadal torsion in females is less common in the pediatric age group, especially prior to puberty, but has been described.[1] When it occurs, it is commonly associated with ovarian pathology (i.e. masses or cysts), although it can occur in an otherwise normal ovary.[1]

- *Pathophysiology*: Testicular torsion occurs when the testicle twists around the spermatic cord, compressing the vasculature and causing ischemia. The two types of testicular torsion are intravaginal and extravaginal.[2–4] Testicles are normally covered by the tunica vaginalis, which is attached to the posterior surface of the testicle. This prevents the testicle from excessive movement. However, about 12 percent of the male population has the "bell clapper" variation, where the tunica vaginalis attaches in a higher position on the testicle.[1] This results in a more horizontal position of the testicle and allows the testicle more mobility around the spermatic cord. This type of torsion is termed intravaginal torsion and occurs at any age after the neonatal period.[2–4] Extravaginal torsion (occurring prenatally and in neonates) is caused by twisting around the spermatic cord proximal to the tunica vaginalis. This occurs during the descent of the testicles from the abdomen into the scrotal sac, where the testicles have more mobility and are thus more predisposed to torsion.[2–4]

  Ovarian torsion similarly occurs when the ovary twists on its pedicle, leading to obstructed lymphatic and venous drainage.[1] This eventually leads to edema and obstructed arterial flow. This may involve the ovary, the fallopian tube, or both. Most torsed ovaries are abnormally enlarged, many greater than 5 cm, but there have been cases of prepubertal girls presenting with torsion.[1]

- *Presentation*: The classic presentation of testicular torsion is acute, severe, unilateral scrotal pain and swelling, with nausea and/or vomiting. Children may present with abdominal pain and vomiting rather than scrotal pain; it is important to keep testicular torsion on the differential for acute lower abdominal pain in pediatric patients.[1,3,5,6] The pain may be unrelenting. Physical examination will vary based on the time of initial presentation. Scrotal erythema and edema are common, and in late presentations may be severe enough to obscure landmarks.[1,3,5,6] Loss of the cremasteric reflex is classically present and is the most reliable finding, but the presence of the reflex does not entirely exclude testicular torsion in the setting of high suspicion.[5] There is usually tenderness to palpation of the testicle (in spermatic cord torsion) or focal tenderness on the superior testis (torsed appendix testis). The torsed testicle may be high-riding and horizontally oriented.

  The presentation for ovarian torsion is also typically one of acute pain, which is usually unilateral although it can be visceral and poorly localized. Pain can be colicky and intermittent, and is often associated with vomiting, nausea, fever, and dysuria.[1] The presentation in girls is often misleading, and diagnosis requires a high index of suspicion.

- *Diagnosis*: The critical evaluation of a child with testicular torsion is a careful history and physical

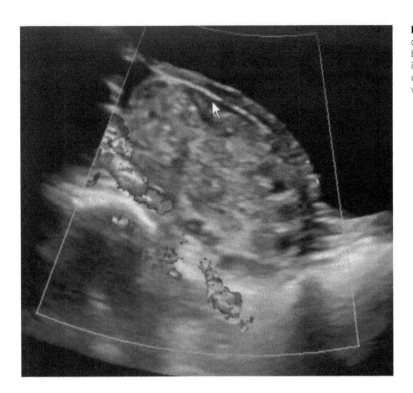

Figure 8.7 U/S of torsed ovary demonstrating decreased internal blood flow, but some evidence of peripheral flow. It is important to image both the affected and the unaffected side for comparison. For the color version, please refer to the plate section.

examination. Key diagnostic elements include acute onset of testicular or abdominal pain and an abnormal testicular/scrotal examination. U/S with color Doppler may show decreased blood flow and coiling of the spermatic cord, but is not sensitive enough to exclude this diagnosis in small infants in whom your index of suspicion is high (lower limit of sensitivity 88 percent).[1,7] In these infants, urology should be consulted, as truly, surgical exploration is the gold standard for diagnosis. Radionucelotide imaging was once the diagnostic study of choice, but is rarely used since the advent of diagnostic U/S. U/A is recommended in order to evaluate for other causes of acute testicular pain, such as epididymitis or orchitis. Bacterial infections may produce pyuria or bacteriuria.

In girls, diagnosis is more challenging and is often delayed, with many girls having misdiagnoses.[1] U/S is the diagnostic test of choice, and is typically performed transabdominally in young girls.[1] Colorflow Doppler alone is not adequate, as the ovary has a dual blood supply (both ovarian and uterine artery) and up to two-thirds of cases of torsion will have evidence of blood flow (Figure 8.7).[1] CT scanning may show an enlarged ovary, but cannot rule out torsion.

- *Treatment*: Gonadal torsion is a surgical emergency. Significant ischemia can occur as early as 4 hours after onset of torsion (with 4–8 hours considered the "golden" window for salvage). Testicular torsion can impair sperm formation later in life even if the testicle is not removed. The likelihood of viability of the gonad is inversely related to the amount of time since the onset of pain. Those undergoing surgical correction within 6 hours have close to 100 percent salvage rate, while those waiting more than 24 hours have virtually no chance of salvage. Surgery should not be delayed in order to complete imaging in a patient with a high suspicion of testicular torsion. Manual detorsion of the testicle may be attempted in the ED, though patients may not be able to tolerate this due to pain. Even if the testicle can be detorsed manually, surgical exploration is still indicated to ensure complete resolution. Surgical correction usually includes detorsion of the testicle and exploration of the contralateral hemiscrotum. Frequently, surgeons will fix the contralateral testis to the scrotal wall in order to prevent recurrent torsion. If the affected testicle is unlikely to be viable, it is removed. If it is viable, it is fixed in a similar fashion to the scrotal wall.

Ovarian torsion obviously cannot be manually detorsed, and requires surgical correction or oophorectomy if the ovary is no longer viable.

- *Disposition*: When the diagnosis of testicular torsion has been made or is highly suspected, an emergent urologic consult should be obtained, or the patient should be transferred emergently to a center where urologic consultation is immediately available.

Historical clues	Physical findings	Ancillary studies
• Severe sudden abdominal pain • Vomiting	• Tender, swollen testicle • Abnormal testicular lie • Absent cremasteric reflex	• Negative U/A • U/S with evidence of torsion

Follow-Up

The patient was taken to the OR for emergent exploration. The left testicle was detorsed, and it regained blood flow and appeared viable. The contralateral hemiscrotum was also explored and both testicles were affixed to the scrotal wall to prevent future torsion. The patient recovered overnight on the pediatric surgery service. Edema and pain resolved within 24 hours, and the patient was sent home with pain control.

References

1. Smith J, Fox SM. Pediatric abdominal pain: An emergency medicine perspective. *Emerg Med Clin N Am* 2016; 34: 341–61.

2. Gatti JM, Murphy JP. Acute testicular disorders. *Pediatr Rev* 2008; 29: 235–41.

3. Goel A, Gaillard F. Testicular torsion. See http://radiopaedia.org/articles/testicular-torsion.

4. Bombiński P, Warchoł S, Brzewski M, et al. Ultrasonography of extravaginal testicular torsion in neonates. *Pol J Radiol* 2016; 81: 469–72.

5. Kadish HA, Bolte RG. A retrospective review of pediatric patients with epididymitis, testicular torsion, and torsion of testicular appendages. *Pediatrics* 1998; 102: 73–6.

6. Pogorelić Z, Mrklić I, Jurić I. Do not forget to include testicular torsion in differential diagnosis of lower acute abdominal pain in young males. *J Pediatr Urol* 2013; 9: 1161–5.

7. Baker LA, Sigman D, Mathews RI, et al. An analysis of clinical outcomes using color Doppler testicular ultrasound for testicular torsion. *Pediatrics* 2000; 105: 604–7.

Case 8

Contributing Author: Donald Jeanmonod

History

A 15-year-old female presents to the ED with her mother for evaluation of abrupt onset of abdominal pain. The patient relates that she has been feeling intermittently unwell over the past 2 weeks, with several episodes of vomiting occurring over that time period. On the day of presentation, the patient was in school in her normal state of health and without complaint when she developed abrupt onset of abdominal pain. The pain is generalized, but seems to be more severe in the lower abdomen. Initially, the patient reported that the pain was sharp, but has now become more achy in nature. The patient reports that the pain seems worse when she is moving around, and is improved with lying still. Additionally, she reports that she has started to feel nauseated and slightly light-headed since the onset of the pain. The patient denies any headache, chest pain, cough, diarrhea, dysuria, urinary frequency, vaginal bleeding, and vaginal discharge. She reports some mild shortness of breath on review of systems. She is unsure as to when her last menstrual period was.

Past Medical History

- None.

Medications

- None.

Allergies

- NKDA.

Physical Examination and Ancillary Studies

- *Vital signs*: T 99.1 °F, HR 115, RR 24, BP 88/62, O_2 sat 98% on room air.
- *General*: Appropriately developed Caucasian female adolescent, lying recumbent on the stretcher. The patient appears slightly pale and appears uncomfortable.
- *HEENT*: Head is normocephalic and atraumatic. Eyes appear normal. Mucous membranes moist, without pharyngeal erythema.
- *Neck*: Unremarkable in external appearance, with full range of motion.
- *Cardiovascular*: Tachycardic and regular, without any M/R/G. Capillary refill 3 seconds.

- *Lungs*: Slightly tachypneic, without accessory muscle use. Lungs are CTA bilaterally. Normal work of breathing.
- *Abdomen*: Non-distended. The patient has generalized tenderness to percussion and palpation. She is most tender in the lower abdomen and suprapubic region.
- *Extremities and skin*: No obvious abnormalities. Full range of motion.
- *Neurologic*: GCS 15. Motor intact throughout. No obvious deficits.

Questions for Thought

- What elements of the history and examination are missing on this patient?
- What is the best way to approach data gathering in this patient?
- Along the spectrum of disease, is this patient sick or not sick?
- What are your initial management steps?
- Given your formulated differential diagnosis, what two tests are essential for making a diagnosis?

Diagnosis

- Ruptured ectopic pregnancy.

Discussion

- *Epidemiology*: Teenage pregnancy (age 15–19) rates have declined by 64 percent since 1991 in the USA, possibly through better education, more abstinence, and improved access to forms of contraception.[1] Despite falling rates of teenage pregnancy, there are still 22.3 live births per 1,000 females in this age group. Since the Pregnancy Mortality Surveillance System was implemented in 1987, pregnancy-related deaths have risen from 7.2 deaths per 100,000 live births to 17.8 deaths per 100,000 live births between 2009 and 2011.[2]

  Ectopic pregnancy is thought to complicate 1–2 percent of all pregnancies in the USA and continues to be an important cause of first-trimester morbidity and mortality in the pregnant patient. Because of the decreased incidence of risk factors for ectopic pregnancy in adolescents, the incidence of ectopic pregnancy in adolescents is less than adults and reported to be 0.3 percent.[3] That said, patients presenting to an ED for evaluation during the first trimester of

pregnancy are at significantly higher risk for complications. A retrospective study of 2,721 women, including 649 adolescents, presenting to an ED for evaluation during the first trimester of pregnancy found the incidence of ectopic pregnancy to be 21.7 percent in adults and 9.7 percent in adolescents.[4]

Risk factors for ectopic pregnancy include a number of conditions which result in tubal scarring, including a history of infection, prior surgery, or prior ectopic pregnancy. Additional risk factors include intrauterine device use and cigarette smoking. When compared to the adult cohort, adolescents are less likely to have had prior ectopic pregnancy or surgery as a risk factor for current ectopic pregnancy and are more likely to have had a history of sexually transmitted infection or active infection at the time of their diagnosis.[4] Patient risk factors, a history of present illness, and symptoms are poorly predictive of the possibility of ectopic pregnancy, with reported likelihood ratios that are less than 1.5.[5]

- *Pathophysiology*: Ectopic pregnancy occurs when a fertilized egg implants somewhere other than the uterine fundus. This implanted embryo, as it grows, can cause tube rupture, hemorrhagic shock, abdominal pain, vaginal bleeding, or even death.
- *Presentation*: Ectopic pregnancies can present in a variety of ways, from asymptomatic to back pain to abdominal pain to shock. In cornual ectopic pregnancy, the pregnacy can proceed for a long time without problems, often well into the second trimester. The clinician needs to maintain a high index of suspicion for ectopic pregnancy in all reproductive-aged girls.
- *Diagnosis*: In 2013, individuals aged 15–24 years represented 15 percent of all ED visits, with 62 percent of these being visits by adolescent and young adult females.[6] Abdominal pain represented the most common reason for ED visit (8.5 percent of visits) and vaginal bleeding represented 2 percent of visits in adolescent and young females.[7] In a nationwide sample of ED visits between 2005 and 2009, only 20.9 percent of those visits included pregnancy testing.[8] In this sample, patients presenting to a pediatric ED were even less likely to receive testing. A retrospective study of female adolescents presenting to an ED found that only 10 percent of patients who were

eventually diagnosed as being pregnant mentioned the possibility of pregnancy in triage, and 10.5 percent denied being sexually active.[9] Obviously, having a high index of suspicion of pregnancy in any post-menarcheal female presenting with nausea, vomiting, abdominal or pelvic pain, or vaginal bleeding or discharge is an important first step to making the diagnosis.

The initial assessment of any patient presenting to the ED should include careful attention to vital signs. A shock index (ratio of heart rate to systolic blood pressure) of > 0.85 in pregnant patients presenting with vaginal bleeding or abdominal pain in the first trimester has been demonstrated to make the likelihood of a ruptured ectopic pregnancy 15 times more likely.[10] After addressing instabilities in the primary survey, urine testing for pregnancy remains the first step in patient evaluation. Although urine pregnancy tests have been touted as being very sensitive in detecting pregnancy, very low concentrations (<45 IU/L) of β-hCG can result in false negative testing,[11] which might prompt serum β-hCG testing if you have a high index of suspicion.

Although ectopic pregnancy has been reported to be the most common cause of first-trimester maternal mortality, an increased awareness, better diagnostic modalities, improved therapeutics, and better resuscitation science have led to a steady decline in mortality rates from 1.15 deaths per 100,000 live births between 1980 and 1984 to 0.5 deaths per 100,000 live births between 2003 and 2007.[12] Because the incidence of ectopic pregnancy increases with age, mortality has been demonstrated to increase with age as well, with women aged 35–39 being 2.5 times more likely to have pregnancy-related mortality, and women aged 40 years and older being 5.3 times more likely to have pregnancy-related mortality, when compared to women in their 20s with ectopic pregnancy. In addition, there are significant racial disparities with African Americans being 6.8 times more likely to die of ectopic-related complications when compared to Caucasians.[12]

Because the incidence of ectopic pregnancy is higher in ED patients presenting with abdominal/pelvic pain or vaginal bleeding than the group of pregnant patients at large, a diagnosis of first-trimester pregnancy should be assumed to be ectopic, until proven otherwise. Transabdominal and transvaginal U/S remain the primary methods to determine the location of pregnancy in the first trimester. Previously reported β-hCG discriminatory thresholds should not be used to determine U/S utility in evaluation of the location of a pregnancy. In a retrospective study of 693 patients presenting with a ruptured ectopic pregnancy, 11 percent were found to have β-hCG levels < 100 IU/L.[13] ED-performed U/S can be used to accurately exclude ectopic pregnancy by demonstrating an intrauterine pregnancy with a negative predictive value of 99.96% (95% CI of 99.6–100%) in a pooled meta-analysis.[14] U/S findings that have been associated with the presence of an ectopic pregnancy include an empty uterus (LR+ 3.95, 95% CI of 2.70–5.77%), adnexal mass (LR+ 7.39, 95% CI 3.63–15.05%), pelvic free fluid (LR+ 6.12, 95% CI of 3.08–12.18%), and obviously a live extrauterine gestation.[15]

- *Treatment*: Management of the patient with a pregnancy of unknown location with no definitive intrauterine pregnancy and no adnexal pregnancy or suggestive adnexal mass remains a predicament with frequently changing guidelines. Studies demonstrate that 5–40 percent of women presenting with complaints in the first trimester will ultimately be diagnosed with a pregnancy of unknown location. Of these patients, between 6 and 20 percent will have an ectopic pregnancy. The majority (50–70 percent) will eventually be diagnosed with failed pregnancies, with falling β-hCG levels, and the remainder (30–47 percent) will be diagnosed with ongoing intrauterine pregnancy.[16] Typically, management includes follow-up with serial β-hCG levels being checked every 48 hours until the location of the pregnancy is confirmed. The minimal rise in β-hCG has consistently fallen over time, with more recent studies suggesting that a rise of at least 35 percent in 48 hours considered the minimal rise consistent with a possible intrauterine pregnancy.[16]

After addressing the primary survey and aggressively managing hemodynamic instability, if present, management of a patient with an ectopic pregnancy should involve consultation with an obstetrician/gynecologist. IV access should be established and laboratory studies

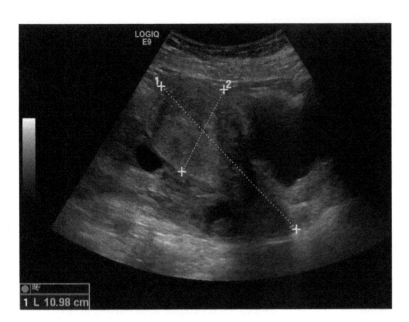

LOGIQ
E9

1 L 10.98 cm

Figure 8.8 U/S demonstrating empty uterus with complex free fluid.

should include a baseline CBC, renal tests and LFTs, a type and screen with crossmatch if unstable, and baseline quantitative β-hCG. Treatment options for the ectopic pregnancy include expectant management, medical abortive therapy, or surgical treatment.

If the patient has signs or symptoms of tubal rupture, immediate surgical intervention is warranted. In general, surgery is the preferred modality in definitive rupture, suspected rupture, and in the presence of a heterotopic pregnancy (concomitant intrauterine and extrauterine pregnancies). Patients who have contraindications to medical therapy, who are suspected of having issues with compliance and follow-up, who have failed medical therapy to terminate the ectopic pregnancy, or have U/S evidence (ectopic mass > 3.5 cm or presence of fetal heart rate) that makes medical therapy unlikely to succeed are also candidates for surgical therapy.[17] Surgical therapies include salpingostomy, where the fallopian tube is incised and the fetal tissue removed, and salpingectomy, where the affected portion of the tube is removed. Both procedures can be performed by either laparoscopy or laparotomy; however, laparotomy is preferred if the patient has ruptured.

With the knowledge that many ectopic pregnancies would spontaneously abort or reabsorb if allowed to run their course, expectant management may be used as a treatment option for patients who are asymptomatic, have low β-hCG levels (< 200 IU/L), and are good candidates for compliance with every-48-hour laboratory draws.

The final method of managing ectopic pregnancy is with medical therapy. Methotrexate is an antimetabolite that binds to the catalytic site on dihydrofolate reductase, leading to inhibition of DNA synthesis and cell replication. Observational studies have reported successful treatment rates of between 71.2 and 94.2 percent,[17] with higher success rates in those with lower β-hCG levels and smaller ectopic mass. Contraindications to methotrexate include immunosuppression, liver disease (including alcohol-induced liver disease), blood dyscrasias, renal disease, pulmonary disease, and peptic ulcer disease. Methotrexate is administered as an IM injection of 50 mg/m^2, with a second dose administered if β-hCG has not declined by 15 percent on repeat testing by day 4 to 7. Fifteen to twenty percent of patients will require a second dose. Because methotrexate affects rapidly dividing tissue, common side effects include nausea, vomiting, diarrhea, and stomatitis.

- *Disposition*: Disposition depends on treatment course and patient presentation. Patients with operative intervention require admission. Those who are hemodynamically stable with reliable

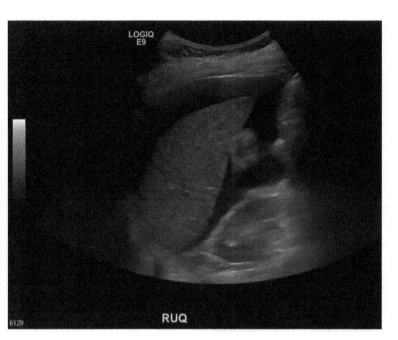

Figure 8.9 Right-upper-quadrant view of Morrison's pouch, demonstrating free fluid.

follow-up, and who are undergoing medical management or observation, may be discharged home with careful return precautions.

Historical clues	Physical findings
• Subacute nausea	• Tachycardic
• Acute lower abdominal pain	• Tachypneic
• Light-headed	• Pale
• Unknown last period	• Hypotensive

Follow-Up

The patient's mother was asked to step out of the room and a sexual and substance abuse history were obtained from the patient. The patient stated that she had had consensual vaginal intercourse on several occasions with a boy in her school and would usually use a condom, but two times had not. She continued to deny vaginal bleeding and discharge. She denied smoking, alcohol use, and drug use.

The patient was identified as requiring resuscitation. IV access was established and resuscitation was initiated with normal saline. The patient was unable to provide a urine specimen for urine β-hCG. Labs were sent for CBC, basic metabolic panel, serum quantitative β-hCG, and type and crossmatch. Bedside U/S was performed and the images demonstrated an empty uterus with complex pelvic free fluid (Figure 8.8), which tracked up the right pericolic gutter to Morrison's pouch (Figure 8.9). A live extrauterine pregnancy

was seen in the left adnexa (Figure 8.10). An emergent obstetrics and gynecology consultation was placed and the patient was taken to the OR where a diagnosis of a ruptured left adnexal ectopic pregnancy was confirmed and managed surgically.

References

1. Hamilton BE, Mathews TJ. Continued declines in teen births in the United States, 2015. *NCHS data Brief, no. 259*. Hyattsville, MD: National Center for Health Statistics, 2016.

2. Centers for Disease Control. Reproductive Health: Pregnancy Mortality Surveillance System. https://www.cdc.gov/reproductivehealth/MaternalInfantHealth/PMSS.html (accessed February 13, 2017).

3. Hoover KW, Tao G, Kent CK. Trends in the diagnosis and treatment of ectopic pregnancy in the United States. *Obstet Gynecol* 2010; 115: 495–502.

4. Menon S, Sammel MD, Vichnin M, Barnhart KT. Risk factors for ectopic pregnancy: A comparison between adults and adolescent women. *J Pediatr Adolesc Gynecol* 2007; 20: 181–5.

5. Crochet JR, Bastian LR, Chireau MV. Does this woman have an ectopic pregnancy? The rational clinical examination systematic review. *JAMA* 2010; 309: 1722–9.

6. Rui P, Kang K, Albert M. National Hospital Ambulatory Medical Care Survey: 2013 Emergency department summary tables. See www.cdc.gov/nchs/data/ahcd/nhamcs_emergency/2013_ed_web_tables.pdf

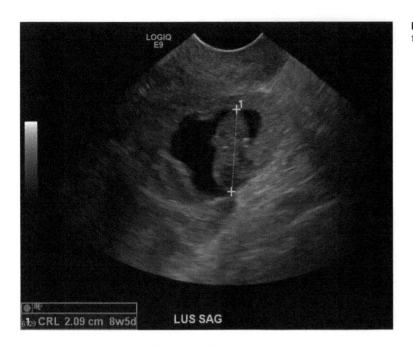

Figure 8.10 Live extrauterine pregnancy in the left adnexa.

7. Ziv A, Boulet JR, Slap GB. Emergency department utilization by adolescents in the United States. *Pediatrics* 1998; 101: 987–94.

8. Goyal M, Hersh A, Luan X, et al. Frequency of pregnancy testing among adolescent emergency department visits. *Acad Emerg Med* 2013; 20: 816–21.

9. Causey AL, Seago K, Wahl NG, Voelker CL. Pregnant adolescents in the emergency department: Diagnosed or not diagnosed. *Am J Emerg Med* 1997; 15: 125–30.

10. Birkhahn RH, Gaeta TJ, Bei R, Bove JJ. Shock index in the first trimester of pregnancy and its relationship to ruptured ectopic pregnancy. *Acad Emerg Med* 2002; 9: 115–19.

11. Greene DN, Schmidt RL, Kamer SM, et al. Limitations in qualitative point of care hCG tests for detecting early pregnancy. *Clin Chim Acta* 2013; 415: 317–21.

12. Creanga AA, Shapiro-Mendoza CK, Bish CL, et al. Trends in ectopic pregnancy mortality: 1980–2007. *Obstet Gynecol* 2011; 117: 837–43.

13. Saxon D, Falcone T, Mascha E, et al. A study of ruptured ectopic pregnancy. *Obstet Gynecol* 1997; 90: 46–9.

14. Stein JC, Wang R, Adler N, et al. Emergency physician ultrasonography for evaluating patients at risk for ectopic pregnancy: A meta-analysis. *Ann Emerg Med* 2010; 56: 674–83.

15. Richardson A, Gallos I, Dobson S, et al. Accuracy of first trimester ultrasound in diagnosis of tubal pregnancy in the absence of an obvious extrauterine embryo: Systematic review and meta-analysis. *Ultrasound Obstet Gynecol* 2016; 47: 28–37.

16. Kirk E, Bottomley C, Bourne T. Diagnosing ectopic pregnancy and current concepts in the management of pregnancy of unknown location. *Hum Reprod Update* 2014; 20: 250–61.

17. Murtaza UI, Ortmann MJ, Mando-Vandrick J, Lee AS. Management of first-trimester complications in the emergency department. *Am J Health Syst Pharm* 2013; 70: 99–111.

Altered Mental Status

Case 1

Contributing Author: Rebecca Jeanmonod

History

A 3-year-old girl is brought to the ED by her mother for confusion. The child did not get up when she usually does for daycare, so mom went to wake her up. She noted that the child was difficult to rouse and seemed sweaty and confused. The child had some odd body jerks that were not rhythmic and not frequent, which mom describes as "spasms." Mom attempted to give the child some juice, but it dribbled out of the child's mouth. EMS was called, and on arrival to the house, they checked the child's glucose, which was 34. An IV line was placed and the child was given dextrose. She is now acting "more normal" per mom, but still "not quite herself." The child's IV line was dislodged during transport.

Past Medical History

- The child was a term neonate with no birth complications. She is a small child, but has been consistent in her growth curve between the 5th and 10th percentile. She is fully immunized and has met all her milestones. She is potty trained. There is no family history of diabetes or inherited metabolic diseases.

Medications

- Multivitamins.

Allergies

- NKDA.

Physical Examination and Ancillary Studies

- *Vital signs*: T 98.6 °F, HR 140, RR 42, BP 110/63, O$_2$ sat 100% on room air.

- *General*: Listless but conscious and interactive toddler, with normal work of breathing and normal perfusion.
- *HEENT*: There are no signs of trauma. PERRL. The child is oriented to person and place. There are no oral lesions. Her mucous membranes are moist. There is no evidence of tongue biting.
- *Neck*: Neck is supple, with no adenopathy or masses.
- *Cardiovascular*: Regular tachycardia, with no M/R/G. Normal capillary refill.
- *Lungs*: Clear bilaterally, with normal effort and good air movement.
- *Abdomen*: Soft, with normal bowel sounds. No masses. No hepatomegaly.
- *Extremities and skin*: Pale. No rashes or signs of trauma.
- *Neurologic*: The child is drowsy but answers questions and follows commands. She has no focal deficits. Her reflexes are intact.
- *Pertinent laboratory values*: CBC normal. Na 138, K 5, Cl 103, bicarbonate 14, BUN 20, Cr 0.33, glucose 64, pH 7.25, 3+ urine ketones.
- *Pertinent imaging*: Head CT negative.

> ### Questions for Thought
> - What is the differential diagnosis for the hypoglycemic toddler?
> - What labs are important to obtain in this child?
> - Should the IV be replaced?
> - If the child continues to be hypoglycemic, how would you manage her?

Diagnosis

- Idiopathic ketotic hypoglycemia.

Discussion

- *Epidemiology*: Idiopathic ketotic hypoglycemia is the most common cause of hypoglycemia in children who do not have diabetes, occuring in about 4 in 100,000 children.[1] It is typically diagnosed between the ages of 18 months and 5 years.[2,3]

- *Pathophysiology*: The exact pathophysiology of this disease process is incompletely understood. Unlike children with true inborn errors of metabolism, these children have intact pathways for glycogenolysis and gluconeogenesis; however, their gluconeogenesis may be inadequate because of low levels of amino acids used in gluconeogenesis.[4,5] These children may also have limited glycogen stores (as the disease is more common in children with low birth weight and who fall under the 50th percentile for height and weight) as a contributor, or they utilize ketone bodies less effectively.[6] These children are usually developmentally normal. As infants, children receive a steady source of glucose with regularly scheduled feeds, which precludes presentation of this disease. Presentation generally occurs when a child begins to forgo night-time feeds or switches to a lower carbohydrate diet. Presentation beyond 5 years of age is rare. Most children with idiopathic ketotic hypoglycemia will outgrow it by age 10.[3]

- *Presentation*: Children with idiopathic ketotic hypoglycemia will classically present in the morning after an overnight fast with altered mental status and hypoglycemia. Seizures are uncommon, but can be a presenting complaint, and ketosis may lead to vomiting as well. Altered mental status may take the form of lethargy, focal neurologic deficits, abnormal vital signs, or confusion. Children may have an infectious process that precipitates their symptoms, or they may be otherwise well. They are classically age 18 months to 5 years and, although most are of a slender build, there are cases reported in larger children. Although this presentation is classic, it is not pathognomonic, and the ED provider should consider inborn errors of metabolism, hyperinsulinemia, endocrine deficiencies, toxins (specifically, oral hypoglycemics and alcohols), and sepsis as part of the differential.

- *Diagnosis*: Because the difference between this child and a child with an inborn error of metabolism may not be readily apparent, the provider should initiate the work-up for inborn errors of metabolism, including serum pH, urine studies for ketones, lactate, glucose testing, ammonia, serum ketones, and electrolytes, and other tubes of blood should be drawn on presentation and held for further testing should the child be suspected of having an inborn error. There is more information on this in Chapter 7 Case 1. When the child is hypoglycemic, with positive blood and urine ketones and a history inconsistent for other items on the hypoglycemia differential, a presumptive diagnosis of idiopathic ketotic hypoglycemia may be made.[1] Diagnosis is confirmed when the child is unable to tolerate a ketogenic diet or a fast.

- *Treatment*: Ill children should be resuscitated, with careful attention to the ABC algorithm. Hypoglycemic children should receive 25% dextrose, 2cc/kg. IV dextrose typically improves the child's symptoms rapidly, in contrast to hypoglycemia from inborn errors of metabolism or intoxicants, where the child may take a long period of time to return to baseline mental status. If the provider is assured that the child has idiopathic ketotic hypoglycemia, the best treatment for the child is to eat a carbohydrate-rich meal. However, if the provider believes the child may have an inborn error of metabolism or is unsure, the child should be made NPO to avoid ongoing metabolism and creation of toxic substances. These children should be placed on dextrose infusion at a rate that prevents catabolism, typically D10 at 1 to 1.5 maintenance.[7,8] Long-term management of children with idiopathic ketotic hypoglycemia involves frequent non-ketotic meals and regular home glucose and urine testing for hypoglycemia and ketonuria.

- *Disposition*: Most children with idiopathic ketotic hypoglycemia warrant an inpatient admission to monitor their blood sugars and ascertain definitive diagnosis. Although this condition is generally benign and self-limited, with spontaneous resolution by age 10, recurrent episodes of hypoglycemia and ketonemia can lead to complications such as brain abnormalities, lowered IQ, and seizures.[9]

Historical clues	Physical findings	Ancillary studies
• Developmentally normal • Low body weight • Toddler age group • No family members with diabetes (i.e. no access to hypoglycemic agents)	• Lethargy • Tachypnea (signaling acidosis)	• Hypoglycemia • Elevated anion gap acidosis • Ketonuria • Negative head CT

Follow-Up

The child was made NPO for concern for inborn errors. She became more lethargic, and an IV line was placed for a glucose of 42. The child was given IV dextrose and was started on a dextrose infusion. She was transferred to a pediatric hospital where a full metabolic evaluation was performed, which was largely unremarkable. She was in the hospital for 10 days while adjustments were made to her diet to prevent recurrent hypoglycemia. She was eventually discharged home, and at 6-month follow-up was doing well with high carbohydrate meals every 4–6 hours.

References

1. Daly LP, Osterhoudt KC, Weinzimer SA. Presenting features of idiopathic ketotic hypoglycemia. *J Emerg Med* 2003; 25: 39–43.

2. Soyka LF, Glass AG, Halldorsson TS. Ketotic hypoglycemia, an important cause of seizures. *Clin Pediatr* 1967; 6: 368–72.

3. Denmark TK. Inborn errors of metabolism. In *Pediatric Emergency Medicine*, Baren J, ed. Philadelphia, PA: Saunders, 2008, pp. 273–6.

4. Pagliara AS, Kari IE, De Vivo DC, et al. Hypoalaninemia: A concomitant of ketotic hypoglycemia. *J Clin Invest* 1972; 51: 1440–9.

5. Haymond MW, Karl IE, Pagliara AS. Ketotic hypoglycemia: An amino acid substrate limited disorder. *J Clin Endocrinol Metab* 1974; 38: 521–30.

6. Huidekoper HH, Duran M, Turkenburg M, et al. Fasting adaption in idiopathic ketotic hypoglycemia: A mismatch. *Eur J Pediatr* 2008; 167: 859–65.

7. Fletcher JM. Metabolic emergencies and the emergency physician. *J Paediatr Child Health* 2016; 52: 227–30.

8. Long D, Long B, Koyfman A. Inborn errors of metabolism: An emergency medicine approach. *Am J Emerg Med* 2016; 34: 317–18.

9. Pollack ES, Pollack CV. Ketotic hypoglycemia: A case report. *J Emerg Med* 1993; 11: 531–4.

Case 2

Contributing Author: Abhishek Chaturvedi

History

The patient is a 5-month-old full-term boy brought to the ED for altered mental status with lethargy, fussiness, and decreased feeding for 3 days. He has been exclusively breastfed since birth but has not been latching well lately. His last bowel movement was 6 days ago despite two glycerin suppositories. According to his mother, he usually stools three to four times a day. Yesterday, he had only four wet diapers compared to his usual eight to ten wet diapers per day. His mother denies any history of fever, vomiting, jaundice, or any sick contacts except that the boy had some congestion and cough 1 month back, which resolved with administration of tea prepared by a family friend. The child lives with his parents and two siblings. They have recently moved to a new neighborhood in California because of mom receiving a promotion at work.

Past Medical History

- He is a developmentally normal, healthy term neonate who is UTD on immunizations.

Medications

- 400 international units of liquid vitamin D daily.

Allergies

- NKDA.

Physical Examination and Ancillary Studies

- *Vital signs*: T 99.1 °F, HR 155, RR 24, BP 80/50, O_2 sat 92% on room air.
- *General*: Awake but lethargic, poorly responsive, overall well-nourished and well-developed.
- *HEENT*: PERRL but sluggish, intact red reflex. Normocephalic, atraumatic, with flat scalp veins and sunken fontanelle. Mucous membranes tacky.
- *Neck*: Supple, with midline trachea and no adenopathy.
- *Cardiovascular*: Slightly tachycardic, with regular rhythm. No M/R/G.
- *Lungs*: CTA bilaterally, with no W/R/R.
- *Abdomen*: Soft, non-tender, non-distended, with no organomegaly. Bowel sounds are decreased.

- *Extremities and skin*: Extremities are flaccid and in extension, with no localizing signs. No rash, trauma, or edema noted.
- *Neurologic*: Markedly decreased tone throughout, with minimal withdrawal to pain. Pupils are sluggish. The baby does not track and has a weak suck, with lack of head control. Deep tendon reflexes are 1+.
- *Pertinent laboratory values*: CBC, comprehensive metabolic panel, CRP, ABG, and CSF analysis are all normal. The child's U/A is only remarkable for a specific gravity of 1.030.
- *Pertinent imaging*: Head CT is normal. An abdominal radiograph was obtained due to his constipation; however, there was no significant stool burden appreciated.

Questions for Thought

- What are the next important resuscitative treatments to be undertaken for this infant?
- What is appropriate further testing?
- What are the conditions that can have similar presentations?
- Why is it important to not delay the administration of the drug for a confirmed diagnosis?
- What is the most feared complication of this condition?

Diagnosis

- Infant botulism.

Discussion

- *Epidemiology*: About 70 cases of infant botulism are reported annually in the USA, although the true incidence is likely higher due to under-recognition of the disease.[1,2] Throughout the world, most cases are reported in the USA, likely due to under-reporting.[2,3] Geographically, the prevalence of infant botulism in the USA is highest in California, Utah, and the eastern Pennsylvania–New Jersey–Delaware area.[2]

  Up to 95 percent of infant botulism cases occur in children younger than 6 months of age.[2] Young children are thought to be at increased risk due to immaturity of their gut flora. Infants living in rural/farm environments and around active construction sites appear to be at higher risk for

contracting botulism, presumably because of higher exposure to dust particles containing clostridium spores.[2,4] Breastfeeding as a risk factor is controversial. Some studies show that it increases risk, whereas others suggest it may protect from rapidly progressive disease.[2] Formula-fed infants tend to develop botulism at earlier ages and may have a more fulminant presentation.[2]

Ingestion of contaminated honey has been implicated in a number of cases of infant botulism. Microbiologic surveys of honey products have reported the presence of *Clostridium botulinum* spores in up to 25 percent of products; however, it is worth noting that in 85 percent of diagnosed cases, a definitive source of *C. botulinum* spores is never identified.[2,4] Corn syrup was previously found to contain *C. botulinum* spores, but no cases of infant botulism to date have been definitively attributed to contaminated corn syrup. Nonetheless, the AAP continues to recommend against feeding unpasteurized corn syrup and honey to infants younger than 12 months of age. Constipation has been shown to represent an independent risk factor for botulism in infants older than 2 months of age. This is presumably because decreased colonic motility allows *C. botulinum* spores further time to germinate in the GI tract and produce toxins.

There are multiple other recognized clinical forms of botulism, including wound botulism, in which wounds become contaminated with *C. botulinum* spores; and foodborne botulism, in which the preformed toxin is ingested from contaminated food sources.

- *Pathophysiology*: *C. botulinum* is a sporulating, obligate anaerobic, Gram-positive bacillus, present in soil and aquatic sediment. The bacteria generate spores that can survive extreme weather and temperature conditions. Unlike the toxin, which is heat-labile, the spores are relatively heat-resistant. Temperatures of 248 °F may be required to kill the spores, although heating at 185 °F inactivates the toxin. Infant botulism occurs when the clostridial spores of *C. botulinum* are inhaled, caught in saliva, and swallowed. The cecum is thought to be the initial site of activity and paralysis of the ileocecal valve might allow the colonizing bacteria to extend into the terminal ileum. In the large intestine, the spores then germinate and multiply (with an incubation period of 3–30 days), allowing the release of botulinum neurotoxin into the bloodstream. Botulinum neurotoxin then irreversibly binds cholinergic receptors in the presynaptic cell membrane of voluntary motor and autonomic neuromuscular junctions, preventing acetylcholine release. This creates the vast array of symptoms with which these infants may present. More than 70 percent of the neuromuscular junctions have to be impaired before impairment of voluntary muscles and autonomic function becomes evident, and when 90 percent are involved, diaphragmatic function becomes impaired, leading to respiratory failure.[2,4]

- *Presentation*: Clinically, botulism infection can cause a wide spectrum of presentations in infants, ranging from mild hypotonia to a combination of bilateral cranial nerve palsies, flaccid paralysis, and diaphragmatic weakness necessitating mechanical ventilation.[2,4] Typically, the first symptom noted in infant botulism is constipation (characterized by 3 or more days without defecation), which is then followed by some combination of lethargy, decreased spontaneous activity, and diminished appetite.[2,4] Infants then go on to experience loss of head control secondary to neck muscle weakness, typically followed by symmetric descending hypotonia and weakness, ultimately progressing to involve the diaphragmatic muscles. Approximately half of patients will require mechanical ventilation at some point during their hospital course. Symmetric cranial nerve palsies (ptosis, sluggishly reactive pupils, diminished gag reflex, bifacial weakness, poor suck, and difficulty swallowing) are often particularly notable. Muscle stretch reflexes are typically preserved. In advanced illness, autonomic disturbances may be present, such as decreased heart-rate variability, dilated and fixed pupils, xerostomia, intestinal ileus, and urinary retention.

- *Diagnosis*: The differential diagnosis for the floppy infant is broad. The neurologic presentation should prompt consideration of myasthenia gravis, Guillain–Barré syndrome, tick paralysis, intracranial mass lesions, cerebrovascular accident, toxins, and encephalitis. The clinician should also consider abuse/shaken baby

syndrome, sepsis, and inborn errors of metabolism. Children with infant botulism are classically afebrile and of normal mental status with motor weakness, but may have altered mental status secondary to dehydration from feeding difficulties, which may make their diagnosis more challenging.

In the ED, diagnosis is clinical, and treatment should not be withheld pending definitive diagnosis. Definitive diagnosis is made by detection of botulinum toxin in the stool.[2] Following the initial exposure, the toxin may continue to be present in the stool for up to several months. Toxin is less commonly found in serum than in the stool and has been detected in only 1 percent of US infants with botulism.

On initial presentation, basic serum studies in the infant with botulism will typically be normal, or they may demonstrate mild perturbations related to dehydration. CSF may show mildly elevated protein, again related to dehydration. These studies are generally only helpful to rule out other conditions. MRI and EEG are generally not indicated, but if obtained, they will usually be unremarkable.

Nerve conduction studies and electromyography can be used to help confirm the botulism diagnosis but are not used in the ED.

- *Treatment*: Supportive care, in particular, monitoring of respiratory function and appropriate use of endotracheal intubation (for airway protection and for mechanical ventilation) are important. Non-intubated patients should be positioned with the head of the bed elevated to 30° above the level of the feet to minimize risks of aspiration. Fluid resuscitation is often necessary. Aminoglycosides should be avoided because their use can lyse bacteria, releasing additional intracellular toxin into the infant gut.

IV botulism immunoglobulin was approved by the US Food and Drug Administration in 2003 and should be given to all infants with suspected botulism prior to confirmatory testing.[5] The half-life of botulism immunoglobulin is about 28 days. It has been shown to reduce the hospital length of stay from a mean of 5.7 weeks to 2.6 weeks.[2,5] In addition, duration of intensive care, mechanical ventilation, and tube or IV feeding are all significantly reduced in patients treated with botulism immunoglobulin.[5]

Gastric decontamination has historically been recommended to remove unabsorbed toxin from the baby's GI tract, but has not been shown to shorten illness duration. If cathartic agents are used, sorbitol is preferable to magnesium salts because the latter may exacerbate neuromuscular blockade. Whole bowel irrigation with polyethylene glycol may have a theoretical role in decontamination and it could be evaluated in severe poisoning. However, these procedures may be difficult and their efficacy may be reduced in the presence of constipation/toxin-induced ileus. In some cases, neostigmine, which inhibits the enzymatic degradation of acetylcholine, appears to be useful in reversing ileus.

Antibiotics to eradicate the infection are contraindicated, as they may cause an increased release of botulinum toxin.[2]

- *Disposition*: All children with suspected infant botulism should be admitted to a monitored setting with access to critical care services.

Historical clues	Physical findings	Ancillary studies
• Refusal to feed • Altered mental status • Constipation • Exposure to high-risk area	• Hypotonia • Bilateral ptosis • Decreased bowel sounds • Decreased reflexes	• Normal laboratory tests • Normal imaging • Clinical dehydration

Follow-Up

The stool sample collected was positive for *C. botulinum* toxin. The baby was transferred to the PICU. He did not require intubation, but was on enteral tube feeds. He received BabyBIG® and physical therapy was consulted for strength and range of motion exercises. He began taking all of his feeds orally and made a gradual but full recovery. He was discharged home from the hospital on hospital day 14.

References

1. Shapiro RL, Hatheway C, Swerdlow DL. Botulism in the United States: A clinical and epidemiological review. *Ann Intern Med* 1998; 129: 221–8.

2. Cox N, Hinkle R. Infant botulism. *Am Fam Phys* 2002; 65: 1388–93.

3. Koepke R, Sobel J, Arnon SS. Global occurrence of infant botulism, 1976–2006. *Pediatrics* 2008; 122: e73–82.

4. Rosow LK, Strober JB. Infant botulism: Review and clinical update. *Pediatr Neurol* 2015; 52: 487–92.

5. Chalk CH, Benstead TJ, Keezer M. Medical treatment for botulism. *Cochrane Database Syst Rev* 2014; 2: CD008123.

Case 3

Contributing Author: Denis R. Pauzé

History

A 3-month-old boy is brought into the ED for persistent crying, fussiness, and poor weight. He was seen twice in the ED over the past 2 weeks for similar complaints and both times diagnosed with colic. His PCP saw him yesterday and told the parents it is colic and "he will get better soon and grow out of it." The parents brought the infant in again because he is now persistently crying.

The parents state that he always cries with feeds and has not gained weight in the past several weeks. The parents state the infant is "sweaty" and is much more irritable, especially with feeds. He has no fevers, bilious vomiting, cough, or rash. He has good tone and is "always hungry" but isn't feeding.

Past Medical History

- Full term, normal spontaneous vaginal delivery, no prenatal complications.

Medications

- Acetaminophen.

Allergies

- NKDA.

Physical Examination and Ancillary Studies

- *Vital signs:* T 100.2 °F, HR 140, RR 40, BP 90/48, O_2 sat 96% on room air.
- *General:* Non-toxic in appearance and in no acute distress. He is not crying.
- *HEENT:* Circumference at 50 percent; no scalp hematoma or facial bruising. Corneas appear normal. PERRL. Mucous membranes moist.
- *Neck:* Normal range of motion. No masses or adenopathy.
- *Cardiovascular:* Normal S1, S2. +S3. No murmurs. Strong and normal distal pulses.

- *Lungs*: Clear bilaterally, with good air movement. No accessory muscle use.
- *Abdomen*: Soft and non-distended. No masses. No hernia. No splenomegaly. Liver feels mildly enlarged.
- *Genitourinary*: Circumcised penis. Testicles descended. No masses or erythema.
- *Extremities and skin*: No rashes. No signs of trauma. Warm and well-perfused.
- *Neurologic*: Intact reflexes, symmetric motor examination, social smile present.
- *Pertinent laboratory values*: WBC 23,000, Hb 12, Plt normal. Na 129, K 3.3, Cl 88, bicarbonate 31. BUN and Cr normal.
- *Pertinent imaging*: CXR reveals cardiomegaly.

Questions for Thought

- What is the differential diagnosis for the colicky baby?
- How is colic defined? How is it diagnosed?
- Is it common for colicky babies to fail to gain or to lose weight?

Diagnosis

- Anomalous left coronary artery with take-off from the pulmonary artery.

Discussion

- *Epidemiology*: "During the second century BC, the Greek physician Galen prescribed opium to calm fussy babies, and during the Middle Ages in Europe, mothers and wet nurses smeared their nipples with opium lotions before each feeding. Alcohol was also commonly given to infants."[1] Colic is a common presentation for many primary care offices and EDs. The exact prevalence is unknown because there are different definitions of colic and not all parents report or see their PCP for colic. Colic has many potential definitions, with a common criteria (Wessel's rule of 3s) being an infant that cries for > 3 hours per day, > 3 days per week, in an infant 3 months of age or younger.[2,3] Crying in infants is common, with the average infant crying 1–2 hours per day. This can be very distressing to parents. Cases of true colic are benign and self-limited. However, for the ED provider, a baby brought in for "persistent crying"

needs a very careful, detailed, and thorough evaluation. Although the vast majority of true colic is caused by benign or unknown factors, it is important to note the more critical diagnoses that cannot be missed. Some potential causes of worrisome crying in the infant include non-accidental trauma, (abusive head trauma and fractures), meningitis, corneal abrasion, hair tourniquets, incarcerated hernias, and testicular torsion.[4,5] Cardiac issues such as supraventricular tachycardia or congenital heart anomalies must also be considered.[6]

- *Pathophysiology*: There is no known etiology for colic. Multiple hypotheses have been postulated, including GI issues such as feeding difficulties, milk or lactose intolerance, and intestinal flora abnormalities. Some have hypothesized that colic is caused by increased serotonin release while others have suggested an infantile migraine as the cause for normal baby crying.[7] Others have postulated maternal smoking and family stress as a cause.

- *Presentation*: Excessive and persistent crying is virtually always the chief complaint in true colic. Infants are usually brought in when the crying is persistent and the parents "don't know what to do" and are at "their wits end." Remember, excessive infant crying is very distressing to the parent.

- *Diagnosis*: In general, the cause of crying is often found in the history and physical examination. Colic is really a diagnosis of exclusion. The cardinal rule for not missing a critical cause of "crying or colic" involves a thorough, complete history and a detailed "head-to-toe" physical examination.

  The history can give specific crucial clues for diagnosis. The EM provider should determine the following: What is the pattern of crying, and how long has it been going on? Does it only happen during certain periods of the day? Have there been any fevers, trauma, or (bilious) vomiting? Are there any new medications or herbal supplement exposures? Has there been adequate weight gain? Any diaphoresis or cyanosis or fatigue with feeds? For instance, a baby with 2 weeks of crying at night time is much different than an infant with a corneal abrasion, who has cried non-stop for the past 8 hours. A child with inadequate weight gain or other symptoms such as vomiting should not be diagnosed with colic; there is something else going on and a broader work-up should be pursued.

- *Physical examination* should be thorough and systematic.

  · *Vital signs* can often help narrow down the diagnosis. A febrile infant could harbor meningitis or infection as a cause for crying. A tachycardic infant may have supraventricular tachycardia. Infants with unequal distal blood pressures may have a coarctation of the aorta.

  · *Head*: Is the head circumference large? Are there any signs of head trauma? Does this infant have any bruises? These are concerning for non-accidental trauma.

  · *Eyes*: Is there any evidence of corneal abrasion or infantile glaucoma?

  · *Cardiovascular*: Any signs of heart failure? Unequal distal pulses? S3 gallop?

  · *Abdomen*: Any evidence of masses, incarcerated hernia, or hepatomegaly? Is the abdomen distended?

  · *Genitourinary*: Is there a bad diaper rash? Anal fissure? Phimosis or paraphimosis? Evidence of testicular torsion? Distended bladder?

  · *Skin*: Any rashes or vesicles? Any bruises that could signify non-accidental trauma? Any hair tourniquets?

- *Treatment*: Treatment varies depending upon what is uncovered in the history and physical examination. When no acute pathology is discovered, different interventions can be discussed with the caregivers. Parents can try soothing techniques, such as pacifier use, using an infant swing, car ride, or noise machines.

  Once a thorough history and physical examination has been performed, it is important to assess the parent/guardian. Persistent crying is a risk factor for and may lead to non-accidental trauma. Parents should understand that in most cases, crying in an infant is normal and will resolve. Providers should emphasize to the caregiver that they are not doing anything wrong to cause the crying. Additionally, parents/caregiver may need a break from a crying child, and it is okay for them to "walk away" from a screaming infant. Additional resources can be found at National Center on Shaken Baby Syndrome (www.dontshake.org).

- *Disposition*: Disposition depends upon the diagnosis. Infants with true colic can be discharged home with close follow-up if their guardians are reliable and are coping well with the crying.

Historical clues	Physical findings	Ancillary studies
• Multiple visits for same complaint • Sweating with feeds • Failure to gain weight	• Abnormal vital signs • Abnormal cardiac examination • Abnormal abdominal examination	• Labs demonstrating dehydration • CXR with cardiomegaly

Follow-Up

Our patient had historical red flags, including numerous visits for the same complaint, sweating with feeds, and failure to gain weight. He had an examination which was remarkable for abnormal vital signs, abnormal cardiac examination, and hepatomegaly. These findings led the EM provider to check laboratory tests and CXR, both of which were abnormal. Because of this, the provider performed an EKG, which revealed large Q waves in the anterior and lateral leads. Pediatric cardiology was consulted and an echocardiogram was performed. The patient was diagnosed with an anomalous left coronary artery with take-off from the pulmonary artery. This coronary artery anomaly in infants can cause pain (especially with "stress testing" such as feeding), myocardial infarction, and heart failure. The patient was admitted to the PICU and had successful corrective surgery the next day.

References

1. From Wikipedia. Their referenced source: Solter A. *Tears and Tantrums: What to Do When Babies and Children Cry.* Goleta, CA: Shining Star Press, 1998.

2. Harb T, Matsuyama M, David M, Hill RJ. Infant colic – what works: A systemic review of interventions for breast-fed infants. *J Pediatr Gastroenterol Nutr* 2016; 62: 668–86.

3. Hall B, Chesters J, Robinson A. Infantile colic: A systematic review of medical and conventional therapies. *J Paediatr Child Health* 2012; 48: 128–37.

4. Jenny C, Hymel KP, Ritzen A, et al. Analysis of missed cases of abusive head trauma. *JAMA* 1999; 281: 621–6.

5. Sugar NF, Taylor JA, Feldman KW. Bruises in infants and toddlers: Those who don't cruise rarely bruise. *Arch Pediatr Adolesc Med* 1999; 153: 399–403.

6. Lardhi AA. Anomalous origin of left coronary artery from pulmonary artery: A rare cause of myocardial infarction in children. *J Family Community Med* 2010; 17: 113–16.

7. Qubty W, Gelfand AA. The link between infantile colic and migraine. *Curr Pain Headache Rep* 2016; 20: 31.

Case 4

Contributing Author: Rebecca Jeanmonod

History

A 5-month-old girl with history of failure to thrive is brought to the ED for "not acting right." Her parents report that she has been "lethargic" and "angry," beginning 4 days ago and getting worse every day. The child has been irritable and difficult to console. She has not had restful sleep, although she seems unusually sedate to them. She has seemed uncomfortable and fussy when receiving feeds through her G-tube and has had high residuals. They have therefore reduced the volume of her feeds and spaced their intervals. She has been having decreased PO, as well. She was hospitalized about 2 weeks ago for fever and was in the hospital for 5 days, during which time she was treated for dehydration and discharged home with resumption of her normal schedule. The child has not had fever since then. She has not been vomiting, and there has been no diarrhea. Her parents report that she is making very few wet diapers, and that they "smell bad." There has been no coughing or difficulty breathing. The parents are most concerned about the G-tube not functioning well, and are requesting surgery be called to evaluate the G-tube.

Past Medical History

- Baby was born at 34 weeks for premature rupture of membranes. She spent 2 weeks in the hospital for feeding difficulties, and went home on nasogastric feeds. She had a percutaneous G-tube placed about 3 months ago for ongoing feeding issues and failure to thrive. The family has tried many different formulations of nutrition and have been seen by a nutritionist as recently as her last hospitalization. The child has, over the last 6 weeks, been feeding somewhat regularly on her own, but still receives regular tube feeds. She has had a metabolic work-up, which has revealed no underlying source of her failure to thrive. The

child has otherwise been meeting her milestones, and is able to sit supported. She is immunized.

Medications

- Metoclopramide.

Allergies

- None.

Physical Examination and Ancillary Studies

- *Vital signs*: T 97 °F, HR 175, RR 70, BP 75/42, O_2 sat 96% on 2 L nasal cannula.
- *General*: The child is conscious and purposeful, pushing at nasal cannula. She is ashen.
- *HEENT*: There are no signs of head trauma. The child's anterior fontanelle is open and sunken. PERRL. Her mucous membranes are dry.
- *Neck*: Supple and non-tender, with no adenopathy.
- *Cardiovascular*: Regular tachycardia, with no M/R/G. Capillary refill 4 seconds.
- *Lungs*: Tachypneic and shallow, but clear bilaterally with no adventitial sounds.
- *Abdomen*: Soft and scaphoid, non-tender/non-distended. G-tube in place with no surrounding erythema or drainage. No organomegaly.
- *Extremities and skin*: Ashen and mottled with no signs of trauma.
- *Neurologic*: The child is purposeful at times, at other times she is listless. Not interactive.
- *Pertinent laboratory values*: Fingerstick glucose 142.

Questions for Thought

- What are the appropriate initial steps to take to stabilize this child?
- What historical information should be elicited to make this diagnosis?
- If you are unable to obtain IV access in this child, what are other options for initiating treatment?

Diagnosis

- Hypernatremic dehydration from receiving concentrated feedings.

Discussion

- *Epidemiology*: Dehydration is a common problem in the pediatric population, with annual admissions of 200,000 in the USA for dehydration related to gastroenteritis alone.[1] Worldwide, diarrheal diseases affect 2 billion people each year, killing about 1.5 million children.[2] The specific contribution of formula preparation mistakes to dehydration burden in children is unknown, but errors during reconstitution of formula are common, with overconcentration being the more frequent error.[3] In the USA, 77 percent of women breastfeed their infants, but this proportion falls to under 50 percent by 6 months.[4]

- *Pathophysiology*: Children are at increased risk for dehydration due to their relatively large body surface areas, resulting in increased evaporative losses from skin, increased respiratory rate with losses due to exhalation of hydrated air, and frequent illnesses which cause increased sensible (diarrhea and vomiting) and insensible losses (tachypnea, fever, sweating). Hypernatremic dehydration in infants is most commonly secondary to diarrheal disease, but receiving hyperconcentrated feeds is another cause.[5] The infant kidney is not able to excrete large sodium loads, nor is it able to dilute as well as the adult kidney. Therefore, hypernatremia may be secondary to relative water depletion, water depletion in excess of sodium depletion, or sodium excess with normal volume status. In ambulatory pediatric and adult patients with access to water, thirst usually prevents significant hypernatremia; however, in small children and bedbound individuals, hypernatremia can be a significant problem.
- *Presentation*: Children with dehydration may appear listless, with dry mucous membranes and decreased tear formation. Children with hypernatremia, regardless of volume status, often have irritability and altered mental status. Children will often present with symptoms from the underlying source of dehydration, such as fever, diarrhea, or respiratory illnesses.
- *Diagnosis*: History is often not helpful in making the diagnosis of dehydration, although it may give important clues to underlying pathology, such as a history of recent diarrheal illness. It is important to obtain a full feeding history, including how the caregiver mixes the formula, as this may be the only clue to the true diagnosis. Different scoops from different brands of formula vary in size, and parents may use a standard spoon rather than the appropriate commercial scoop, thus unwittingly altering the electrolyte and carbohydrate concentration in the child's food. The diagnosis of dehydration is clinical, and the most accurate and reproducible finding in dehydration is reduction of body weight.[1] Unfortunately, the EM provider may not have access to the child's prior weights, and scales may not be appropriately calibrated. Without knowing the child's weight changes, the most accurate physical signs for dehydration are decreased capillary refill, abnormal skin turgor, and abnormal respirations.[6] The diagnosis of hypernatremia is made on laboratory chemistry studies, but may be suspected in irritable infants in whom a history of inappropriately prepared feeds is elicited.

- *Treatment*: In dehydrated infants, the appropriate therapy is a weight-based bolus of isotonic crystalloid fluid at 20 cc/kg. For maintenance fluid, studies demonstrate that isotonic (and not the traditional hypotonic) crystalloid with dextrose is the preferred fluid in both general pediatric patients and in the PICU.[7,8] If IV access is unable to be obtained, IO access (or umbilical access) is acceptable.[9] In children with moderate to severe dehydration with a working gut (without intractable vomiting), nasogastric resuscitation is as successful as IV.[9] Therefore, it is not unreasonable to resuscitate a child through a nasogastric tube, or in this case, a G-tube, when IV access is not available. Hypernatremia should be corrected slowly, no quicker than 0.5 mEq/hour, as more rapid correction may result in cerebral edema and further complications.
- *Disposition*: Sick children should be resuscitated according to the ABC algorithm. Most children with mild dehydration can be discharged home with instructions for oral hydration with appropriate fluids (NOT sports drinks with high sugar contents) and close follow-up and return precautions. Children with moderate or severe dehydration with unreliable follow-up, who cannot take oral fluids, should be admitted for IV fluid therapy. Hypernatremic infants should be admitted for sodium correction and further evaluation to determine the underlying cause of hypernatremia (such as adrenal or renal disease), if the source is unclear.

Historical clues	Physical findings	Ancillary studies
• Reduced tube feeds • Decreased PO • Reduced wet diapers	• Mottled skin • Abnormal vital signs • Poor capillary refill • Sunken fontanelle	• Normal glucose

Follow-Up

ED nursing was initially unable to obtain an IV, so the PICU nursing team was called. During the 90 minutes it took to obtain IV access, the child suffered cardiac arrest. Her initial laboratory chemistries during her code demonstrated the following: Na 165, K 7.3, Cl 118, bicarbonate 22. The child received full ACLS protocol, IV fluid bolus, and treatment of hyperkalemia with calcium, insulin, and glucose. She had return of spontaneous circulation after 17 minutes of cardiac arrest. After review of the family's discharge instructions and notes from the child's prior admission, it became clear that there had been miscommunication between the parents and the nutritionist regarding feeding preparation, and that this error had likely been responsible for her prior admission, as well. She was admitted to the PICU for a prolonged period and was ultimately discharged to a rehabilitation facility with spastic quadraparesis secondary to anoxic brain injury and hypernatremia.

References

1. Canavan A, Arant BS. Diagnosis and management of dehydration in children. *Am Fam Phys* 2009; 80: 692–6.

2. Diarrhoeal Disease Fact Sheet. Geneva: World Health Organization, 2009.

3. Renfrew MJ, Ansell P, Macleod KL. Formula feed preparation: helping reduce the risks; a systematic review. *Arch Dis Child* 2003; 88: 855–8.

4. National Center for Chronic Disease Prevention and Health Promotion, Division of Nutrition, Physical Activity, and Obesity. Breastfeeding Report Card United States/2013. See www.cdc.gov/breastfeeding/pdf/2013breastfeedingreportcard.pdf (accessed October 2016).

5. Leung C, Chang W-C, Yeh S-J. Hypernatremic dehydration due to concentrated infant formula: Report of two cases. *Pediatr Neonatol* 2009; 50: 70–3.

6. Steiner MJ, DeWalt DA, Byerley JS. Is this child dehydrated? *JAMA* 2004; 291: 2746–54.

7. Padua AP, Macaraya JRG, Dans LF, et al. Isotonic versus hypotonic saline solution for maintenance intravenous fluid therapy in children: A systematic review. *Pediatr Nephrol* 2015; 30: 1163–72.

8. Almeida HI, Mascarenhas MI, Loureiro HC, et al. The effect of NaCl 0.9% and NaCl 0.45% on sodium chloride, and acid–base balance in a PICU population. *J Pediatr (Rio J)* 2015; 91: 499–505.

9. Rouhani S, Meloney L, Ahn R, et al. Alternative rehydration methods: A systematic review and lessons for resource-limited care. *Pediatrics* 2011; 127: e748–57.

Case 5

Contributing Authors: Tom Williams, Emily Miller, and Denis R. Pauzé

History

A 9-day-old is brought into the ED by his parents for "not acting like himself." He was born full term, without complications, and was discharged home. The previous week at home had been completely uneventful. Tonight, he started making funny noises and looked gray and pale to them. They tried to suction his nose, but he seemed limp and they did not like his breathing, so they brought him immediately to the ED. On arrival to the ED, the parents are screaming "my baby looks gray!" The child is immediately brought into a room where he is noted to be obviously mottled with grunting respirations. He is ashen-gray in appearance. As the baby is placed on the monitor and nursing works on IV access, you immediately start resuscitating the child. Your medical student asks the parents a few quick questions. You establish that there have been no known fevers or vomiting episodes and that the child was eating normally up until tonight.

Past Medical History

• Born at 39 weeks, normal vaginal delivery. Normal prenatal screening. No birth complications. Discharged from the hospital on day 2.

Medications

• None.

Allergies

• None.

Physical Examination and Ancillary Studies

• *Vital signs*: T 99 °F, HR 170, RR 70 and labored, BP in the right arm 70 systolic, unable to obtain lower extremity BP, O_2 sat 92% in right arm, 79% in left arm.

- *General*: He appears mottled and ashen-gray. He has grunting respirations.
- *HEENT*: There are no signs of head trauma. Fontanelle soft. Sclera normal.
- *Neck*: Trachea midline.
- *Cardiovascular*: Tachycardic. Unable to palpate femoral pulses.
- *Lungs*: Accessory muscle use and obvious distress. Bilateral rhonchi.
- *Abdomen*: Soft and non-distended. No masses. No appreciable hepatomegaly.
- *Extremities and skin*: Mottled. No rash or vesicles. There is delayed capillary refill.
- *Neurologic*: Listless.
- *Pertinent laboratory values*: WBC 14,000, Cr 1.1, bicarbonate 14, Na 130, urine and blood culture sent.
- *Pertinent imaging*: CXR reveals early pulmonary edema. There is no obvious cardiomegaly, pneumonia, or rib fractures.

Questions for Thought

- What is the differential diagnosis for the neonate in shock?
- What medications should be started, even without a definitive diagnosis?
- What are your management priorities?

Diagnosis

- Critical ductal dependent coarctation of the aorta.

Discussion

- *Epidemiology*: Congenital heart defects occur at a rate of somewhere near 8 in every 1,000 live births, depending on the specific definition of congenital heart disease (CHD).[1-4] About 1 in 1,000 of patients with CHD will be discharged home with a critical obstructive left heart process.[1,2] Coarctation of the aorta occurs at a rate of roughly 4 in 10,000 live births and accounts for approximately 5–8 percent of all congenital heart defects.[5] Of these, approximately 60 percent are male. While advances in prenatal screening and U/S are enhancing our ability to

diagnose congenital heart defects in the prenatal period, less than 50 percent of coarctations are diagnosed before birth.[5]

- *Pathophysiology*: In utero, the fetus has a unique circulation that differs in several important ways from that of the infant. Oxygenated blood from the placenta travels to the fetal heart via the umbilical veins and right atrium. A large proportion of this oxygenated blood is shunted directly to the left atrium through the foramen ovale, allowing oxygenated blood to flow to the body's tissues. Some of the blood from the right atrium enters the right ventricle and is pumped into the pulmonary artery. As the lungs are not ventilated in utero, blood flow to the pulmonary circuit is largely unnecessary. Pulmonary blood is shunted from the pulmonary artery to the aorta via the ductus arteriosus. At birth, the pulmonary circuit opens up as the foramen ovale and ductus arteriosus begin to close. The pressure difference between the left and right atrium should snap the foramen ovale shut within the first few breaths, while ductus arteriosus closure is more gradual.

As mentioned, the ductus arteriosus connects the pulmonary artery and the aorta. Some patients with congenital heart lesions are dependent upon an open and functioning ductus arteriosus in order to survive. These lesions are called ductal dependent lesions and come in two general categories: ductal dependent pulmonary blood flow lesions (right-sided obstructive lesions) and left-sided obstructive lesions.

Ductal dependent pulmonary blood flow lesions compromise right-sided blood flow to the pulmonary circuit. These lesions rely on retrograde flow through the ductus arteriosus from the aorta to supply blood to the pulmonary artery. These lesions can be seen in anatomic variants such as pulmonary atresia, critical pulmonary stenosis, and Tetralogy of Fallot with pulmonary atresia.

Left-sided obstructive lesions include anatomic lesions that impede flow of blood through the aorta and to the peripheral circulation. These patients become dependent on the patent ductus arteriosus to bypass the obstruction and supplement the systemic circulation. Examples include hypoplastic left heart syndrome, critical coarctation of the aorta, critical aortic stenosis, and interrupted aortic arch.

For our patient with a critical coarctation of the aorta, once the ductus arteriosus closes, blood can no longer bypass this severe obstruction. This increases the left ventricle afterload, thus causing a decrease in the left ventricle ejection fraction. As cardiac output diminishes, manifestations of poor perfusion can be seen as infants develop signs and symptoms of shock, including mottled skin, cool extremities, decreased urine output, and central cyanosis.[6,7]

- *Presentation*: Ductal dependent lesions typically share common aspects of history and presentation. The degree of clinical distress depends a great deal on the severity of the underlying lesion. For instance, the clinical presentation of coarctation depends on the degree of stenosis. Ductal dependent lesions may present anywhere along the spectrum of illness from non-specific and mild symptoms to frank heart failure.[1,6-8] Neonates may present with poor feeding and fussiness, or may be seen with more drastic symptoms such as irritability, tachypnea, or cyanosis.[1,6,7] In the extreme, they may present with hypotension, mottled skin, frank shock, or cardiac arrest.[1,6-8] About 40 percent of patients with coarctation are symptomatic within the first 2 days of life. Therefore, the majority will present outside of the hospital in offices or EDs. Others may present later in life, with claudication, headaches, and hypertension. It should be noted that coarctations can present at any age.

Neonatal cardiogenic shock may easily be confused for septic shock.[8] In the extreme, it can be incredibly difficult to tell these two etiologies apart. Additionally, some infections may exacerbate a cardiac lesion. Therefore, all infants less than 2 weeks old with shock should be considered to have a ductal dependent congenital heart lesion and be treated with prostaglandin E1 (PGE1) until a confirmatory echocardiogram can be performed by pediatric cardiology.[1,7] These infants should also undergo full septic evaluation and be treated with broad-spectrum antibacterial agents as well as antivirals.

- *Diagnosis*: The diagnosis of a ductal dependent lesion is suggested by history, physical examination, and clinical suspicion. Confirmation is made by imaging, typically an echocardiogram.

While there are findings on physical examination that can strongly suggest a ductal dependent lesion, the spectrum of ductal dependent systemic blood flow and ductal dependent pulmonary blood flow lesions is variable and not all findings may be present.[1-4] However, a focused physical examination can uncover findings that should alert the examiner to the presence of a cardiac anomaly. On cardiovascular examination, one may palpate a hyperactive precordium, auscultate a systolic heart murmur, or find a single S2 or the presence of an S3. When palpating central and peripheral pulses, a critical ductal dependent systemic blood flow lesion will produce weakened, or even absent, pulses in the lower extremities. However, a ductal dependent pulmonary blood flow lesion has no impediment to systemic flow and thus will have intact peripheral pulses. Generally, however, these children are cyanotic.

Use your vital signs! A key finding in diagnosing coarctation is a difference in oxygen saturation between the right upper extremity and the lower extremities. With the ductal dependent systemic blood flow lesion in coarctation, the preductal flow will produce a normal oxygen saturation in the right upper extremity while post-ductal flow, which is supplemented with deoxygenated blood, will produce a reduced oxygen saturation level in the lower extremities. Four-extremity pulse oximetry has become a life-saving neonatal screening that should happen in all well-baby nurseries.[2] Pre- and post-ductal oxygen saturation and BP gradients are non-invasive and incredibly informative.

A CXR is always indicated if you suspect cardiac or pulmonary disease. In the case of cardiac defects, CXR can reveal helpful clues. Increased vascular markings can indicate pulmonary congestion and heart failure while the cardiac silhouette may show classic findings such as cardiomegaly or the "boot shape" of Tetralogy of Fallot (very rare). While not always present, there are some X-ray findings that may be seen with coarctation. The "3" sign of coarctation is formed by the pre-stenotic aortic dilation, followed by the indentation of the stenotic lesion, followed by the post-stenotic aortic dilation. Notching of the inferior rib margins may be seen as collateral intercostal vessels enlarge to help supply the post-ductal portion of the aorta, eroding the associated rib margins as they grow (this isn't seen in infants, only older patients who have had time to develop collaterals). In reality, the clinician should focus on looking for pulmonary congestion or cardiomegaly because these are likely the only abnormalities on CXR. Additionally, cyanotic CHD should be considered if there is persistent hypoxia but the lungs are clear. CHD is discussed further in Chapter 3, Case 7.

EKG may also be useful in suspected CHD. Evidence of ventricular hypertrophy or hypoplasia or conduction abnormalities may give clues to underlying pathology.

The definitive diagnosis of cardiac defects is made by echocardiography, in which the lesion is visualized using either a transthoracic or transesophageal approach.[1] However, a formal, detailed echocardiogram may not be practical or feasible during the initial ED presentation. ED point-of-care U/S is growing in availability, quality, and extent of use and can guide the ED work-up. One particular approach is to use the BLEEP examination, in which the ED provider examines the inferior vena cava, observes the quality of myocardial contractility, and evaluates for the presence and extent of pericardial effusion.[1] Imaging the arch is extremely challenging and definitive diagnosis should be done by pediatric cardiology.

- *Treatment*: ED management of a patient with a ductal dependent lesion does not need to wait for definitive diagnosis. The initial management of any patient in undifferentiated shock should obviously focus on the ABC algorithm.[1] One particular treatment challenge for these unstable infants is vascular access. The shock state will leave the neonate clamped down and hypoperfused. Potential sites include umbilical vein access and IO access. Scalp veins may also be a potential site of access.

For the neonate, it may be difficult in the initial stages to differentiate between cardiogenic shock and septic shock, particularly in children with left-sided ductal dependent lesions, who may not be hypoxic.[8] They appear similar to infants with shock from dehydration, trauma, or inborn errors of metabolism. Therefore, as mentioned, work-up and management should address many potential etiologies, especially infectious diseases and CHD. These infants should expediently be given antibiotics (ampicillin–gentamycin or ampicillin–cefotaxime as well as acyclovir). PGE1 treatment should be started immediately to open and maintain the ductus arteriosus and must not be delayed for a definitive diagnosis. The dose used to open the duct is 0.05–0.1 mcg/kg per minute while the dose to maintain an open duct is 0.01 mcg/kg per minute. The response to treatment should be swift and is measured by improvement of femoral pulses in the case of ductal dependent systemic blood flow lesions and improvement of cyanosis in ductal dependent pulmonary blood flow lesions. Potential side effects of PGE1 include respiratory depression, apnea, hypotension, bradycardia, fever, and rash.[9] While the extent of respiratory depression is dose-dependent, it is often recommended to intubate the patient prior to initiation of PGE1 to secure the airway and avoid significant episodes of hypoxia from apnea. Neonates on PGE1 who need to be transferred should be intubated prior to transfer. Hypotensive children should be given pressor support, such as dobutamine or dopamine.

- *Disposition*: Once a patient has been stabilized, he/she should be admitted for further evaluation and definitive diagnosis. The level of care under which the patient will be admitted, whether it is an ICU (for infants in shock) or lower level of monitoring, will depend on the individual patient, his or her clinical status, and local protocol (NICU vs. PICU). Pediatric cardiology will need to be engaged to diagnose and delineate the lesion. Once the diagnosis is confirmed, pediatric cardiothoracic surgery becomes involved for surgical management.

Many of these patients will need to be transferred to a children's hospital with the appropriate specialists. It should be emphasized that these are fragile infants with highly complex and unusual physiology, with a high probability for serious decompensation. They require 1:1 nursing care with attention to minutiae. These neonates should be transported by experienced neonatal or pediatric transport teams, whenever possible. Ventilator settings, oxygen, fluids, and sedation must be finely titrated to maintain stability and prevent an unexpected decompensation.

Historical clues	Physical findings	Ancillary studies
• Sudden deterioration • Rapid, shallow breathing • Altered mental status	• Tachycardia • Hypotension • Respiratory distress • Absent femoral pulses • Discordant O_2 sat • Abnormal lung examination	• CXR with pulmonary edema

Follow-Up

The patient was immediately intubated. Fortunately, a nurse was able to obtain IV access. A blood and urine culture as well as laboratory tests were sent. An LP was not performed because of the instability of the patient. Ampicillin, cefotaxime, and acyclovir were started. PGE1 was also initiated in the ED. After 30 minutes of PGE1, the infant's color improved dramatically. A call was made to the pediatric cardiologist and the child was admitted to the PICU. Shortly thereafter, an echocardiogram revealed a coarctation of the aorta.

References

1. Strobel AM, Nu LN. The critically ill infant with congenital heart disease. *Emerg Med Clin N Am* 2015; 33: 501–18.

2. Liske MR, Greeley CS, Law DJ, et al. Report of the Tennessee Task Force on Screening Newborn Infants for Congenital Heart Disease. *Pediatrics* 2006; 118: e1250–6.

3. Brown K. The infant with undiagnosed cardiac disease in the emergency department. *Clin Pediatr Emerg Med* 2005; 6: 200–6.

4. Hoffman JIE, Kaplan S. The incidence of congenital heart disease. *J Am Coll Cardiol* 2002; 39:1890–900.

5. Centers for Disease Control and Prevention. Facts about coarctation of the aorta. See www.cdc.gov/ncbddd/heartdefects/coarctationofaorta.html (accessed January 2017).

6. Savitsky E, Alejos J, Votey S. Emergency department presentations of pediatric congenital heart disease. *J Emerg Med* 2003; 24: 239–45.

7. Lee YS, Baek JS, Kwon BS, et al. Pediatric emergency room presentation of congenital heart disease. *Korean Circ J* 2010; 40: 36–41.

8. Ramby AL, Nguyen N, Costello JM. Cardiogenic shock masquerading as septic shock. *Clin Pediatr Emerg Med* 2014; 15: 140–8.

9. Sharma M, Sasikumar M, Karloopia SD, et al. Prostaglandins in congenital heart disease. *Med J Armed Forces India* 2001; 57: 134–8.

Case 6

Contributing Author: Rebecca Jeanmonod

History

An 11-year-old boy is brought to the ED by EMS with his mother for acting strangely. Mom states that the child didn't come down to dinner, and when she went up to his room to retrieve him, she found him sitting on the floor with his eyes closed, his hands grasping at the air. There was vomit on his shirt. She called his name, but he didn't respond to her voice, so she shook him. He felt sweaty to her. He opened his eyes and seemed startled, stated "I am made of wood," and closed his eyes again. She could not get him to accompany her down the stairs to the car to bring him in for evaluation, so she called EMS. EMS reports that the child has been tachycardic en route, with a heart rate of about 125, and had a normal blood glucose. He was otherwise "fine for us," stable and not combative. Mom states she has never seen the child like this before. He had been previously healthy, and is a 6th grader who generally gets Bs in school. He had been playing video games in his room throughout the day today with several friends, but his friends went home an hour before mom found him. The child provides no meaningful history.

Past Medical History

- Healthy and developmentally normal, has received all immunizations.

Medications

- None.

Allergies

- None.

Physical Examination and Ancillary Studies

- *Vital signs*: T 99.6 °F, HR 132, RR 22, BP 100/62, O_2 sat 100% on room air.
- *General*: The child is sitting upright on the stretcher with his eyes closed, picking at the air. He is not in any obvious distress.
- *HEENT*: There are no signs of head trauma. The child's pupils are small, but reactive. When he opens his eyes, his eye movements are generally roving, but he occasionally seems to fixate on his mother. His mucous membranes are moist. His oropharynx is clear.

- *Neck*: Supple and non-tender, with no adenopathy.
- *Cardiovascular*: Regular tachycardia, with no M/R/G. Capillary refill is brisk.
- *Lungs*: CTA bilaterally.
- *Abdomen*: Soft, without distension or tenderness. No masses or organomegaly. Normal genitalia.
- *Extremities and skin*: Diaphoretic, warm, and well-perfused, no signs of trauma.
- *Neurologic*: The child resists movements of his extremities and does not follow commands. He does move his extremities spontaneously and symmetrically. His face is symmetric. His sensory examination, cerebellar examination, and gait are unable to be assessed due to his mental status.
- *Pertinent laboratory values*: Fingerstick glucose 81.

Questions for Thought

- What sort of laboratory and ancillary tests are important to get in this patient?
- Are there medications that should be given to this child?
- If the child returns to his baseline, can he be discharged home? Why or why not?

Diagnosis

- Dextromethorphan overdose.

Discussion

- *Epidemiology*: In the USA, there are over 5 million poisonings each year.[1] Seventy-five percent of these are acute ingestions, while 25 percent represent chronic toxicity or remote ingestion.[1] Ingestions may be accidental or intentional, and may be recreational or as an attempt at self-harm. Ingestions account for 5–10 percent of all ED visits, but the majority of overdose patients are released to home, with an admission rate of only about 5 percent.[1,2] The patients who get admitted, however, may be quite ill. Intoxicated patients account for more than 5 percent of ICU admissions. The most common intentional overdoses involve pain medications, such as over-the-counter NSAIDs or prescription narcotics, but psychiatric medications, illegal drugs, vitamins, and cardiac medications are also common. Dextromethorphan, a compound in many over-the-counter cough and cold medications, accounts for about 13,000 cases of

poisonings annually presenting for treatment.[3] Almost half of these patients are between the ages of 12 and 20, with the majority of poisonings intentional (for the purpose of getting high), although some are suicide attempts.[3]

- *Pathophysiology*: Poisoning is ultimately a matter of dosing. Even substances that are non-toxic, like water, can be intoxicating and even fatal in high doses. Because children are generally smaller than adults, they are at increased risk of toxicity when ingesting substances because the substance distributes through a smaller total volume. This is why a single tablet of a calcium channel blocker or a beta blocker may be fatal in a small child. Many over-the-counter medications have not been studied in children, and most dosing guidelines for children are based on child age, rather than size, even though size can vary widely for a given age. For these reasons, the AAP states that children age 6 and younger should not receive over-the-counter cough or cold preparations.[4]

  Dextromethorphan and its metabolites have a host of pathophysiologic effects, including NMDA receptor antagonism, inhibition of catecholamine reuptake, and agonism of serotonin receptors.[3] Additionally, dextromethorphan is usually combined with other agents in a given cold preparation, most commonly pseudoephedrine, acetaminophen, or anticholinergics. This can make these overdoses harder to recognize, as anticholinergic findings or catecholamine excess may predominate in the clinical picture.

  The pathophysiology for how any given toxin works depends on what the toxin is. A complete discussion of all intoxicants is beyond the scope of this book; however, the clinician should be aware of the major classes of toxidromes: sympathomimetic, anticholinergic, opioids, sedatives, and cholinergics. These are described in Table 9.1.

- *Presentation*: Presentations for intoxication vary with the agent ingested. Patients may present with local GI irritation (vomiting and diarrhea) from an agent that may not have systemic harm (such as rhododendron). They may present with a toxidrome related to specific effects of the agent on neurotransmitters in the CNS and systemically (Table 9.1), such as diphenhydramine, cocaine, or selective serotonin reuptake inhibitors. They may present with non-specific altered mental status,

Table 9.1 Examination findings with specific toxidromes

	HR	RR	BP	T	Pupils	Skin
Sympathomimetics	Elevated	Elevated	Elevated	Elevated	Mydriasis	Moist
Anticholinergics	Elevated	Either	Either	Elevated	Mydriasis	Dry
Opioids	Decreased	Decreased	Decreased	Decreased	Miosis	Dry
Sedatives	Decreased	Decreased	Decreased	Decreased	Either	Dry
Cholinergics	Either	–	Either	–	Miosis	Moist

either on the sedation spectrum or the agitation spectrum, such as with zolpidem. They may present with hemodynamic instability (common in cardiac medications), hypoglycemia (with oral hypoglycemics, beta blockers, or insulin), or hallucinations (as with anticholinergics, LSD, phencyclidine, or dextromethorphan). Because of the wide variety of possible presentations, the clinician should at least consider the possibility of poisoning during formulation of the differential for *virtually all chief complaints*. Most diagnoses are ultimately based on history, but there are clues that may be provided on physical examination or on laboratory evaluation.

- *Diagnosis*: History is the mainstay of diagnosis of a specific intoxicant. Obtaining a history from family members and friends, reviewing details of the scene with EMS, calling pharmacists to ascertain the patient's medication lists, and review of the medical record may all prove valuable in narrowing down the toxin involved. Vital signs, pupil examination, and assessment of skin is helpful in making diagnosis of a toxidrome (Table 9.1). A careful neurologic examination may reveal clonus (pathognomonic for serotonin syndrome) or rigidity (which may occur with neuroleptics), as well as evidence of hallucinations (patient responding to internal stimuli) or seizures. Visual and tactile hallucinations are more likely to be toxic in etiology, while auditory hallucinations are more likely to be psychiatric. Serum electrolytes may be helpful, as in cases where a patient displays an elevated anion gap acidosis (anion gap >12), calculated as [sodium – (chloride + bicarbonate)]. Methanol, ethylene glycol, salicylates, paraldehyde, iron, isoniazid, carbon monoxide, and cyanide can all cause an elevated anion gap. Measurement of serum osmolarity and calculation of an osmolar gap may be helpful, as methanol, ethanol, ethylene glycol,

and isopropyl alcohol may cause an elevated osmolar gap (calculated as [laboratory osmoles – (2Na) – (glucose/18) – (BUN/2.8)], abnormal being >10 or < –10). Low glucose can occur from alcohols, oral hypoglycemics, insulin, or beta blockers. A host of toxins may cause renal failure or liver failure. Anemia can suggest iron toxicity or isopropyl alcohol ingestion. An EKG with a wide QRS or a prolonged Q–T should raise concern for ingestion of psychiatric medications (such as tricyclics or antipsychotics), antihistamines (diphenhydramine), or cardiac medications (type 1a and 1c anti-arrhythmics or amiodarone). Urine tests are available for a host of intoxicants, including methadone, benzodiazepines, cocaine, and marijuana. Specific blood tests are available to identify many toxins, such as acetaminophen, salicylates, ethanol, toxic alcohols, cardiac glycosides, and many seizure medications, but further toxicologic testing is often not available in real time in the ED for the purpose of making clinical decisions.

- *Treatment*: For most intoxicants, including dextromethorphan, treatment is quite simply supportive care. This includes the ABC algorithm, establishment of an IV line, and fluid resuscitation. Symptomatic patients with an ingestion should be placed on a monitor and observed. Agitated and hallucinating patients like this patient should have external stimuli minimized and may be given benzodiazepines for further symptom control. If the ingestion was within 1 hour of evaluation, the believed substance is harmful and known to adsorb to charcoal, and the patient has an intact airway, activated charcoal at a dose of 1 g/kg should be given.[2] There has been no demonstrated benefit and some harm to whole bowel irrigation, gastric lavage, or forced vomiting, and these practices are generally not indicated in intoxicated pediatric patients.

Table 9.2 Specific poisons and their antidotes

Poison	Antidote
Acetaminophen	N-acetyl-cysteine
Narcotic analgesics	Naloxone
Benzodiazepines	Flumazenil
Methanol and ethylene glycol	Fomepizole, ethanol
Isopropyl alcohol	Dialysis
Diphenhydramine (and other agents that widen the QRS complex)	Sodium bicarbonate
Oral hypoglycemics	Glucose, octreotide for sulfonylureas
Beta or calcium-channel blockers	Glucagon, high-dose insulin and glucose therapy
Digoxin or other cardiac glycosides	Digoxin-specific antibody (Fab) fragments
Iron	Deferoxamine
Mercury, lead	Dimercaprol, EDTA
Organophosphates	Pralidoxime
Cyanide	Hydroxocobalamin
Isoniazid	Pyridoxine
Local anesthetics and dapsone (cause methemoglobinemia)	Methylene blue

Some intoxicants have specific antidotes, the most notable of which is acetaminophen. Acetaminophen is a common co-ingestant and may cause fatal hepatotoxicity, which is completely preventable with treatment with N-acetyl-cysteine within 12 hours of the ingestion. Likewise, salicylates and toxic alcohols may be treated with dialysis, digoxin is treated with digoxin-specific antibody (Fab) fragments, and heavy metals are treated with chelation therapy (see Table 9.2 for a list of poisons with their antidotes). For this reason, in the patient with an unknown intoxicant, it is important to check levels of substances that would require a change in therapy, especially in the critically ill patient, as failure to treat appropriately may result in death.

- *Disposition*: Sick children should be resuscitated according to the ABC algorithm. In most patients with a known ingestion, who are asymptomatic, an assessment for suicidal ideation (possibly with psychiatric consultation in the right clinical scenario) and observation for 4–6 hours is appropriate. However, substances that are sustained-release, controlled-release, have long half-lives (such as methadone), or delayed effects (such as bupropion) should prompt admission for observation. If the clinician is unfamiliar with the substance or has any questions about the management of the child, he or she should call the Poison Control Hotline for recommendations.

Historical clues	Physical findings	Ancillary studies
• Age group	• Active hallucinations • Tachycardia • Diaphoresis	• Normal glucose

Follow-Up

The child seemed to be having visual hallucinations, and was medicated with lorazepam for his symptoms. Mom was able to provide the phone number to the child's friends, who provided the history that the child had been drinking cough syrup in order to get high earlier in the day, and they had left when he "started acting weird." The child's laboratory tests did not show any significant electrolyte or renal abnormalities, and his LFTs were normal. The child had a negative serum toxicology screen for ethanol, salicylates, and acetaminophen, and had a negative urine toxicology screen. His EKG showed sinus tachycardia with normal intervals and no ectopy. The child was admitted for observation, and his sensorium improved over the following 8 hours. The child admitted to taking the syrup recreationally, and stated that he had not done it before, but had heard it was fun from an older child on the school bus. He denied suicidal intent. He was evaluated and cleared by the crisis staff. The child was ultimately discharged home with his parents, after observation, and has had no further problems.

References

1. Watson WA, Litovitz TL, Rodgers GC Jr, et al. 2004 Annual report of the American Association of Poison Control Centers Toxic Exposure Surveillance System. *Am J Emerg Med* 2005; 23: 589–666.
2. Chyka PA, Seger D, Krenzelok EP, et al. Position paper: Single-dose activated charcoal. *Clin Toxicol (Phila)* 2005; 43: 61–87.
3. Chyka PA, Erdman AR, Manoguerra AS, et al. Dextromethorphan poisoning: An evidence-based consensus guideline for out-of-hospital management. *Clin Toxicol (Phila)* 2007; 45: 662–77.

4. Lowry JA, Leeder JS. Over-the-counter medications: Update on cough and cold preparations. *Pediatr Rev* 2015; 36. See http://pedsinreview.aappublications.org/content/36/7/286 (accessed November 2016).

Case 7

Contributing Author: Kinsey Leonard

History

A 7-month-old male is brought to the ED by his parents. He is sleeping in his mother's arms. His parents state that they have not been able to wake him up for the last 3 hours. He typically takes a 1.5-hour afternoon nap. Today, after 1.5 hours, mom tried to wake him but was unsuccessful. She figured the infant was tired and let him sleep longer. When she couldn't arouse him after an additional 1.5 hours, she became concerned. She states that the infant was acting normally earlier in the day. Mom states that he had taken a bottle every 3 hours, he had been making normal wet diapers, and he had a normal bowel movement in the morning.

On review of systems, mom states that he is a healthy male and denies recent illness. She denies fevers, rhinorrhea, cough, decreased PO intake, diarrhea, vomiting, melena, hematochezia, or decreased urination. She denies increased fussiness. The infant is UTD on all immunizations. He is breast fed. He has met all developmental milestones. He does not attend daycare, mom stays at home with the infant and his older brother.

Past Medical History

- Normal spontaneous vaginal birth at 39 weeks' gestation, no medical problems, UTD on immunizations.

Medications

- Vitamin D.

Allergies

- NKDA.

Physical Examination and Ancillary Studies

- *Vital signs*: T 99 °F, HR 110, BP 90/60, RR 30, O$_2$ sat 100% on room air.
- *General*: The patient is asleep in his mother's arms. Unarousable. Withdrawals from painful stimuli.
- *HEENT*: Normocephalic and atraumatic. Anterior fontanelle is soft and flat. PERRL.
- *Neck*: Supple, with a midline trachea.
- *Cardiovascular*: Regular rate, with no M/R/G.
- *Lungs*: Clear and equal, with no W/R/R.
- *Abdomen*: Soft, non-distended. Palpable mass in the right lower quadrant. Guaiac positive.
- *Extremities and skin*: Skin is warm and dry. Capillary refill < 3 seconds. No rash. No bruises, lacerations, or other signs of trauma.
- *Neurologic*: Patient withdraws all extremities to painful stimuli. Examination appears non-focal.
- *Pertinent laboratory values*: Fingerstick glucose is normal. Toxicology screen is negative. Electrolytes and divalents are normal. WBC 17,000.
- *Pertinent imaging*: CT head normal.

Questions for Thought

- What are the appropriate initial steps in managing this child?
- What ED work-up is necessary to diagnose this entity and exclude other entities?
- How does this condition usually present?
- What is the definitive treatment for this condition?
- What is the disposition of this patient?

Diagnosis

- Intussusception.

Discussion

- *Epidemiology*: Children are at greatest risk for intussusception before the age of 3 years, although it can occur at any age. Males are at an increased risk compared to females. Intussusception is the leading cause of intestinal obstruction in children.
- *Pathophysiology*: Intussusception occurs when a proximal segment of bowel "telescopes" into a more distal segment. The most common location is ileocolic. The proximal segment and the associated mesentery become edematous due to decreased venous return, which can result in ischemia. Seventy-five percent of cases are idiopathic. Intussusception has been postulated to be caused by viral illness, with increase lymphoid tissue at Peyer's patches acting as the lead point. Intussusception has also been linked to Meckel's

diverticulum, polyps, duplication cysts, lymphomas, and hematomas from Henoch–Schönlein purpura. Some studies report increased risk of intussusception in children with cystic fibrosis, celiac disease, and Crohn's disease.[1-3]

- *Presentation*: Most commonly, children present with colicky abdominal pain and vomiting. More information on this presentation is present in the chapter on vomiting. The triad of intermittent abdominal pain, emesis, and currant-jelly stool is seen in about 20 percent of presentations. Both vomiting and grossly bloody stool occur as a later complication of intussusception; however, guaiac testing is most often positive even in early presentations. A palpable, "sausage-shaped," abdominal mass is found in the majority of cases, but the absence of an abdominal mass should not be falsely reassuring.

  In 10–20 percent of cases, lethargy, or altered mental status may be the sole presenting complaint or a component of the presentation, as in this case.[4]

- *Diagnosis*: Diagnosing intussusception is easier when the patient presents with the typical triad. In this presentation, the clinician may only want to order U/S to confirm the suspected diagnosis. U/S not only diagnoses the condition (demonstrating a "target sign," in which loops of bowel are seen invaginated within one another), it can also confirm the location and whether or not a pathologic lead point exists. If the history is extremely suggestive of intussusception and the physical examination supports the diagnosis, some institutions recommend proceeding directly to air enema, which will simultaneously confirm the diagnosis and treat the condition.

  If the child presents atypically, as in this case with altered mental status, a more comprehensive work-up is indicated, to exclude other pathology. Evaluation for metabolic, endocrine, infectious, neurologic, traumatic, and toxicologic sources of altered mental status should be undertaken. In children with altered mental status of unclear etiology, the clinician should consider performing U/S of the abdomen as part of the child's evaluation.

  Plain films of the abdomen are not specific for the diagnosis of intussusception and may be entirely normal. Intussusception may be diagnosed on CT scan, but this is not the modality of choice due to the risks of radiation exposure and the expense of the modality.

- *Treatment*: The child should be resuscitated with IV fluids and close attention to the ABC algorithm. A nasogastric tube is often used to decompress the stomach before the child has an air contrast enema performed. The treatment of choice for intussusception is a pneumatic enema, using either air or carbon dioxide, rather than a hydrostatic enema, which has a higher risk of perforation, although either may be used. The enema is usually performed under U/S or fluoroscopic guidance to confirm reduction of the intussusception, with U/S being the preferred modality. Perforation occurs in about 1 percent of cases that are treated with enemas.[5]

- Surgery is indicated in cases where the pneumatic or hydrostatic enema is unsuccessful, when there are multiple recurrences, when perforation is suspected, or when the patient is hemodynamically unstable or has a peritoneal abdomen. A pediatric surgeon should be consulted in all intussusception cases in case surgery needs to be performed.

- *Disposition*: Children are usually observed for 24 hours after reduction. Intussusception recurs in about 10 percent of children.[6] In these cases, enema reduction can be attempted again. If the intussusception keeps recurring, surgical treatment is indicated.[6,7]

Historical clues	Physical findings	Ancillary studies
• Age 3 months to 3 years	• Mass in the abdomen • Guaiac positive	• Leukocytosis • Negative metabolic, trauma, and toxic work-up

Follow-Up

The child had IV fluid resuscitation and was admitted to the hospital for observation. On hospital day 2, he became less stable and underwent CT which demonstrated intussusception and free fluid in the abdomen. An example of a CT with intussusception is shown in Figure 9.1. He was flown to a pediatric center where he underwent exploratory laparotomy during which he had the necrotic bowel excised. His post-operative course was uncomplicated and he was discharged after 7 inpatient days.

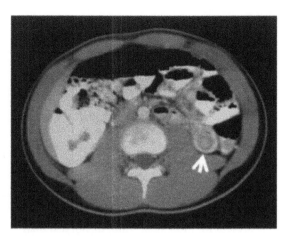

Figure 9.1 CT of the abdomen showing intussuscepted bowel (white arrow) in the left lower quadrant.

References

1. Holmes M, Murphy V, Taylor M, et al. Intussusception in cystic fibrosis. *Arch Dis Child* 1991; 66: 726–7.

2. Mushtaq N, Marven S, Walker J, et al. Small bowel intussusception in celiac disease. *J Pediatr Surg* 1999; 34: 1833–5.

3. Cohen DM, Conard FU, Treem WR, et al. Jejunojejunal intussusception in Crohn's disease. *J Pediatr Gastroenterol Nutr* 1992; 14: 101–3.

4. Kleizen KJ, Hunck A, Wijnen MH, et al. Neurological symptoms in children with intussusception. *Acta Paediatr* 2009; 98: 1822–4.

5. Maoate K, Beasley SW. Perforation during gas reduction of intussusception. *Pediatr Surg Int* 1998; 14: 168–70.

6. Yang CM, Hsu HY, Tsao PN, et al. Recurrence of intussusception in childhood. *Acta Paediatr Taiwan* 2001; 42: 158–61.

7. Weihmiller SN, Buonomo C, Bachur R. Risk stratification of children being evaluated for intussusception. *Pediatrics* 2011; 127: e296–303.

Case 8

Contributing Author: Kinsey Leonard

History

A 15-year-old male presents to the ED with altered mental status. The patient's parents state that he became very agitated at home and punched the television set, injuring his hand. The parents report that they have heard the patient talking to the television and also speaking out loud as if in conversation with someone when he is alone in his room. The patient denies drug or alcohol use, but does not answer further questions. His parents report that he is a healthy male and deny any recent illness. Mom states that he had several friends at his high school, but has not been hanging out with them for the past few months. To the best of her knowledge, she concurs that he does not use drugs, drink alcohol, or smoke cigarettes.

Past Medical History

- Asthma.
- UTD on immunizations.

Medications

- Albuterol.

Allergies

- NKDA.

Physical Examination and Ancillary Studies

- *Vital signs*: T 98.2 °F, HR 73, BP 120/70, RR 18, O_2 sat 100% on room air.
- *General*: The patient is awake and alert.
- *HEENT*: Normocephalic and atraumatic. PERRL. There is no nystagmus. Oropharynx clear.
- *Neck*: Supple, with a midline trachea.
- *Cardiovascular*: Regular rate, with no M/R/G.
- *Lungs*: Clear and equal, with normal work of breathing.
- *Abdomen*: Soft, with no tenderness, distension, rebound, or guarding.
- *Extremities and skin*: Skin is warm and dry. Superficial lacerations to the second-fourth metacarpophalangeal joints on the right hand. Bleeding well controlled.
- *Neurologic*: Alert and oriented × 4. No focal neurologic deficits. Patient ambulated into the ED with a normal gait.
- *Psychiatric*: The patient appears anxious. He is looking around the room and seems to be listening to something because he keeps shaking his head. He seems agitated, is moving rapidly and unexpectedly. He demonstrates echolalia when he is asked questions directly.
- *Pertinent laboratory values*: Urine toxicology is negative. Ethanol level is undetectable.

Diagnosis

- Acute psychosis.

Discussion

- *Epidemiology*: The prevalence of schizophrenia is about 1 percent, with equal prevalence in females and males.[1,2] A strong genetic predisposition has been found. The prevalence of bipolar disorder in the pediatric population is 2–3 percent.[2,3] The prevalence of depression ranges depending on age of the child, with less than 1 percent in children under 5 years and about 4 percent in late adolescence.[2,3]
- *Pathophysiology*: Psychosis can be caused by many underlying problems beyond primary psychiatric disease. The clinician should consider underlying medical causes, such as metabolic/electrolyte derangements, toxins, CNS disease and infections, seizures, autoimmune disease, and vitamin deficiencies. Primary psychiatric disease should only be considered once these other processes are eliminated through history, physical examination, and ancillary studies as indicated.

  Psychiatric disease often has its first presentation as psychosis in the ED. There is usually a history of progressively worsening symptoms over several weeks to months.[1,2] The most common psychiatric diseases with psychotic features are depression with psychotic features, bipolar disorder, brief psychotic disorder, schizophreniform, schizophrenia, and schizoaffective disorder.[2] Personality disorders and conduct disorder can also present with psychosis. These are each described in brief below.

  - *Depression with psychotic features*: The patient meets criteria for major depressive disorder and has delusions or hallucinations during the mood disorder. The mood disorder occurs at times without psychosis.
  - *Bipolar disorder*: During manic episodes, the patient may have delusions of grandeur that may appear to the clinician as psychosis.
  - *Brief psychotic disorder*: Delusions, hallucinations, or disorganized speech is present acutely for less than 1 month. The child completely recovers back to baseline after the episode. An acute stressor precipitates the episode.
  - *Schizophreniform*: Diagnosis requires two of the following five symptoms – hallucinations, delusions, disorganized thoughts, abnormal/catatonic behavior, and/or negative symptoms, present for more than 1 month, but less than 6 months.
  - *Schizophrenia*: Continuation of the psychotic disturbance for at least 6 months, with two of the five symptoms (hallucinations, delusions, disorganized thoughts, disorganized/catatonic behavior, negative symptoms) present for the majority of 1 month.
  - *Schizoaffective disorder*: two of the five criteria for schizophrenia are present, with intermittent mood disorder, either bipolar or major depression, for at least 1 month. The psychotic symptoms of the illness are present for at least 2 weeks without the mood disorder.
  - Schizoid and schizotypal personality disorder also may have psychotic features.

- *Presentation*: An abrupt, acute onset of psychosis in children is more likely secondary to an underlying medical/organic cause, while a more gradual onset is more likely psychiatric in origin. Most patients with primary psychiatric disease will have normal vital signs. They typically have an unremarkable physical examination, with normal neurologic examination, level of alertness, and orientation. The only abnormal findings on examination are typically psychiatric: evidence of abnormal thinking, hallucinations, a tangential thought process, pressured speech, disorganized or catatonic behavior, and agitation. Patients with hallucinations from a psychiatric cause are typically auditory, while those from an underlying medical/toxic process are more commonly visual or tactile.[2]
- *Diagnosis*: In the ED, if there is any doubt that the child's psychosis is psychiatric in origin, alternative medical causes should be sought.

Glucose testing, electrolytes, divalents, thyroid studies, and LFTs may all be indicated for a newly psychotic child. All children with psychosis should undergo toxicology screening, and appropriately aged female patients should have a pregnancy test done. If toxins are suspected, EKG should also be performed to look for evidence of QRS widening or dysrhythmias. Neuroimaging and LP might be indicated in the right clinical setting.

If a psychiatric cause is suspected, the evaluation should be tailored to determining the patient's risk as an immediate threat to him/herself or someone else. This includes an assessment of suicidal or homicidal ideation. It is important to remember that a child may be a threat to him/herself without being suicidal. A psychotic patient who is unable to interact with and attend to his/her environment in an appropriate way may be at risk for accidental death (for example, walking into traffic) or self-harm. Either scenario necessitates inpatient hospitalization. The majority of newly psychotic children should have a psychiatric/crisis evaluation, and admission versus close outpatient treatment should be decided in concert with psychiatric professionals.

- *Treatment*: Acutely psychotic patients should be placed in a quiet area of the ED, with decreased stimulation, preferably in an area designed for such patients. They should be provided with verbal redirection and de-escalation. Sedatives such as benzodiazepines or antipsychotics may be necessary for the violent psychotic patient, and physical restraints may also be required to preserve the safety of the ED staff and other patients. Providers should be familiar with their state's laws concerning the restraint and involuntary admission of psychiatric patients, as these laws vary in different regions. Crisis/psychiatric consultation should be obtained, and social workers may also assist in disposition issues and follow-up.

- *Disposition*: If the child is in a safe environment with reliable follow-up and poses no harm to him/herself or others, he/she may be discharged with close follow-up. All others require inpatient admission.

Historical clues	Physical findings	Ancillary studies
• Auditory hallucinations • Gradual onset	• Normal vital signs • Normal neurologic examination • Normal eye examination	• Negative urine toxicology • Negative ethanol

Follow-Up

The child was admitted to psychiatry, where he was ultimately diagnosed with schizophrenia. He is currently on a stable drug regimen that allows him to function, and has returned to school.

References

1. Holder SD, Wayhs A. Schizophrenia. *Am Fam Phys* 2014; 90: 775–82.

2. Griswold KS, Del Regno PA, Berger RC. Recognition and differential diagnosis of psychosis in primary care. *Am Fam Phys* 2015; 91: 856–63.

3. American Psychiatric Association. *Diagnostic and Statistical Manual of Mental Disorders*, 5th edition. Washington (DC): American Psychiatric Association, 2013.

Chapter 10

Head and Neck Pain

Case 1

Contributing Author: Sonika Raj

History

The patient is a 14-year-old girl who was brought to the ED immediately after her mother found her unconscious on the bedroom floor. The patient had been complaining of headache and dizziness for 1 day, but thought it was "just stress" for an upcoming examination. Shortly after arrival, the child suffers cardiopulmonary arrest; after a short course of CPR and resuscitative efforts, she regains cardiac function but remains unconscious. While you prepare for endotracheal intubation, she regains consciousness and starts to complain of nausea and a headache.

The mother states she has had no recent illnesses, fevers, or other complaints. According to her mother, the patient is a happy, generally healthy young teenager, with a good support system of family and friends. She earns top grades in school and her mother often finds her working late into the night on school assignments. There is no history of drug or alcohol use, depression, being bullied, or suicide attempts.

Past Medical History

- Tension headaches, approximately 1 per month since the start of the school year.
- Immunizations UTD.

Medications

- Ibuprofen 200 mg PO every 6 hours as needed for tension headaches.

Allergies

- NKDA.

Physical Examination and Ancillary Studies

- *Vital signs*: T 100.4 °F, HR 113, BP 97/50, RR 25, O_2 sat 98% on room air.
- *General*: Teenage female lying supine and in distress secondary to headache. She is intermittently somnolent.
- *HEENT*: Normocephalic and atraumatic. PERRL. No photophobia. No pharyngeal erythema or exudates.
- *Neck*: Supple, with midline trachea.
- *Cardiovascular*: Tachycardic and regular. No M/R/G.
- *Lungs*: CTA bilaterally, with no W/R/R.
- *Abdomen*: Soft, non-distended, non-tender, with normoactive bowel sounds and no hepatosplenomegaly.
- *Extremities and skin*: Pale, mildly cyanotic extremities with no edema.
- *Neurologic*: She has generalized difficulty concentrating during the examination. Somnolent but responsive. Cranial nerves II–XII intact. Muscle strength 4/5 and symmetric throughout. Sensory and vibratory examinations intact and symmetric throughout. Reflexes 3+ and symmetric throughout. Patient has significant difficulty with rapid alternating movements, heel-to-shin test, and finger-to-nose test. Positive Romberg test. Negative pronator drift. When asked to demonstrate gait, patient refuses due to fatigue.
- *Pertinent laboratory values*: Fingerstick glucose 110. Na 140, K 5, Cl 106, bicarbonate 11. Thyroid and drug screen negative. EKG shows sinus tachycardia.
- *Pertinent imaging*: Head CT unremarkable.

Diagnosis

- Carbon monoxide (CO) poisoning.

Discussion

- *Epidemiology*: Thousands of patients visit the ED each year for CO poisoning. It is a leading cause of death by accidental poisoning, and accounts for several thousand hospital admissions each year. In a national study of adolescent poisoning deaths in the USA between 1979 and 1994, CO inhalation caused 38.2 percent of the deaths, and 65.1 percent of these were suicides.[1] The true incidence of CO toxicity is unknown, as symptoms may be mild (and patients do not seek care) as well as vague (resulting in misdiagnoses). Sources of exposure include house fires, fuel-burning devices which are inadequately vented (i.e. inhalation of car exhaust in a closed garage), and damaged heating units (i.e. space heaters or gas radiators). While CO toxicity is more common in the winter when people use alternate heat sources, it can occur at any time of the year.

- *Pathophysiology*: CO is an odorless and colorless gas that is absorbed into the pulmonary vascular bed where it attaches to hemoglobin. Since hemoglobin has a much stronger affinity for CO than oxygen, most hemoglobin molecules will attach to CO. This shifts the oxygen–hemoglobin saturation curve to the left, which in turn reduces oxygen delivery to peripheral tissues. This produces tissue hypoxia and, secondarily, lactic acidosis. CO also causes anoxia by integrating into the intracellular oxygen–cytochrome oxidase system, where it blocks cellular oxidation. The sequelae are the sequelae of hypoxia: seizure, cardiopulmonary arrest, and death.

- *Presentation*: Acute CO toxicity may present with a range of symptoms. The most common symptom is headache.[2,3] Additional complaints include dizziness, fatigue, and visual changes.[2,3] Neurologic symptoms include changes in memory/concentration, disorientation, and coma.[2,3] Cardiovascular (chest pain secondary to myocardial ischemia), GI (nausea/vomiting), or pulmonary symptoms (shortness of breath) may also be seen.

  Some patients may have long-term, undiagnosed exposure to CO. These patients may present with a myriad of non-specific symptoms, such as cognitive decline, sleep problems, memory difficulty, and emotional lability.[2,3]

- *Diagnosis*: Diagnosing CO toxicity requires a high index of suspicion, as well as careful questioning regarding potential sources for CO exposure (the patient's work environment, heat sources in the home, and recreational activities). Household members with similar symptoms represent another diagnostic clue.

  Venous carboxyhemoglobin levels are helpful in confirming the diagnosis of CO poisoning, although it is important to remember that this test has limitations.[2,3] Patients may be exposed to CO at their house, then have their levels decrease when they leave the source. By the time they reach the ED for diagnostic testing, which may be several hours later, their CO levels can normalize. Information from the fire service/EMS at the scene with environmental CO measurements is important to obtain for CO evaluation, when possible. Pulse oximetry has no role in screening for CO poisoning.

  In patients with confirmed CO poisoning, other tests may be useful. Blood glucose testing may reveal hypoglycemia, creatine kinase levels may demonstrate secondary rhabdomyolysis from tissue hypoxia, and EKG/troponin may show cardiac ischemia or infarction. For those patients in whom exposure was secondary to house or chemical fire, evaluation for cyanide toxicity is also very important.

  In the undifferentiated teen with altered mental status, toxicologic screening and other laboratory tests may rule out other metabolic and toxic sources of mental status changes. CT imaging may help rule out other central causes, such as subarachnoid hemorrhage or mass. In severe cases of CO toxicity, CT may show hypodensities in the basal ganglia.[2,3] The detection of such changes within 24 to 48 hours of the poisoning is associated with a poor prognosis.

- *Treatment*: The initial treatment for CO toxicity is to remove the patient from the source and immediately start 100 percent oxygen via a non-rebreather mask;[2,3] 100 percent oxygen should be administered until symptoms have resolved and the carboxyhemoglobin level is below 10 percent. Tracheal intubation should be performed when clinically indicated.

  Hyperbaric oxygen significantly decreases the half-life of CO. Indications for hyperbaric oxygen therapy include patients who are unconscious, those with a neurologic deficit, those with EKG changes and/or infarction, and those with a carboxyhemoglobin level greater than 25 percent.[2,3] Because fetal hemoglobin has an especially high affinity for CO, pregnant patients with a carboxyhemoglobin level greater than 20 percent should be considered for hyperbaric therapy.[2,3]

  Rhabdomyolysis, seizures, and myocardial ischemia should be treated as indicated.

  CO poisoning may be intentional, and each patient should be evaluated by a psychiatrist if clinically indicated.

- *Disposition*: Asymptomatic patients with elevated carboxyhemoglobin levels should be treated with high-flow oxygen therapy until their levels normalize. Symptomatic patients who do not meet criteria for hyperbaric therapy should be admitted for high-flow oxygen therapy and monitoring. Patients who meet criteria for hyperbaric therapy should be transferred to a facility with capability for this therapy, when possible.

Historical clues	Physical findings	Ancillary studies
• Loss of consciousness • Headache and nausea • Use of space heater	• Abnormal vital signs • Abnormal neurologic examination	• Negative head CT • Negative tox screen • Anion gap acidosis • Elevated carboxy-hemoglobin level

Follow-Up

Upon further questioning, it was discovered that the child was using a space heater in her room, with the door closed at night to keep warm. The child's carboxyhemoglobin level was checked, and measured 20 percent. Given her neurologic symptoms, she underwent hyperbaric oxygen therapy, which was successful. Her headache, nausea, and disorientation resolved. She was instructed to avoid using the space heater with inadequate ventilation. She has no lasting neurologic deficits secondary to this isolated exposure.

References

1. Shepherd G, Klein-Schartz W. Accidental and suicidal adolescent poisoning deaths in the United States, 1979–1984. *Arch Pediatr Adolesc Med* 1998; 152: 1181–5.

2. Colomb-Lippa D. Acute carbon monoxide exposure: Diagnosis, evaluation, treatment. *J Am Acad Phys Assist* 2005; 18: 41–6.

3. Weaver LK. Carbon monoxide poisoning. *N Engl J Med* 2009; 360: 1217–25.

Case 2

Contributing Author: Rebecca Jeanmonod

History

A 15-year-old boy is brought to the ED complaining of headache. The child was at school, where he is a sophomore, when he began to complain of a severe headache. He was sent to the nurse where he was noted to be diaphoretic and pale. He vomited twice, and was sent by EMS from the school. He is accompanied by a school representative, who states that the nurse was concerned enough about the boy that she did not wait for his parents to transport him. The boy has an action plan in place at the school for an underlying condition of migraine headaches. He has been having intermittent severe headaches for the last 2 years, and his pediatrician has been managing him with NSAIDs and sumatriptan. The child's headaches are episodic and severe, occipital in location, pounding in character, and usually accompanied by vomiting, pallor, and diaphoresis. The child states that he occasionally has palpitations and "sometimes I feel like I can't breathe because I'm vomiting so hard." This headache is similar in character to his typical headaches, but more severe. The child denies trauma. He has not had fevers or chills. He denies abdominal pain or diarrhea. His review of systems is otherwise negative.

Past Medical History

- Immunizations UTD.
- Migraine headaches.
- Occasional marijuana use.

Medications

- Sumatriptan.
- Ibuprofen.

Allergies

- Penicillin.

Physical Examination and Ancillary Studies

- *Vital signs*: T 99.6 °F, HR 125, RR 24, BP 223/128, O_2 sat 100% on room air.
- *General*: He is anxious. He has a receptacle for vomit on his lap. He is pale and diaphoretic and looks dyspneic and uncomfortable.
- *HEENT*: No signs of head trauma. PERRL. Extraocular movements intact. Papilledema present. Slightly dry mucous membranes. Oropharynx clear.
- *Neck*: Supple, with no adenopathy or JVD.
- *Cardiovascular*: Regular tachycardia, with no M/R/G. Patient has delayed capillary refill.
- *Lungs*: Clear bilaterally. Patient is tachypneic.
- *Abdomen*: Soft, non-tender/non-distended, no masses or organomegaly. Normal genitourinary examination.
- *Extremities and skin*: Diaphoretic and generally pale. No deformity.
- *Neurologic*: Normal cranial nerves, strength, sensation, reflexes, and coordination
- *Pertinent imaging*: Head CT normal.

Questions for Thought

- What should be the treatment priorities in this patient?
- Does the child require further diagnostic imaging or blood work?
- What is your differential for this presentation?
- Do you need to wait for his parents to be present to initiate treatment?

Diagnosis

- Hypertensive emergency secondary to pheochromocytoma.

Discussion

- *Epidemiology*: Hypertension in children, defined as a blood pressure higher than the 95th percentile for age, is increasing in incidence in the USA, mostly secondary to increasing obesity.[1,2] The current incidence is estimated to be approaching 4 percent.[2] That said, hypertension in a child should never be considered essential hypertension without a work-up, as most hypertension in children is secondary to underlying disease, typically renal/renovascular or endocrine.[1] Pheochromocytoma is exceedingly rare, with about 0.3 cases in a million in the general populous, and only 10–20 percent presenting in the pediatric age group.[3] These are associated with a specific genetic mutation or familial syndrome (such as von Hippel–Lindau and multiple endocrine neoplasia) in 40–56 percent of pediatric patients.[3,4]
- *Pathophysiology*: Although patients frequently state that they get headaches from having elevated blood pressure, it may well be that in most cases, the pain of the headache precipitated the hypertension, and not the other way around. Generally, in a patient without chronic hypertension, cerebral autoregulation keeps cerebral blood flow constant at mean arterial pressures (calculated as [diastolic BP + 1/3(systolic BP – diastolic BP)]), anywhere from about 60–120. When blood pressure climbs above that level, however, cerebral autoregulation fails, which results in increased cerebral blood flow and cerebral edema. Therefore, in patients with no history of hypertension who complain of severe headache with mean arterial pressures above 120, the provider should consider the diagnosis of malignant hypertension. Malignant hypertension is diagnosed when severe hypertension causes any end-organ damage, and this damage is generally secondary to failure of autoregulatory mechanisms in the affected organ. For the purposes of most patients, these presentations involve hypertensive encephalopathy (cerebral edema, sometimes confusion or focal neurologic deficits, headache), cardiac damage (acute

myocardial infarction or acute congestive heart failure secondary to pressure overload), and renal failure.

Pheochromocytoma causes malignant hypertension through secretion of catecholamines, most commonly norepinephrine. These catecholamines activate both alpha- and beta-adrenergic receptors. Alpha activation leads to vascular constriction in the brain, GI tract, kidney, and skin, which causes cool, pale extremities in the setting of severe hypertension. Beta activation leads to increased heart rate as well as stroke volume, increased renin secretion, and increased glucagon secretion. Therefore, the hypertension caused by a secretory pheochromocytoma is multifactorial; not only secondary to vascular constriction, but also due to increased cardiac output and activation of the renin–angiotensin system. Because of longstanding vasoconstriction in most of these patients, they are commonly very volume depleted in spite of their hypertension.

- *Presentation*: Patients with malignant hypertension present with elevated blood pressure and signs of end-organ damage. Patients with hypertensive encephalopathy may have headache, vomiting, altered mental status, and focal neurologic deficits. Their head CTs may be normal or may show regional or generalized edema or intracranial hemorrhage. Patients with cardiac involvement may have complaints of chest pain, shortness of breath, palpitations, or peripheral edema. Their examinations and ancillary studies may demonstrate rales, jugulovenous distension, hepatomegaly, EKG changes (ischemia or evidence of ventricular hypertrophy or conduction abnormalities), elevated troponin, or elevated BNP. Those with renal involvement may present with edema or laboratory evidence of renal failure.

For malignant hypertension secondary to pheochromocytoma, most patients present with headache (70–90 percent), palpitations (50–70 percent), and diaphoresis (60–90 percent).[5] Because neurotransmitter secretion may be episodic, the hypertension +/– tachycardia that occurs with pheochromocytoma may also be episodic. These patients may present dramatically, with cardiovascular collapse secondary to extremely high vascular tone and profound volume depletion, or may present more subtly, with intermittent non-specific symptoms.

- *Diagnosis*: The diagnosis of hypertensive emergency, although supported through laboratory studies, EKG, and radiographic studies, is generally a clinical one. In emergency medicine, it is easy to overlook a BP that is not low, but it is critically important to recognize the high value that is outside the range of the body's autoregulation, especially in more subtle presentations. The differential in a teenager with malignant hypertension should include renovascular hypertension and endocrine syndromes, but toxins (such as sympathomimetics, some prescribed psychiatric medications) pre-eclampsia/eclampsia, coarctation of the aorta, and underlying lung disease should also be considered.[1]

For a definitive diagnosis of pheochromocytoma, biochemical testing of urine (24-hour urine metanephrines) and blood (fractionated metanephrines) is the initial step. This may be performed as an outpatient in stable, asymptomatic adult patients with good follow-up, but, in general, children with suspected pheochromocytoma or significant hypertension should undergo evaluation as an inpatient.[6] If blood work suggests pheochromocytoma, imaging studies should be performed to locate the tumor. There is debate as to whether CT or MRI is the preferred imaging modality. CT exposes the child to significant radiation, but MRI has inferior spatial resolution for this entity and is more expensive.[7] Tagged radioisotope studies using iodine-131 MIBG (which resembles norepinephrine) have a 77–90 percent sensitivity and 95–100 percent specificity for identification of pheochromocytoma.[7,8]

- *Treatment*: The diagnosis of the specific cause of malignant hypertension can be time- and resource-consuming. That said, this is a dangerous diagnosis that needs aggressive initial management. Initial therapy should follow the ABC algorithm. In patients with pheochromocytoma or with malignant hypertension from toxins or renovascular causes, the blood pressure should be treated initially with an alpha-adrenergic blocker, such as hydralazine or nicardipine. Monotherapy with beta-adrenergic blockade is contraindicated, as this can cause decreased cardiac output with no reduction in the actual vascular tension, and can result in unopposed alpha effect and cardiovascular collapse. If the patient additionally has significant tachycardia, beta-blockade can be undertaken after adequate alpha-blockade has been achieved. If the hypertension is believed to be secondary to congenital heart disease, your best course of action is to consult with cardiology regarding medication choices. In undifferentiated malignant hypertension, initial medical management can be attempted with nicardipine or nitroprusside. It is important to remember that many of these patients are profoundly dehydrated, and all require IV fluid resuscitation, usually with several weight-based boluses of crystalloid.

The long-term treatment of these patients is initially with oral alpha-blockade, most commonly with phenoxybenzamine, which binds the alpha-receptor irreversibly. Oral beta-blockade may be added after adequate alpha-blockade. Most patients undergo resection of their tumors, but resection is not performed until the child is adequately resuscitated and has adequate alpha- and beta-blockade. Typically, the resection is performed in an elective fashion and the child is observed in an ICU setting before and immediately after the procedure. All children with pheochromocytoma should undergo evaluation for inherited endocrine syndromes.

- *Disposition*: Children with malignant hypertension should be admitted to an ICU setting where they have appropriate monitoring. Children with asymptomatic hypertension require close outpatient follow-up to determine causes of secondary hypertension. Hypertension in children always requires an evaluation, and should never be presumed to be primary in etiology.

Historical clues	Physical findings	Ancillary studies
• Episodic headaches	• Marked hypertension	• Negative head CT
• Diaphoresis	• Tachycardia	
• Vomiting	• Diaphoresis	
• Palpitations	• Dyspnea	

Follow-Up

The child's medical record was reviewed, and it was noted that he had incidental hypertension on numerous unrelated visits for sports injuries. He was started on a nicardipine drip for his hypertension and was fluid resuscitated with 2 L normal saline. The provider did not wait for his parents to arrive, as his entire evaluation was considered a "screening examination for medical emergency" as required by law, and in his case, his condition was found to constitute a medical emergency warranting immediate treatment and stabilization. The patient's symptoms improved with BP control. He was admitted to the ICU for further testing. The child's metanephrine levels were high, and he had a negative renovascular evaluation. He underwent CT scanning, which demonstrated a concerning mass in his pelvis. He was discharged home and returned for elective surgery after 3 weeks. The mass was identified as an extra-adrenal malignant pheochromocytoma. The child has since had the mass resected and is undergoing chemotherapy.

References

1. Brady TM, Feld LG. Pediatric approach to hypertension. *Semin Nephrol* 2009; 29: 379–88.

2. Riley M. High blood pressure in children and adolescents. *Am Fam Phys* 2012; 85: 693–700.

3. Waguespack SG, Rich T, Grubbs E, et al. A current review of the etiology, diagnosis, and treatment of pediatric pheochromocytoma and paraganglioma. *J Clin Endocrinol Metab* 2010; 95: 2023–37.

4. Havekes B, Romijn JA, Eisenhofer G, et al. Update on pediatric pheochromocytoma. *Pediatr Nephrol* 2009; 24: 943–50.

5. Adullah I, Cossey K, Jeanmonod R. Extra-adrenal pheochromocytoma in an adolescent. *West J Emerg Med* 2011; 12: 258–61.

6. Eisenhofer G, Goldstein D, Walther M, et al. Biochemical diagnosis of pheochromocytoma: How to distinguish true- from false-positive test results. *J Clin Endocrinol Metab* 2003; 88: 2656–66.

7. Guller U, Turek J, Eubanks S, et al. Detecting pheochromocytoma: Defining the most sensitive test. *Ann Surg* 2006; 243: 102–7.

8. Ilias I, Pacak K. Current approaches and recommended algorithm for diagnostic localization of pheochromocytoma. *J Clin Endocrinol Metab* 2004; 89: 479–91.

Case 3

Contributing Authors: Tom Dittrich, Denis R. Pauzé, and Matthew Adamo

History

The patient is a 16-year-old male who fell from his skateboard approximately 30 minutes prior to arrival. He was riding the skateboard when the board came out from under him and he fell backwards, striking the back of his head on concrete. He was not wearing a helmet. The fall was from a standing height and he briefly lost consciousness. An ambulance was called. He was awake and alert and vomited once during transport. He complained of a severe headache described as pressure, originating from the posterior of the occiput. He reports neck pain. He repeatedly asks for an emesis bag throughout the ride to the hospital. He denies chest pain, shortness of breath, abdominal pain, extremity pain, visual changes, or dizziness.

Past Medical History

- UTD on immunizations.

Medications

- None.

Allergies

- NKDA.

Physical Examination and Ancillary Studies

- *Vital signs*: T 98.6 °F, HR 112, BP 128/74, RR 16, O_2 sat 99% on room air.
- *General*: Healthy-appearing 16-year-old male, somnolent but easily arousable.
- *HEENT*: Round abrasion and hematoma on the posterior occiput, about 4 cm in diameter, no lacerations or active bleeding. No skull depressions or Battle's sign. Face and jaw non-tender. Teeth intact.
- *Neck*: No step-offs, tender at C6, c-collar in place.
- *Cardiovascular*: Regular, with no M/R/G.
- *Lungs*: Clear bilaterally, with no W/R/R, no chest-wall tenderness.
- *Abdomen*: Soft and non-tender, with no distension or signs of trauma.
- *Extremities and skin*: No thoracic or lumbar midline tenderness. Pelvis is stable, all peripheral joints ranged and palpated with full range of

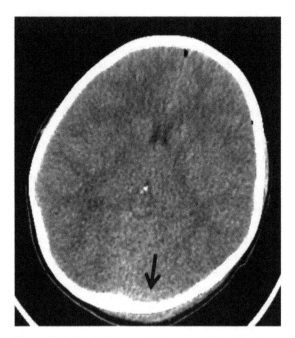

Figure 10.1 Head CT demonstrating an occipital epidural hematoma.

motion and no tenderness on examination. Superficial abrasions over the right posterior thorax.
- *Neurologic*: Child is sleepy but rouses easily. No focal deficits.
- *Pertinent laboratory values*: WBC 17,000, Hb 14, complete metabolic panel normal.
- *Pertinent imaging*: CXR and CT neck normal. Head CT shown in Figures 10.1 and 10.2.

Questions for Thought

- When is a head CT indicated in the pediatric patient?
- What are the diagnostic studies this patient should receive in the ED?
- What are the treatment options for this condition in the ED? What are options for consultants?
- What are important management strategies in patients with traumatic brain injury (TBI)?

Diagnosis

- Occipital epidural hematoma.

Discussion

- *Epidemiology*: Head injuries, including falls with "bump on the head," concussions, and TBIs are

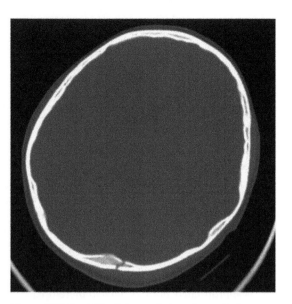

Figure 10.2 Head CT with bone windows demonstrating an occipital skull fracture.

commonly encountered scenarios for the EM clinician. It is estimated that more than 1.5 million TBIs occur annually, with a resultant more than 50,000 yearly deaths.[1,2] From 2001 to 2010, TBI ED visits, hospitalizations, and deaths have increased, with 715 TBI-related visits per 100,000 population in 2010.[1,2] Children age 0–4 have had the greatest frequency of TBI, with a rate more than double that of any other age group.[1,2] This high-risk age group also has the greatest increase in injury rate, with an approximately 50 percent increase in ED visits for TBI between 2001 and 2010.[1,2] Common causes of TBI in children aged 0–14 include motor vehicle crashes, falls, and assault.

TBI encompasses a wide range of brain injury, including edema, bleeding, herniation, and contusions. Epidural hematomas represent a small subset of TBIs. Causative factors will vary by age. Falls and abusive head trauma are more prevalent in the younger patient, while motor vehicle crashes account for the most common cause in the teenage population. Epidural hematomas that are promptly diagnosed and treated often have an excellent outcome.

- *Pathophysiology*: Epidural hematomas typically arise from trauma to the temporal or occipital regions of the head. The skull is fractured, causing damage to an underlying vessel (such as the middle meningeal artery), which subsequently bleeds in the extradural space between the dura and the skull. As blood fills this space the hematoma tends to thrust inwards, displacing the brain. This yields the classic convex appearance of blood visualized on CT imaging. If left untreated, this bulging can lead to the brain herniating through the foramen magnum at the skull base, leading to death. Symptoms are related to the pressure from the bleeding site.
- *Presentation*: The presentation for an epidural hematoma varies considerably by age group. In patients younger than 12 months, the open fontanelles may allow for expansion of bleeding in the skull. This is important to note, as active bleeding may result in a large amount of blood accumulation in the skull, even before signs of clinical deterioration. Initially, these infants may present with non-specific symptoms, such as vomiting, fussiness, irritability, or lethargy.[3] Seizure and unresponsiveness may also be seen. Physical examination should pay particular attention to signs of head trauma, which includes scalp bruising, hematoma, or cephalohematoma. Although a late clinical finding, a large and bulging fontanelle may also be seen. Classic changes of bradycardia and pupillary changes are also delayed findings. The commonly described "lucid interval" for temporal epidural hematoma is often absent in children younger than 12 months.[3] Rather, infants may present with vomiting, irritability, or hemorrhagic shock from blood loss in the brain. It is important to note that, in cases of non-accidental head injury, there may be no history of trauma provided.

Varied presentations exist in older children, and may be related to the size and location of the bleed.[3] History may reveal a loss of consciousness and/or a lucid interval. Headaches with nausea/vomiting are common complaints. Patients with persistent bleeding may be confused or altered. Anisocoria, hemiparesis, or hemiplegia are late clinical findings and indicators of significant bleeding and eventual herniation. Cushing's triad of hypertension, bradycardia, and respiratory depression may be seen in this age group.

- *Diagnosis*: Not all children with head injuries need imaging. Certainly, an obtunded pediatric patient or one with a diminished GCS does not present as a diagnostic dilemma, as imaging is clearly needed. The indications for imaging include considering the mechanism of the injury, the location of the head injury, neurologic examination, and features such as a loss of consciousness, irritability, lethargy, vomiting, or seizures. Clinical decision rules have been developed to help aid the clinician as to when appropriate CT imaging in children with a TBI is indicated. Examples of clinical decision rules for pediatric head injuries include CHALICE, CATCH (Canadian Assessment of Tomography for Childhood Head Injury), and PECARN.[4] The PECARN decision rule is discussed in detail in Chapter 2, Case 2, and Table 2.2.

When the decision is made to use radiographic imaging, the diagnosis of an epidural hematoma is made in the ED with a non-contrast head CT. Classically, a biconvex area of hematoma is seen between the inside of the skull and the brain. Features to note include midline shift, effacement of ventricles, "swirling" within the hematoma suggestive of active bleeding, and evidence of herniation. Cranial U/S is not an appropriate diagnostic study to evaluate for an epidural hematoma, even in very young infants where cranial U/S is used for other purposes. MRI may be used, but has a limited role in many institutions secondary to its lack of availability. LP is contraindicated for the theoretical risk of inducing herniation.

Patients with a suspected epidural hematoma typically also meet criteria for imaging of the c-spine. Patients with multi-trauma, altered mental status, or a complaint of pain and bony tenderness should be strongly considered for c-spine imaging. Further discussion of c-spine imaging may be found in Chapter 2, Case 3.

- Treatment: The goal of treatment in the ED is to prevent secondary brain damage caused by the initial TBI. Secondary brain damage leads to increased intracranial pressure, cerebral edema, and subsequently poor neurologic outcomes.[5-7] Therefore, maintaining and optimizing blood perfusion throughout the brain is a paramount component of therapy for TBI, as hypoxia and hypotension lead to worse outcomes.[5-7] Special attention to oxygenation, blood pressure, carbon

dioxide status, and glucose levels are paramount to optimize treatment in the brain-injured child. For patients with epidural hematomas, goals include making the correct diagnosis, finding additional injuries such as c-spine pathology, timely neurosurgical consultation and care, and, if needed, airway protection. These will each be considered below.

- Airway and oxygenation: Maintaining oxygenation and ventilation during care remains a high priority, as hypoxia worsens secondary brain injury. Patients with a poor GCS (typically less than 9) or with rapidly declining mental status should be intubated for airway protection. Special attention should be placed on maintaining oxygen saturation and preventing desaturation. Making sure the child is appropriately pre-oxygenated therefore remains a crucial component of care. Remember, children are rapid oxygen metabolizers and will desaturate quickly. A nasal cannula before and during intubation is recommended. Etomidate may be used as an induction agent, as it may decrease intracranial pressure and improve cerebral perfusion pressure.[8,9] Intubated patients should be ventilated to maintain a $PaCO_2$ of 35–40 to keep the intracranial pressure relatively low.[5] Once intubated, the bed should be placed with the head elevated to 30 degrees.
- Cerebral perfusion pressure and systolic blood pressure: As previously mentioned, when cerebral blood flow is compromised, harmful secondary brain injury results. Therefore, maintaining blood perfusion through the brain is of paramount importance. Cerebral perfusion pressure is measured by the mean arterial pressure minus the intracranial pressure ($CPP = MAP - ICP$). Thus, optimizing blood pressure is another vital component to maintaining appropriate cerebral perfusion pressure.[8] It is estimated that an episode of hypotension during the first 6 hours after the initial TBI is a predictor of poor neurologic outcome. It is therefore recommended that blood pressure be maintained at least at the 75 percent range for the patient's age. Fluid resuscitation and/or pressors to maintain mean arterial pressures

should be implemented in order to maintain cerebral perfusion.

- *Hyperosmolar solution*: If signs of herniation are present, then treatment with hyperosmolar solution such as 3% saline or mannitol may be indicated. Although debatable, 3% saline may be a more favorable option, especially in the hypotensive patient.[9]
- *Neurosurgical consultation*: All patients with epidural hematomas require consultation with a neurosurgeon as early as possible. Operative management is recommended for patients with a poor GCS or rapidly declining mental status, focal neurologic deficits such as signs of impending herniation, a midline shift on CT, or relatively large hemorrhages. The procedure involves opening the skull and evacuating the hematoma. In the event that a neurosurgeon is not available at the treating hospital, transfer to a trauma center with appropriate capabilities is required.
- *Burr hole*: Very rarely, the EM provider may need to perform a burr hole. Certainly, this is a procedure that the vast majority of EM physicians do not do, have never done, and are not trained to do. A scenario exists where a child comes into the ED, is diagnosed with a large epidural hematoma, and has deteriorating mental status that subsequently requires airway protection and intubation. If the hospital has no neurosurgical availability and transfer is necessary, it is possible that a long transport time is required to get to the nearest trauma center with neurosurgical capabilities. Unfortunately, the child described in this scenario may not survive a prolonged transport time. Active bleeding could cause herniation in a short period of time. This could certainly occur at a rural hospital, many miles away from a trauma center. Bad weather could also prevent evacuation by helicopter and thus force a lengthy ground transport. Faced with this difficult and unusual scenario of a time-sensitive procedure and long transport time, the EM provider should consider a burr hole when herniation or death is likely. Descriptions of this technique are available in the article Emergency burr holes: "How to do it."[10]

- *Disposition*: All patients with an epidural hemorrhage should be admitted to an ICU for close monitoring of their neurologic status. If not available, transfer to a capable trauma center is needed. Neurosurgery consultation is also indicated.

Historical clues	Physical findings	Ancillary studies
• Trauma • Vomiting • Loss of consciousness	• Signs of trauma • Sleepiness	• Head CT with epidural hematoma and skull fracture

Follow-Up

The patient had an isolated occipital epidural hematoma and an otherwise unremarkable trauma work-up. His blood pressure and oxygen saturation were consistently within normal limits. Neurosurgery was consulted. He was made NPO and started on IV fluids. He was deemed to be a candidate for non-operative management and was admitted to the PICU. He maintained a GCS of 15 throughout his hospital course and had an uneventful recovery without requiring surgical evacuation of the hematoma.

References

1. Centers for Disease Control and Prevention. Rates of TBI-related emergency department visits, hospitalizations, and deaths – United States, 2001–2010. See www.cdc.gov/traumaticbraininjury/data/rates.html (accessed January 2017).

2. Centers for Disease Control and Prevention. Annual number of TBIs. See www.cdc.gov/traumaticbraininjury/pdf/tbi_blue_book_annualnumber.pdf (accessed January 2017)

3. Rocchi G, Caroli E, Raco A, et al. Traumatic epidural hematoma in children. *J Child Neurol* 2005; 20: 569–72.

4. Lyttle MD, Crowe L, Oakley E, et al. Comparing CATCH, CHALICE, and PECARN decision rules for paediatric head injuries. *Emerg Med J* 2012; 29: 785–94.

5. Kochenek PM, Carney N, Adelson PD, et al. Guidelines for the acute medical management of severe traumatic brain injury in infants, children, and adolesscents: Second edition. *Pediatr Crit Care Med* 2012; 13 Suppl 1: S1–82.

6. Vavilala MS, Bowen A, Lam AM, et al. Blood pressure and outcomes after severe pediatric traumatic brain injury. *J Trauma* 2003; 55: 1039–44.

7. Chaiwat O, Sharma D, Udomphorn Y, et al. Cerebral hemodynamic predictors of poor 6-month Glasgow Outcome Score in severe pediatric traumatic brain injury. *J Neurotrauma* 2009; 26: 657–63.

8. Allen BB, Chiu YL, Gerber LM, et al. Age specific cerebral perfusion pressure thresholds and survival in children and adolescents with severe traumatic brain injury. *Pediatr Crit Care Med* 2014; 15: 62–70.

9. Shein SL, Ferguson NM, Kochanek PM, et al. Effectiveness of pharmacological therapies for intracranial hypertension in children with severe traumatic brain injury. *Pediatr Crit Care Med* 2016; 17: 236–45.

10. Wilson MH, Wise D, Davies G, et al. Emergency burr holes: "How to do it." *Scand J Trauma Resusc Emerg Med* 2012; 20: 24.

Case 4

Contributing Authors: Anst Gelin and Janet Young

History

The patient is a 4-year-old male, who is presenting to the ED, accompanied by his mother, for headaches. The patient's mother reports that for approximately 1 week the patient has been complaining of intermittent headaches. However, he has been "doing fine" in terms of eating, sleeping, and playing with his older sister (2 years older than the patient). Initially, she was not concerned because the child appeared to be acting normally. After a week, she became concerned for several reasons: in the prior 24 hours, the patient had bumped into the doorway twice as he was coming out of his room, and he once appeared to be drifting to his left side when running during playtime. The mother reports that the patient is usually very agile, and the imbalance is very unusual for him.

Past Medical History

- Full-term vaginal delivery with no complications.
- Vaccinations UTD.

Medications

- None.

Allergies

- NKDA.

Physical Examination and Ancillary Studies

- *Vital signs*: T 98.6 °F, HR 90, BP 98/56, RR 20, O_2 sat 100% on room air.
- *General*: Patient is calm, not distressed, but points to his head as he says "it hurts."
- *HEENT*: Tympanic membranes are clear without erythema. No discharge. No rhinorrhea. No tonsillar erythema or abscess. PERRL. Pain with extraocular movements. Funduscopic examination not performed due to patient's lack of cooperation.
- *Neck*: Supple, without masses or adenopathy.
- *Cardiovascular*: Regular rate and rhythm, with no M/R/G.
- *Lungs*: Normal work of breathing, clear bilaterally. No W/R/R.
- *Abdomen*: Soft. No tenderness or distension. Positive bowel sounds.
- *Extremities and skin*: No bruising, tenderness, or rash.
- *Neurologic*: The patient is alert and oriented. He follows commands without difficulties. Positive dysmetria. Positive Romberg. No focal weakness noted.
- *Pertinent laboratory values*: CBC, comprehensive metabolic profile, toxicologic screens all normal or negative.
- *Pertinent imaging*: CT head with IV contrast shows a posterior fossa mass, which is located in the midline with homogeneous contrast enhancement.

Questions for Thought

- What symptoms are concerning for intracranial mass?
- What are some options for treatment?
- What is the likelihood that this child will be alive and doing well in 10 years?

Diagnosis

- Medulloblastoma.

Discussion

- *Epidemiology*: In pediatric patients, brain tumors make up approximately one-fifth of solid tumors;

of those, medulloblastomas are the most common.[1] They account for approximately 20 percent of all intracranial tumors in children. They are most commonly seen in children between the age of 1 and 10 years, with peak incidence occurring from 3 to 5 years of age.[1,2] Over 250 children are diagnosed with this disease every year. As is true in most cases of brain tumors, the causes are unknown. There may be a rare hereditary association with isochromosome 17q, which is reported to be present in one-third to one-half of the cases, and it is thought that some cases may be secondary to radiation exposure.[2]

- *Pathophysiology*: Medulloblastomas are usually found in the cerebellum, and usually extend to the fourth ventricle. Although pressure can build up in the intracranial space from a mass effect with tumor growth, CSF obstruction at the fourth ventricle is usually the cause of the increased intracranial pressure that leads to papilledema and the clinical findings that are seen. Although rare, a tumor can metastasize to the spinal cord and, less commonly, to the bone marrow. There is more discussion of pathophysiology of brain tumors in general in Chapter 7, Case 6.

- *Presentation*: Like other brain lesions in children, the initial presentation of a medulloblastoma can be vague and non-specific. Considering the push to limit unnecessary radiation in children, the examiner must perform a very thorough history and physical examination to include brain tumors in the differential diagnosis. The most common symptoms include headaches, vomiting, clumsiness, ataxia, loss of fine motor functions, and cognitive decline.[3,4] As in other tumors of the posterior fossa, early-morning or post-nap headaches and vomiting is a classic presentation. Other reported symptoms include back pain, visual disturbance, seizures, somnolence, and urinary and stool incontinence.[3,4] Other non-specific symptoms can be social in nature, such as behavioral changes and sleeping disturbances. Many of the symptoms listed are due to intracranial hypertension.

- *Diagnosis*: The diagnosis of a medulloblastoma relies on historical clues and physical examination findings, which should lead a provider to consider the diagnosis. The history as provided by the parent or other care provider is very important, given the subtle changes that may be noticed by someone who knows the patient well.

On physical examination, ataxia can be noted; abnormal gaze can also be found. Papilledema will be seen in the setting of elevated intracranial pressure, which may be seen in the setting of headaches, ataxia, and other complaints. Utilization of bedside U/S may non-invasively diagnose papilledema, if the patient will tolerate it. Once the possibility of intracranial lesion is considered, CT and MRI are both useful for diagnostic and treatment planning.[5] While MRI is superior to CT, the cost, rapidity, and availability of CT makes it a valuable tool in the initial evaluation of intracranial masses. MRI of the spine may be necessary to evaluate for metastatic disease preoperatively.

- *Treatment*: In the acute presentation, treatment efforts should be focused on symptomatic management and decreasing the intracranial pressure to prevent herniation. Dexamethasone should be given (1 mg/year of age, maximum dose of 10 mg). An actively seizing patient should receive appropriate dosing of benzodiazepines in addition to the consideration of cerebral diuretics (mannitol), antihypertensives (carbonic anhydrase inhibitors, loop diuretics), or hypertonic (3%) saline.

Definitive treatment in the absence of metastasis involves resection followed by radiation and/or chemotherapy. With the current treatments available, the survival rate for the disease is estimated to reach 80 percent in mild cases and approximately 60 percent in patients with metastatic spread. Younger patients do have higher mortality as compared to older children. One important factor affecting survival is the ability for a complete surgical resection of the tumor.

Tumor recurrence is a concern that exists, with one study reporting survival around 65 percent at 30 years of age for a patient diagnosed at age 0–19 years.[6] A large portion of those deaths were due to primary tumor recurrence and other malignancies.[6]

Seizures can be seen in patients who have been treated for brain tumors.[7] However, the incidence of seizures in medulloblastomas is much less when compared to other intracranial tumors such as glioneuronal tumors, high-grade gliomas, and oligodendrogliomas.[7] Long-term antiepileptic medications can be considered in consultation with a neurologist.

- *Disposition*: Patients diagnosed with medulloblastomas or other unknown brain lesions should be admitted for evaluation and multidisciplinary planning with neurosurgery, oncology, and radiation oncology.

Historical clues	Physical findings	Ancillary studies
• Headache • Bumping into wall • Gait instability	• Positive Romberg • Dysmetria	• Head CT with posterior fossa mass

Follow-Up

The child was admitted to the hospital for neurosurgical consultation and malignancy staging. He underwent primary resection and radiation therapy, and is currently in remission.

References

1. Johnson KJ, Cullen J, Barnholtz-Sloan JS, et al. Childhood brain tumor epidemiology: A brain tumor epidemiology consortium review. *Cancer Epidemiol Biomarkers Prev* 2014; 12: 2716–36.

2. Wrensch M, Minn Y, Chew T, et al. Epidemiology of primary brain tumors: Current concepts and review of the literature. *Neuro Oncol* 2002; 4: 278–99.

3. Purdy RA, Kirby S. Headaches and brain tumors. *Neurol Clin* 2004; 22: 39–53.

4. Wilne S, Collier J, Kennedy C, et al. Progression from first symptom to diagnosis in childhood brain tumours. *Eur J Pediatr* 2012; 171: 87–93.

5. Toriori-Donati P, Fondelli MP, Rossi A, et al. Medulloblastoma in children: CT and MRI findings. *Neuroradiology* 1996; 38: 352–9.

6. Ning MS, Perkins SM, Dewees T, et al. Evidence of high mortality in long term survivors of childhood medulloblastoma. *J Neurooncol* 2015; 122: 321–7.

7. Ullrich NJ, Pomeroy SL, Kapur K, et al. Incidence, risk factors, and longitudinal outcome of seizures in long-term survivors of pediatric brain tumors. *Epilepsia* 2015; 56: 1599–604.

Case 5

Contributing Authors: Christine M. George and Melanie K. Prusakowski

History

The patient is a 5-year-old girl who presents with 3 days of headache. It began with a generalized headache, which improved with ibuprofen. The child developed a fever 2 days ago to 101 °F. She still complained of the headache, and was less active and more irritable. Yesterday, she continued with her symptoms and also vomited twice. Her mother has been alternating ibuprofen and acetaminophen every few hours with minimal relief. This morning her headache became worse. She has associated photophobia, intermittent abdominal pain, and multiple episodes of non-bilious emesis. Her mother also notes she has been very tired and "not herself." There is no reported seizure activity. Her mother believes a few children at daycare were recently sick but cannot provide further details. Mom reports no recent travel or known head trauma.

Past Medical History

- Healthy and UTD on immunizations.

Medications

- Ibuprofen last taken 3 hours ago.
- Acetaminophen last taken 7 hours ago.

Allergies

- NKDA.

Physical Examination and Ancillary Studies

- *Vital signs*: T 99.3 °F, HR 97, RR 20, BP 103/55, O_2 sat 99% on room air.
- *General*: Well-developed girl, laying on stretcher in moderate distress. Upsets easily throughout examination and continually complains of headache.
- *HEENT*: Normocephalic and atraumatic. Mucous membranes are dry. Tympanic membranes are clear. No oropharyngeal exudate or erythema. No oral ulcers. Unable to perform funduscopic examination due to poor patient cooperation. PERRL, although child complains of increased head pain when light is shined into her eyes. No

conjunctivae discharge. No scleral erythema or icterus.

- *Neck*: No cervical lymphadenopathy. Range of movement and nuchal rigidity difficult to assess secondary to patient cooperation.
- *Cardiovascular*: Regular rate and rhythm. No murmur. Brisk capillary refill.
- *Lungs*: Effort normal. CTA bilaterally.
- *Abdomen*: Bowel sounds are normal. Soft, non-tender, no mass, no organomegaly.
- *Extremities and skin*: Normal range of motion. No joint swelling, redness, or tenderness. Erythematous, blanchable, papular rash on the chest, without extremity or face involvement.
- *Neurologic*: Very irritable but able to answer questions appropriately after being consoled by mother. Extraocular movements are intact. Facial muscles activate symmetrically. Tongue midline. Palate elevates symmetrically. Spontaneously moves all four extremities equally, without obvious focal weakness. She is able to ambulate with a steady gait.
- *Pertinent laboratory values:*
  - WBC 7,600, with a normal differential;
  - Glucose 92;
  - U/A with 40+ ketones and trace protein, otherwise normal;
  - CSF:
    - Glucose 56 mg/dL;
    - CSF protein: 54 mg/dL;
    - Tube 1: WBC 253, RBC 1,489;
    - Tube 3: WBC 333, RBC 15;
    - WBC differential: neutrophils 68%, lymphocytes 26%, mononuclear cells 6%, and absolute neutrophils 226.4/mm3;
    - Gram's stain: 2+ WBC, no organisms seen.

Questions for Thought

- How does the clinical presentation of this condition vary by patient age?
- What other laboratory tests could help narrow the diagnosis?
- How do the typical laboratory findings in this condition vary by etiology?
- What are some indications for the use of radiographic diagnostic modalities?
- What treatment should be initiated in the ED?

Diagnosis

- Meningitis, most likely enteroviral.

Discussion

- *Epidemiology*: Meningitis is inflammation of the leptomeninges and subarachnoid space, and is most often the result of an infectious agent. In the USA, bacterial meningitis is much more rare than other kinds of meningitis, and has a mortality of about 10 percent.[1-4] In developing nations where routine immunization is less common, bacterial meningitis affects 1 of 250 children in his or her first year of life.[2,3] Since the successful introduction of conjugate vaccines for *Haemophilus influenzae* type b (Hib) and *Streptococcus pneumoniae*, the incidence of bacterial meningitis in the USA has decreased.[2] Peak incidence occurs in infants less than 2 months of age (80.69 cases per 100,000 population in 2006–2007).[1,5] Patient age and host immunity likely have the greatest effect on the etiology of bacterial meningitis.[4] For example, lack of immunization, asplenia, sickle cell disease, HIV infection, otitis media, sinus infection, and cochlear implants are predisposing risk factors for pneumococcal and Hib meningitis. Immunodeficiency and diabetes mellitus are risk factors for *S. pneumoniae* and *Listeria monocytogenes* meningitis. Terminal complement deficiency and living in certain environments (e.g. dormitory or military barracks) are risk factors for *Neisseria meningitidis* meningitis, which has a peak incidence in older adolescence.

  Aseptic meningitis refers to inflammation of the meninges without the presence of visible microorganisms on routine CSF Gram's stain. The causative agent may be viral, fungal, or parasitic. It may also be secondary to atypical bacteria that are not well seen on Gram's staining, such as *Mycobacterium* or *Borrelia*. Viral meningitis is more common than bacterial meningitis and all other causes of aseptic meningitis combined.[1,4] Enteroviruses, such as echovirus, Coxsackie virus B, and enterovirus-71, account for more than 80 percent of all cases of viral meningitis in the USA, with a majority of these occurring in children less than 5 years of age.[1,4] In temperate climates, the incidence of enteroviral meningitis peaks in the summer and early fall.

- *Pathophysiology*: Pathogens enter the CNS via hematogenous spread or as a direct extension from a contiguous site, such as the inner ear or sinuses. Direct communication with the CSF can occur in cases of trauma and in patients with cochlear implants. Ventriculoperitoneal shunts, and/or congenital dural defects, such as dermal sinus or meningomyelocele, are also causative factors. In neonates, pathogen exposure most often occurs after contact with maternal secretions during delivery. The most common bacterial pathogens associated with neonatal meningitis include *Streptococcus agalactiae* (group B streptococcus), *Escherichia coli*, and *Listeria monocytogenes*.[2-4] In infants and children, organisms often spread after first colonizing the upper respiratory tract and then crossing the blood–brain barrier. The presence of infectious organisms results in the release of cytokines, which can cause fever, subarachnoid inflammation, and altered blood flow. These pro-inflammatory mediators ultimately manifest as meningismus and impaired cerebral glucose metabolism. This may lead to vasculitis, seizures, coma, and potentially may progress to death.

- *Presentation*: The clinical presentation of meningitis can vary significantly based on the causative pathogen, patient age, duration of illness, and host response to infection. Infants younger than 1 month of age who have either viral or bacterial meningitis often present with a constellation of non-specific, "sepsis-like" signs, including fever or hypothermia, lethargy, irritability, and poor feeding.[2] Older infants and young children may instead demonstrate signs and symptoms of meningeal inflammation and increased intracranial pressure, including paradoxical irritability (does not wish to be handled and prefers to remain motionless), vomiting, apnea, and seizures.[2,6] Older children and adolescents with meningitis more often experience malaise, headache, photophobia, and neck stiffness.[6] Bulging fontanelle, neck stiffness, or seizure can occur. Some patients may exhibit a petechial or purpuric rash. Cranial nerve palsy (most often III, IV, and/or VI) can be present with bacterial and Lyme meningitis. In general, a child with viral meningitis does not appear as critically ill as a child with bacterial meningitis. Although it is important to recognize these findings, any specific finding suffers from either poor sensitivity or poor specificity or both, and clinician gestalt is still an important predictor for meningitis.[2,6]

- *Diagnosis*: Initial laboratory evaluation should include a CBC with differential, peripheral glucose, and blood culture(s). CSF should evaluate the WBC with differential, RBC, glucose, protein, and Gram's stain. A CSF culture should also be obtained. CRP should not be used as a screening tool for meningitis.

LP with CSF examination is indicated for all patients with suspected meningitis, unless contraindicated due to clinical instability, coagulopathy, or suspicion of a space-occupying intracranial lesion. Head CT should be confirmed prior to LP if the patient is immunocompromised, has a history of CSF shunt placement, hydrocephalus, prior neurosurgery, or if there are concerns for a CNS space-occupying lesion.[2] Patients with papilledema or a focal neurologic deficit (other than cranial nerve VI or VII) on physical examination should also have a radiographic study prior to LP.[2] Initiation of empiric antibiotic therapy should not be delayed if LP must be deferred. Early antibiotics decrease morbidity and mortality, and should not be delayed for any reason whatsoever.

The *Bacterial Meningitis Score* has been utilized for augmenting clinical distinction of bacterial from viral meningitis.[7] Bacterial meningitis is very unlikely in children without:

- Bacteria on Gram's stain;
- CSF protein > 80 mg/dL;
- Peripheral absolute neutrophil count > 10,000 cells/mm^3;
- CSF absolute neutrophil count > 1,000 cells/mm^3;
- Seizures.

If any of these criteria are present, meningitis cannot be ruled out and empiric antibiotics should be continued.[7] These criteria are less reliable in children with recent antibiotic use, which has been shown to increase CSF glucose and protein levels as well as the likelihood of a positive CSF culture.

For children with a CSF pleocytosis, additional testing should be dictated by the clinical scenario. Enteroviral PCR testing can confirm a viral infection and shorten the duration of hospitalization and IV antibiotics.[8,9] HSV PCR testing should be considered in neonates.[10] Lyme meningitis is a consideration in children with CSF pleocytosis who live in Lyme endemic areas, such as the northeast, mid-Atlantic and upper midwest of the USA. However, it can often be difficult to distinguish between Lyme meningitis and other causes of aseptic meningitis in the ED. One validated clinical prediction rule to help identify children at low risk for Lyme meningitis is the "rule of 7s": less than 7 days of headache, less than CSF 70 percent mononuclear cells, and no (including seventh) cranial nerve palsy (sensitivity 96 percent, specificity 41 percent, negative likelihood ratio 0.1).[11,12] Lyme serology and CSF antibodies should be ordered if Lyme meningitis is suspected. There is more information on Lyme disease in this chapter, Case 7, and Chapter 6, Case 5.

- *Treatment*: Treatment of meningitis begins with an assessment of respiratory, circulatory, and neurologic status. Fluid resuscitation may be required in patients with shock. Airway protection may also be needed. Empiric antimicrobial therapy for suspected bacterial meningitis varies based on patient age and specific predisposing conditions. In neonates, empiric therapy consists of ampicillin plus cefotaxime or an aminoglycoside. In older infants and children, empiric treatment is a third-generation cephalosporin (ceftriaxone or cefotaxime) plus vancomycin. Empiric therapy in the setting of penetrating trauma, recent neurosurgery, or a CSF shunt is vancomycin plus cefepime, ceftazidime, or meropenem. If the patient is unimmunized and Hib meningitis is suspected, the administration of dexamethasone prior to antimicrobial therapy is associated with less severe hearing loss, but does not consistently affect mortality or the risk of other serious neurologic sequelae.[13] Dexamethasone is thus indicated in cases of suspected or confirmed Hib meningitis (e.g. the unimmunized child) if the patient is 6 weeks of age or older and the steroid can be administered just before or concurrently with the first dose of antimicrobial therapy.[13] The efficacy of corticosteroid use in children with meningitis caused by organisms other than Hib is controversial.

In general, there is no specific therapy for viral meningitis. Mainstays of treatment include IV fluids, analgesics, and antiemetics. For patients with suspected HSV meningitis, empiric IV acyclovir should be initiated pending CSF HSV PCR results.

- *Disposition*: Infants and young children with meningitis should be admitted to the hospital for definitive diagnosis, treatment, and supportive care. Children should be admitted to a PICU if they have focal neurologic findings, signs of impending neurologic collapse, or signs of shock or respiratory compromise. Older children and teenagers with confirmed viral meningitis will have a self-limited illness and may be appropriate for discharge home.

Historical clues	Physical findings	Ancillary studies
• Headache • Fever • Vomiting • Irritability • Photophobia	• Photophobia • Irritability	• Elevated WBC in CSF • Negative Gram's stain

Follow-Up

The child received IV antibiotics in the ED for bacterial meningitis and was admitted for IV fluids, antibiotics, and observation. The child's PCR came back positive for enterovirus, and the child's antibiotics were stopped. She was discharged home after 3 days and had a full recovery.

References

1. Thigpen MC, Whitney CG, Messonnier NE, et al. Bacterial meningitis in the United States, 1998–2007. *N Engl J Med* 2011; 364: 2016–25.

2. Dorsett M, Liang SY. Diagnosis and treatment of central nervous system infections in the emergency department. *Emerg Med Clin N Am* 2016; 34: 917–42.

3. Tacon CL, Flower O. Diagnosis and management of bacterial meningitis in the pediatric population: A review. *Emerg Med Int* 2012; 2012: 320309.

4. Centers for Disease Control and Prevention. Meningitis. See www.cdc.gov/meningitis/ (accessed January 2017).

5. Nigrovic LE, Kuppermann N, Malley R, et al. Children with bacterial meningitis presenting to the emergency department during the pneumococcal conjugate vaccine era. *Acad Emerg Med* 2008; 15: 522–8.

6. Bilavsky E, Leibovitz E, Elkon-Tamir E, et al. The diagnostic accuracy of "classic meningeal signs" in children with suspected bacterial meningitis. *Eur J Emerg Med* 2012; 20: 361–3.

7. Nigrovic LE, Kuppermann N, Macias CG, et al. Clinical prediction rule for identifying children with cerebrospinal fluid pleocytosis at very low risk of bacterial meningitis. *JAMA* 2007; 297: 52–60.

8. King RL, Lorch SA, Cohen DM, et al. Routine cerebrospinal fluid enterovirus polymerase chain reaction testing reduces hospitalization and antibiotic use for infants 90 days of age or younger. *Pediatrics* 2007; 120: 489–96.

9. Lyons TW, McAdam AJ, Cohn KA, et al. Impact of in-hospital enteroviral polymerase chain reaction testing on the clinical management of children with meningitis. *J Hosp Med* 2012; 7: 517–20.

10. Long SS, Pool TE, Vodzak J, et al. Herpes simplex virus infection in young infants during 2 decades of empiric acyclovir therapy. *Pediatr Infect Dis J* 2011; 30: 556–61.

11. Garro AC, Rutman M, Simonsen K, et al. Prospective validation of a clinical prediction model for Lyme meningitis in children. *Pediatrics* 2009; 123: e829–34.

12. Cohn KA, Thompson AD, Shah SS, et al. Validation of a clinical prediction rule to distinguish Lyme meningitis from aseptic meningitis. *Pediatrics* 2012; 129: e46–53.

13. Brouwer MC, McIntyre P, Prasad K, et al. Corticosteroids for acute bacterial meningitis. *Cochrane Database Syst Rev* 2013; 6: CD004405.

Case 6

Contributing Author: Carl Daniel

History

The patient is a 12-year-old male who presents to the ED with a headache. The headache was preceded by a loss of vision in his left eye's field of vision, which he described as "snow on a TV." This lasted for approximately 15 minutes. As it resolved, a right temporal crescendo headache started. It was accompanied by nausea, photophobia, and phonophobia. He has never had a headache like this before, and given the nausea he went to the school nurse's office. His father brought him to the ED for further evaluation.

He describes that he has been under significantly more pressure at school lately, with several tests and projects in one week, as well as increased track practice. No recent illnesses or sick contacts. No fevers,

chills, rash, neck complaints, cough, or respiratory complaints. Mom has a history of migraine headaches.

Past Medical History

- None. Immunizations are UTD.

Medications

- Multivitamins.

Allergies

- NKDA.

Physical Examination and Ancillary Studies

- *Vital signs*: 98.8 °F, HR 82, RR 18, BP 114/72, O_2 sat 100% on room air.
- *General*: The patient is well-appearing, non-toxic, and in no acute distress.
- *HEENT*: Atraumatic and normocephalic. PERRL. Extraocular movements intact. Sclera unremarkable. Funduscopic examination unremarkable. Moist mucous membranes without oropharyngeal lesions.
- *Neck*: Supple, no cervical lymphadenopathy. No nuchal rigidity. Full range of motion.
- *Cardiovascular*: Regular rate and rhythm, with no M/R/G.
- *Lungs*: Clear bilaterally, with no W/R/R.
- *Abdomen*: Soft, non-tender, non-distended, no flank tenderness present, no rebound or guarding, bowel sounds present. No masses palpated.
- *Extremities and skin*: No rashes, petechiae, or deformity. Normal capillary refill and good pulses.
- *Neurologic*: Awake and alert. Cranial nerves II–XII intact. Speech fluent. Gait normal. 5/5 upper extremity and lower extremity strength. Child is alert and oriented, with intact memory and insight. No suicidal ideation.

Questions for Thought

- What are the dangerous diagnoses you should consider?
- What is the most likely diagnosis?
- Does this child need imaging or laboratory studies?
- What are two treatment strategies for this diagnosis?
- How would management change if he was febrile? If he had right-arm and right-leg weakness?

Diagnosis

- Migraine headache.

Discussion

- *Epidemiology*: Headaches are a common complaint among children, with a prevalence of 70–80 percent in children under the age of 16 years.[1,2] Headaches are classified into primary headache disorders and secondary headache disorders, which are caused by underlying pathology. Of the primary headache disorders (tension, cluster, migraine, and chronic daily headaches), migraine is the most common in children.[1,2] Prior to the age of 12, migraines are more common in males, and after age 12, females tend to have more migraines.[1-3] Migraines can occur in any age range, and there is evidence linking migraine to episodic syndromes such as colic.[4]

- *Pathophysiology*: The exact pathophysiology of migraines is not clearly defined and remains unknown. Although evidence exists for a genetic etiology, or at least a genetic component, the true pathophysiology of migraine headaches is likely multifactorial. Clinicians and researchers have postulated a multitude of potential causes, including a "hyperexcitable" brain, vasodilation of blood vessels, alteration of cerebral blood flow, serotonin release, elevation of specific neuropeptides, stimulation of specific neurons, neurogenic inflammation, and even cardiac shunting.[5,6]

- *Presentation*: Patients with migraine headache may present in a variety of ways. Episodic migraines have different presentations than chronic migraines. Some migraines may have an aura, such as visual changes (scotomas, loss of vision, bright lights), paresthesias, or hallucinations. Other migraine headaches do not have an aura involved. Headache description can also vary, and may be dull, heavy, vice-like, or throbbing. The headache itself can be unilateral or bilateral and can evolve over the course of hours to days. Children may present with a known prior diagnosis of migraine, or with a first attack.

- *Diagnosis*: The diagnosis of migraine headache is made largely by the history and physical examination. Most patients will present with a history of headaches or as someone with a previous diagnosis of migraine. Indeed, to carry a diagnosis of migraine, a child must have a history of at least five prior headaches.[3] Other diagnostic requirements include two of the following: bilateral or unilateral frontal or temporal location, pulsating quality, moderate to severe intensity, or aggravated by routine physical activities.[3] The headache should be accompanied by either nausea/vomiting or photophobia/phonophobia.[3]

If the patient presents with a first-time headache or is having recurrent headaches without a confirmed etiology, a thorough history and physical examination should be performed, looking for any clues or red flags that indicate significant underlying pathology. Establishing the initial diagnosis of "migraine" is not of paramount importance for the EM provider. This can certainly be completed in follow-up by a neurologist. Rather, the EM provider should focus on ruling out dangerous secondary causes of headaches.[7]

The EM provider should evaluate for "red flags" of headache that could harbor significant and even deadly pathology. Some examples of dangerous causes of secondary headaches include brain tumor, subarachnoid hemorrhage, meningitis, encephalitis, carotid artery dissection, carbon monoxide poisoning, and traumatic brain injury. In these patients, a careful and thorough history and physical examination will guide the need for further diagnostic evaluation. Sudden and severe headaches ("thunderclap" or "worst headache of life," associated with cerebrovascular events), headaches that are worse upon waking and associated with vomiting (concerning for increased intracranial pressure and brain tumor), headaches with neurologic deficits (concerning for mass lesions or strokes), headaches with fever (concerning for infectious and autoimmune causes), headaches with visual symptoms (concerning for pseudotumor cerebri or glaucoma), and headaches in the very young child are all concerning for significant underlying pathology. Physical examination should focus on abnormal vital signs, a careful neurologic examination to look for focal deficits, a funduscopic examination, visual fields, careful eye examination, head circumference (in young infants), and an assessment of skin (for toxidromes as well as for rashes suggestive of systemic pathology). In the child with a reassuring history and physical examination, it is not necessary to perform laboratory tests and neuroimaging.

- *Treatment*: Treatment should begin by placing the patient in a quiet and dark room, and removing stimuli. Migraines characteristically are improved by sleep.[3] Medical therapy includes IV fluids, acetaminophen, and NSAIDs.[3,7]

  Triptans, which are serotonin receptor agonists, are a potential treatment option for the acute migraine, with good efficacy.[7] They are available as an injectable or nasal spray, and orally. Rizatriptan is approved for children aged 6 or older. The combination of a triptan and anti-inflammatory is found in sumatriptan–naproxen (Treximet®). This medication remains a viable option and is approved for children of 12–17 years of age.

  Antiemetics are also part of the armamentarium for the treatment of acute migraine. Promethazine is an option, but should be used with extreme caution. There is a "US black box warning" for pediatric respiratory depression and potential fatality. Because it may cause significant respiratory depression, it should not be given to children less than 3 years of age. Promethazine also has a "black box warning" for causing serious tissue injury. Prochlorperazine is another option and may be used for migraine treatment in children greater than 7 years of age. Metoclopramide may also be used but, as also with the above mentioned phenothiazines, dystonic reactions may occur. When metoclopramide is used, slow infusion over 15 minutes will usually reduce the incidence of akathisia. Prophylaxis with diphenhydramine is not needed if slow infusion takes place. Diphenhydramine has not been shown to decrease migraine severity. Other pharmacologic options include ergotamine drugs, such as dihydroergotamine and IV valproate. Opioids generally should not be utilized.

- *Disposition*: Children whose symptoms can be controlled can be discharged home with follow-up with neurology. Children and parents should be counseled regarding headache triggers, and should be encouraged to keep a headache diary. Lack of sleep, stress, loud noises, bright lights, and dehydration may all be triggers. Dietary factors may also contribute, such as alcohol, caffeine, chocolate, cheese, and shellfish.

  Prophylaxis of migraine headaches in children initially involves regular sleep and meal patterns, avoidance of triggers, and regular exercise. If these do not cause significant improvement, pharmacotherapy can be introduced. This is best done by a neurologist who specializes in migraine care.

Historical clues	Physical findings
<ul><li>Headache</li><li>Classic scotoma</li><li>Family history</li><li>Crescendo headache</li><li>Nausea</li><li>Phonophobia</li></ul>	<ul><li>Normal neurologic examination</li><li>Normal eye examination</li><li>Normal neck examination</li><li>Normal vital signs</li></ul>

Follow-Up

The child was placed in a dark, quiet room. An IV line was inserted, and he was given IV fluids, ketorolac, and metoclopramide. Imaging was not performed. Over the next few hours, his pain completely abated. A diagnosis of probable migraine was given. He was asked to follow up with his pediatrician and the local pediatric neurologist.

References

1. Parisi P, Vanacore N, Belcastro V, et al. Clinical guidelines in pediatric headache: Evolution of quality using the AGREE II instrument. *J Headache Pain* 2014; 15: 57.

2. Abu-Arefeh I, Russell G. Prevalence of headache and migraine in schoolchildren. *BMJ* 1994; 309: 765–9.

3. Lewis DW. Headaches in children and adolescents. *Am Fam Phys* 2002; 65: 625–33.

4. van Hemert S, Breedveld AC, Rovers JM, et al. Migraine associated with gastrointestinal disorders: Review of the literature. *Front Neurol* 2014; 5: 241.

5. Malhotra R. Understanding migraine: potential role for neurogenic inflammation. *Ann Indian Acad Neurol* 2016; 19: 175–82.

6. Burstein R, Noseda R, Borsook D. Migraine: Multiple processes, complex pathophysiology. *J Neurosci* 2015; 35: 6619–29.

7. Damen L, Bruijn JK, Verhagen AP, et al. Symptomatic treatment of migraine in children: A systematic review of medication trials. *Pediatrics* 2005; 118: e295–302.

Case 7

Contributing Authors: Michael Leonard and Rebecca Jeanmonod

History

The patient is a 12-year-old female who comes to the ED with a headache for the last 6 days. The child states that she believed she had "slept wrong" while traveling with her parents on a hiking vacation in the southwest USA (the child lives in Pennsylvania), first noticing the pain upon awaking in a hotel room. The pain began behind her left ear and is constant and aching, made worse by moving her head, and associated with nausea. The patient subsequently developed low-grade fevers, and her parents noticed that she had some swollen lymph nodes in her neck. They started her on ibuprofen every 6 hours for her symptoms, which seemed to help. The child had a single episode of vomiting on day 2 of her illness, and has had a poor appetite throughout. She had never complained of headache before. There has been no trauma. The child was out of school for spring break and traveling with her parents and three siblings, two of whom developed fever, vomiting, and diarrhea during the trip. The parents did not bring the child in earlier because they believed she had the same viral infection as her siblings and that it would get better on its own. Yesterday, prior to flying home, the child awoke and stated "I think my face is starting to get paralyzed." Her parents noted at that time that she seemed to have some left-sided facial weakness. Today, the child complains of inability to drink from a glass, a watery and painful eye, and ongoing head and neck pain.

Past Medical History

- The child has a history of vasovagal syncope. She is fully immunized and developmentally normal.

Medications

- Ibuprofen every 6 hours.

Allergies

- Dogs.

Physical Examination and Ancillary Studies

- *Vital signs*: T 98.9 °F, HR 75, RR 18, O_2 sat 100% on room air.

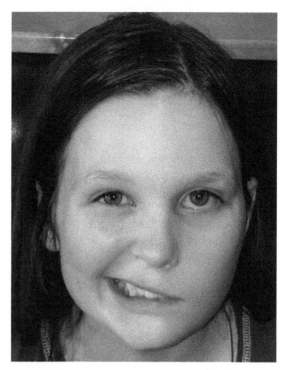

Figure 10.3 Photograph of child's face, demonstrating profound left-sided facial palsy.

- *General*: The patient appears well, without signs of distress.
- *HEENT*: Normal ear examination, without evidence of erythema or bulging of the tympanic membrane, normal funduscopic examination, PERRL, extraocular movements intact.
- *Neck*: Supple, with several tender prominent lymph nodes in the cervical chain.
- *Cardiovascular*: Regular rate, with no M/R/G. Child has brisk capillary refill.
- *Lungs*: Clear bilaterally, with good air movement.
- *Abdomen*: Soft and non-tender, with no masses, rebound, or guarding.
- *Extremities and skin*: No signs of trauma. Beneath the child's hair, there is a faint 6-cm blanching macule surrounding the left ear, with no central clearing.
- *Neurologic*: The child is alert with age-appropriate interactions. She has a complete left facial palsy that includes the forehead (Figure 10.3). She has decreased taste on the left. On hearing testing, she complains of "double hearing" in her left ear. Her neurologic examination is otherwise completely normal.

Diagnosis

- Lyme disease, early disseminated, with facial nerve palsy.

Discussion

- *Epidemiology*: It is estimated approximately 329,000 cases of Lyme disease are diagnosed each year in the USA.[1] Because there are differences in the methods of diagnosis – clinical observation versus laboratory diagnostics – the reporting rate is highly variable. Although the disease is concentrated in a select number of northeastern and upper midwestern states (see Table 10.1), it accounts for the fifth most commonly nationally reported disease.[2]

  The number of cases of Lyme disease diagnosed in the USA appears to have plateaued between 2010 and 2014 but the number of counties with reported cases continues to increase, representing an expanding area – though continuing to be geographically localized.[2] According to the CDC, pediatric males between 5 and 9 years old account for the largest number of reported cases between 2001 and 2010, but all age groups and both genders are susceptible.[3] Lyme disease occurs far more frequently in the summer (June–August) with an increase in outdoor activities, and has a reduced incidence in the winter (December–March).[3]

- *Pathophysiology*: Lyme disease is a common tick-borne illness transmitted primarily by the spirochete *Borrelia burgdorferi* in North America – although a second species, *Borrelia mayonii*, has recently been identified as being

associated with Lyme disease in a cluster in the Minnesota and Wisconsin area. The spirochete uses the blacklegged tick (*Ixodes scapularis*) in the northeastern and upper midwestern USA and the western blacklegged tick (*Ixodes pacificus*) as vectors. There are a number of ticks in the USA that are not vectors for Lyme disease, although identification of ticks can be challenging when they are engorged. Lyme disease is not considered to be transmittable between persons or from pets, although persons or pets may act as a vector for infected ticks.

- *Presentation*: Lyme disease presents variably based upon the stage of the illness:
  - Early localized disease;
  - Early disseminated disease;
  - Late disease.

  Although the characteristic rash of Lyme disease, erythema migrans, is the most common finding – and the only finding that allows clinical diagnosis – fatigue and headache are the next most common findings in the early stages of disease, with the benchmark study of 201 children in Connecticut indicating that 42 percent of patients with *early localized disease* and 70 percent of patients with early disseminated disease have these complaints.[4] Even in children diagnosed early, most did not have a known tick bite within the past month, making diagnosis more elusive.

  If Lyme disease is not diagnosed in the early localized stage, the pathogen enters the bloodstream and spreads throughout the body including the CNS. Consequently, *early disseminated disease* commonly presents with multiple lesions of the characteristic rash and generalized non-specific systemic symptoms including headache, fatigue, arthralgia, and fever. Although the rash is common, it is not universal, and, as stated above, many patients have no known history of tick bite, making diagnosis elusive in those without rash. During this stage, a child may also develop some of the more characteristic findings of Lyme disease, including facial palsy (9 percent), aseptic meningitis (1 percent), and carditis (1 percent).[3] Children may also develop Lyme arthritis, which is dealt with further in Chapter 6, Case 5.

  Facial palsy in a child is not pathognomonic for Lyme disease, but a study of 313 children

Table 10.1 States accounting for 96 percent of the reported cases of Lyme disease in the USA[3]

Connecticut	Pennsylvania	New Jersey	Maine
Maryland	Delaware	Rhode Island	Minnesota
New Hampshire	Massachusetts	Wisconsin	New York
Virginia	Vermont		

presenting to the ED with facial palsy in an endemic area found Lyme as the source in 34 percent of cases.[5] This study identified the onset of symptoms between June through October, presence of fever and headache, and absence of herpetic lesions as clinical predictors of Lyme disease.[5] Other sources of facial weakness to consider include infections with herpes viruses, Guillain–Barré syndrome (particularly when associated with Zika virus), other tick-borne encephalitides, mycoplasma, HIV, intracranial mass lesions, parotid and acoustic tumors, leukemia, trauma, botulism (most commonly in infants), and myasthenia gravis. Although limited to case reports, Lyme disease has been reported to be among the rare contributors to bilateral facial droop.[6]

Lyme meningitis presents as an aseptic meningitis. In patients with aseptic meningitis of unclear etiology, recognition and treatment when secondary to Lyme disease improves outcomes.[7] For children with aseptic meningitis without clinical signs of Lyme disease, who live in endemic areas, rapid identification is challenging as serologic testing may require additional time for completion. A "rule of 7s" was developed as a clinical prediction rule for children to identify low risk for Lyme meningitis to limit treatment, which includes: less than 7 days of headache, less than 70 percent CSF mononuclear cells, and absence of seventh nerve or other cranial palsy.[8] Those meeting all criteria had a less than 2 percent chance of Lyme meningitis.[8] Certainly, the finding of erythema migrans is pathognomonic for Lyme disease, and points to the correct diagnosis when present in a child with clinical meningitis.

Carditis, which most commonly occurs in *late disease*, usually presents as complete heart block. It is a rare presentation for Lyme in children.[4] Partial heart block may be more common but is likely unrecognized due to the lack of clinical manifestation. Most cases of Lyme carditis are self-limited and rarely require a temporary pacemaker.[9]

It is important for the clinician to remember that the vectors that spread the spirochete involved in Lyme disease are host to a number of other transmittable diseases, including anaplasmosis, babesiosis, deer tick virus, Ehrlichiosis, and *Borrelia miyamotoi*.

Co-infections should be considered in patients with unexplained symptoms or those with persistent symptoms after treatment.

- *Diagnosis*: The diagnosis of early Lyme disease may be made clinically when erythema migrans is identified. At this stage in the disease, laboratory testing is typically falsely negative. Once the patient progresses to early disseminated Lyme disease, serologic testing is useful for diagnosis. Laboratory testing of Lyme disease is completed as a two-step method.[3] The initial test is an enzyme immunoassay or immunofluorescence assay, which is highly sensitive in appropriately selected patients (those demonstrating signs of disseminated disease), but is not very specific. If this testing is equivocal or positive, a second set of testing for IgM and IgG is completed as a Western blot, to improve diagnostic accuracy.[3] If symptoms have been persistent for more than 30 days, only the IgG component is necessary. If these tests are negative and symptoms have been present for greater than 2 weeks, alternative diagnoses should be considered as it is unlikely the patient has Lyme disease. Individuals who have previously been diagnosed with Lyme disease have unpredictable antibody titers that variably decline over time.[10] As such, repeat testing for individuals previously diagnosed is generally not necessary and clinical diagnosis is recommended.

For patients with concerns for Lyme meningitis, LP may be useful to guide early treatment. The decision to perform an LP can be complicated. The Infectious Disease Society of America (IDSA) recommends LP in patients with symptoms consistent with strong clinical suspicion of CNS involvement, such as severe headache or nuchal rigidity.[11] In cases of diagnostic uncertainty, as previously discussed, the proportion of mononuclear leukocytes in the CSF can assist in distinguishing viral meningitis versus Lyme meningitis to guide early treatment.[8] Serologic testing of CSF is challenging due to limitations in laboratory quality control to reliably handle PCR testing and is not universally recommended unless appropriate facilities can be identified.[11] That said, in the setting of known Lyme disease, diagnosis of Lyme meningitis may not alter the course of treatment and may therefore not add any additional benefit to patient care.

- *Treatment*: The IDSA recommends that treatment of Lyme disease in children is based upon the clinical stage. For early Lyme disease, treatment is amoxicillin or cefuroxime (for children less than 8 years old) or doxycycline (for children greater than 8 years old without a known allergy). For those with isolated facial nerve palsy and without abnormal LP results, the IDSA guidelines recommend treatment as in early Lyme disease for 14–21 days.[11] The cranial nerve palsy usually resolves within a few weeks regardless of antibiotic treatment but therapy prevents later complications and should be initiated in all cases.[11] These children require close follow-up with outpatient providers, who can carefully monitor response to therapy.

  For children with neurologic manifestations of meningitis or any abnormal CSF results, treatment with parenteral antibiotics is currently the standard of care in the USA (ceftriaxone, cefotaxime, or penicillin G). Patients exhibiting papilledema may require treatment with additional measures. Expert consultation is warranted to ensure optimal treatment based on the most recent evidence, considering the rarity of the condition. All children requiring treatment with parenteral antibiotics likely warrant admission and monitoring. There is evidence that oral doxycycline may be as effective as parenteral antibiotics for the treatment of Lyme meningitis, as doxycycline has excellent CSF penetration, but this evidence is from Europe where different *Borrelia* species are prevalent.[12] Nevertheless, this represents a reasonable alternative when parenteral therapy is not an option or is refused.

- *Disposition*: Lyme is generally treated as an outpatient except in cases of meningitis or carditis.

Historical clues	Physical findings
• Lives in endemic area • Outdoor activities • Fever • Headache	• Erythema migrans • Facial nerve palsy (including chorda tympani, with taste deficits and hyperacusis)

Follow-Up

The child was diagnosed with early disseminated Lyme disease based on her classic presentation. Her parents declined LP. She was treated with doxycycline for 3 weeks. The child had resolution of her rash and headache within 24 hours of starting therapy, but her

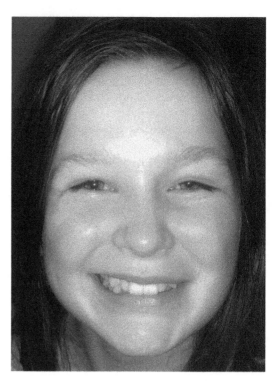

Figure 10.4 Photograph of child's face 6 months after treatment, demonstrating marked improvement in facial weakness.

facial palsy has not completely resolved at 6 months, although it is greatly improved (Figure 10.4).

References

1. Nelson CA, Saha S, Kugeler KJ, et al. Incidence of clinician-diagnosed Lyme disease, United States, 2005–2010. *Emerg Infect Dis* 2015; 21: 1625–31.

2. Adams DA, Thomas KR, Jajosky RA, et al. Summary of notifiable infectious diseases and conditions: United States, 2014. *MMWR Morb Mortal Wkly Rep* 2016; 63: 1–152.

3. Centers for Disease Control and Prevention. Lyme disease. See www.cdc.gov/lyme/index.html (accessed Novemeber 2016).

4. Gerber MA, Shapiro ED, Burke GS, et al. Lyme disease in children in southeastern Connecticut. Pediatric Lyme Disease Study Group. *N Engl J Med* 1996; 335: 1270–4.

5. Nigrovic LE, Thompson AD, Fine AM, et al. Clinical predictors of Lyme disease among children with a peripheral facial palsy at an emergency department in a Lyme disease-endemic area. *Pediatrics* 2008; 122: e1080–5.

6. Mlodzikowska-Albrecht J, Zarowski M, Steinborn B, et al. Bilateral facial nerve palsy in the course of neuroborreliosis in children: Dynamics, laboratory

tests and treatments. *Rocz Akad Med Bialymst* 2005; 50 Suppl 1: 64–9.

7. Halperin JJ. Diagnosis and treatment of the neuromuscular manifestations of Lyme disease. *Curr Treat Options Neurol* 2007; 9: 93–100.

8. Cohn KA, Thompson AD, Shah SS, et al. Validation of a clinical prediction rule to distinguish Lyme meningitis from aseptic meningitis. *Pediatrics* 2012; 129: e46–53.

9. Costello JM, Alexander ME, Greco KM, et al. Lyme carditis in children: Presentation, predictive factors, and clinical course. *Pediatrics* 2009; 123: e835–41.

10. Feder HM Jr, Gerber MA, Luger SW, et al. Persistence of serum antibodies to *Borrelia burgdorferi* in patients treated for Lyme disease. *Clin Infect Dis* 1992; 15: 788–93.

11. Wormser GP. Clinical practice. Early Lyme disease. *N Engl J Med* 2006; 354: 2794–801.

12. Mygland A, Ljøstad U, Fingerle V, et al. EFNS guidelines on the diagnosis and management of European Lyme neuroborreliosis. *Eur J Neurol* 2010; 17: 8–16.

Case 8

Contributing Author: Jason Schwaber

History

The patient is a 3-year-old boy who is sent from a retail-based walk in clinic with his head held in a "funny position." His parents state that he had been well until 3 days ago when he began "clearing his throat," which his parents thought was due to a sore throat. They note that today he is holding his neck tilted to the left and refuses to bend his neck to look upwards. He had a cold 7 days ago, but today he developed a fever. He has been eating less, complaining that swallowing is painful, and has a voice that "sounds funny." The family denies emesis, rash, or swelling of the hands or feet. The urgent care had given him a dose of acetaminophen, performed a rapid strep test (negative), and referred him to the ED.

He was born vaginally at 38 weeks. He is developmentally normal. He lives at home with his parents and an 8-year-old brother. He attends nursery school 3 days a week. His immunizations are UTD for age. The family has a pet turtle and two cats.

Past Medical History

- Otitis media.
- Seasonal allergies.

Medications

- Loratadine as needed.

Allergies

- Amoxicillin causes a rash.

Physical Examination and Ancillary Studies

- *Vital signs*: T 102.9 °F, HR 158, BP 95/70, RR 30, O_2 sat 97% on room air.
- *General*: Well-developed, well-nourished boy, sitting in his mother's lap with noticeable head tilt. Mildly uncomfortable. No drooling. Mild inspiratory stridor is heard.
- *HEENT*: The head is angled to the left with rotation of the chin to right. There is marked limitation of neck extension and mild limitation of neck flexion. He uses his eyes to look upwards, limiting his neck motion. The head is normocephalic, without plagiocephaly. PERRL, extraocular movements intact. The oropharynx is erythematous. The right tympanic membrane is bulging and injected, with white pus behind it.
- *Neck*: There are several 0.5–1.0-cm tender mobile lymph nodes in the left anterior cervical chain. There is no tenderness over the sternocleidomastoid muscles.
- *Cardiovascular*: Tachycardic, but regular, with capillary refill < 2 seconds.
- *Lungs*: CTA bilaterally, without W/R/R.
- *Abdomen*: Soft, non-tender and non-distended. Normoactive bowel sounds.
- *Extremities and skin*: Warm and well-perfused, without rash, or edema.
- *Neurologic*: Motor, sensory, gait, and cranial nerves are intact and symmetric.
- *Pertinent laboratory values*: WBC 22,000 with 91% neutrophils.

Questions for Thought

- What is the differential diagnosis of pediatric torticollis?
- What is the role of advanced imaging in the management of this patient? What factors need to be considered?
- What is the role of antibiotics versus surgery in this patient?

Diagnosis

- Retropharyngeal abscess with inflammatory torticollis. There is further discussion of this disease entity in Chapter 5, Case 9.

Discussion

- *Epidemiology*: Retropharyngeal abscess is a relatively uncommon head and neck infection occurring primarily in children less than 5 years old.[1] The incidence is estimated at 4 per 100,000, with most cases presenting in the winter or spring.[1] It exists as a spectrum of illness, ranging from pharyngitis and deep neck cellulitis to life-threatening airway obstruction, with septic complications throughout the neck, mediastinum, and chest.

- *Pathophysiology*: In young children, infections of the nasopharynx, eustachian tubes, and adenoids are common. Lymph nodes draining these areas pass through the retropharyngeal space, and can suppurate, causing a cellulitis, phlegmon, or localized abscess. The swelling and mass effect can cause obstruction of the airway. An abscess can rupture into the airway, causing aspiration pneumonia. The infection can spread, causing mediastinitis, jugular vein thrombophlebitis, and sepsis. Retropharyngeal infections are typically polymicrobial and include group A streptococci, anaerobes, and *Staphylococcus aureus*.[2] MRSA may also be an etiology.

- *Presentation*: Early presentation of retropharyngeal abscess may be non-specific, often resembling a pharyngitis, with fever and decreased oral intake. Children may also have an antecedent URI. Torticollis, neck stiffness, and refusal to move the neck should heighten the index of suspicion.[3] As upper-airway obstruction progresses, muffled voice and stridor may develop. Most older children have a prior penetrating trauma to their pharynx. Other infections such as peritonsillar abscess, bacterial tracheitis, or epiglottitis should be considered. Advanced croup, anaphylaxis, and foreign bodies are additional causes of airway obstruction. There have been a few case reports describing rare entities such as Kawasaki disease and cervical tuberculosis, mimicking retropharyngeal abscess.

- *Diagnosis*: As these infections usually take place in small children who may not be verbal, diagnosis can be challenging. Neck pain or stiffness should prompt the clinician to consider referred pain (from head injury or shoulder injury), meningeal irritation (from subarachnoid hemorrhage or meningitis), oropharyngeal infection (tonsillitis, epiglottitis, tracheitis, uvulitis), deep neck-space infections (peritonsillar, parapharyngeal, and retropharyngeal abscesses), ENT infection (mastoiditis), malignancy, dissection, and musculoskeletal pain (post-traumatic torticollis). Therefore, it is important to do a complete head, neck, eye, neurologic, and musculoskeletal examination. If the child has abnormal vital signs or any other findings on examination, the clinician should not assume the neck pain is musculoskeletal. Although many of these items can be assessed with history and examination alone, children with concerning findings warrant further testing and imaging.

  The diagnosis of retropharyngeal abscess is confirmed with imaging. Lateral neck X-rays may show a widening of the soft tissues anterior to the vertebrae (see Figure 5.5). These films should be taken during inspiration, if possible. Typically, the width of the retropharyngeal space is less than that of the adjacent vertebral body at C2 or C3. A CT scan with IV contrast has better sensitivity to detect retropharyngeal abscess and is the preferred study to clearly delineate the extent of the infection within the neck or beyond (see Figure 5.6).[3] However, some abscesses well identified on CT scan do not always yield purulent material at the time of surgery. The risk of airway impingement should be considered prior to sending a child with stridor or drooling to CT, as the imaging results may not significantly change the immediate management.

- *Treatment*: Treatment options are based upon the size and location of the abscess. All patients with suspected retropharyngeal abscess should receive antibiotics to cover typical oropharyngeal pathogens. Ampicillin–sulbactam or clindamycin are good options.[2] Coverage against MRSA with vancomycin should also be considered. For patients with airway compromise, immediate involvement with ENT is needed as airway protection and surgical drainage may be required.

Children with a phlegmon or small retropharyngeal abscess on imaging may be treated with IV antibiotics while being closely observed for progression or resolution of their symptoms.

- *Disposition*: All children with suspected retropharyngeal abscess should be admitted to the hospital. ENT should be involved as surgical drainage is required in about half of these cases. Patients with concerns for airway compromise require monitoring in an ICU.

Historical clues	Physical findings	Ancillary studies
• Recent URI • Difficulty eating • Voice change • Fever • Negative strep swab	• Fever • Tachycardia • Torticollis • Otitis media	• Elevated WBC with left shift

Follow-Up

The patient had a CT scan of the neck with IV contrast, which revealed a 2-cm retropharyngeal phlegmon, without extension into the lateral pharyngeal space or posterior mediastinum. The patient was treated with IV fluids, pain control, and clindamycin. He was admitted to a monitored bed. ENT evaluated him and recommended outpatient adenoidectomy with tympanostomy tube placement. After 48 hours of IV antibiotics his neck stiffness and odynophagia had improved, and he was transitioned to oral clindamycin to complete a 14-day course at home. At outpatient follow-up his torticollis had resolved.

References

1. Woods CR, Cash AM, Smith MJ, et al, Retropharyngeal and parapharyngeal abscesses among children and adolescents in the United States: Epidemiology and management trends, 2003–2012. *J Pediatr Infect Dis Soc* 2016; 5: 259–68.

2. Hoffman C, Pierrot S, Contencin P, et al. Retropharyngeal infections in children. Treatment strategies and outcomes. *Int J Pediatr Otorhinolaryngol* 2011; 75: 1099–103.

3. Craig F, Schunk J, Retropharyngeal abscess in children: Clinical presentation, utility of imaging, and current management. *Pediatrics* 2003; 111: 1394–8.

Case 9

Contributing Authors: Jamaine Ortiz Jr., Rebecca Jeanmonod, Carl Daniel, Denis R. Pauzé, and Matthew Adamo

History

A lethargic 7-year-old female is brought into the ED by a local EMS crew. She is accompanied by both of her parents. The parents state that the child was having a push-up contest with her older brother approximately 30 minutes ago when suddenly, she started to scream and complain of having a severe headache. The patient put her hands up to her head and cried out to her parents "My head! It hurts!" The child has no prior history of having migraines. The patient's mother attempted to help relieve the pain by giving her a dose of acetaminophen and having her rest in bed. However, soon after the mother gave the medication, the child began to vomit. The mother states she was washing the vomit off the patient's face when the child started to "talk extremely weird and slur her words like she was drunk." At that point, the parents called 911. While en route to the hospital, the child had one other episode of vomiting. She remained rousable to stimuli, and complains of head pain when prompted. She has been quite lethargic. Parents deny that the child experienced any trauma, fevers, chills, vomiting, diarrhea, or abdominal pain prior to this.

Past Medical History

- Attention deficit–hyperactivity disorder.
- Asthma.
- UTD on immunizations.

Medications

- Adderall extended release.
- Albuterol rescue inhaler.

Allergies

- NKDA.

Physical Examination and Ancillary Studies

- *Vital signs*: T 97.8 °F, HR 100, RR 20, BP 147/88, O₂ sat 98% on room air.
- *General*: Pale and diaphoretic. Vomit is present on chest and arms. Drowsy but rousable.

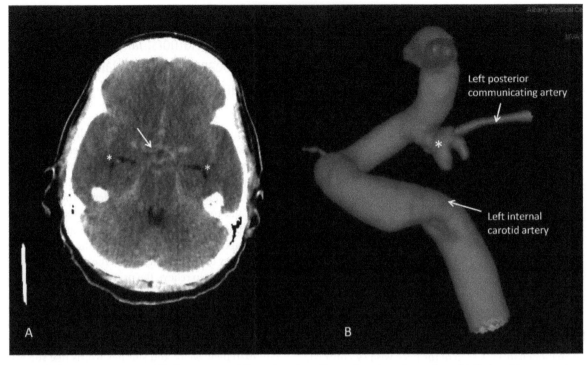

Figure 10.5 (A) Non-contrast axial CT, demonstrating diffuse subarachnoid hemorrhage (arrow) as well as mild dilation of the temporal horns of the lateral ventricles (asterisks). (B) Three-dimensional angiography image of the left posterior carotid wall aneurysm (asterisk) associated with the left posterior communicating artery. For the color version, please refer to the plate section.

- *HEENT*: No external signs of head trauma. Tympanic membranes normal. Pupils sluggish but reactive.
- *Neck*: Supple, with no adenopathy, midline trachea.
- *Cardiovascular*: Normal rhythm, with no M/R/G. Brisk capillary refill.
- *Lungs*: Clear and equal bilaterally, with no W/R/R.
- *Abdomen*: No distension or masses. Normal bowel sounds.
- *Extremities and skin*: No signs of trauma. No rashes.
- *Neurologic*: Responsive to pain, opens eyes to voice, unreliable following commands.
- *Pertinent laboratory values*: CBC and electrolytes normal.
- *Pertinent imaging*: CT head shown in Figure 10.5.

Questions for Thought

- Would any additional laboratory tests or diagnostic imaging be of use in this patient, and why?

- What are your treatment priorities in this patient?
- What are the potential underlying causes of this diagnosis in a pediatric patient?

Diagnosis

- Subarachnoid hemorrhage.

Discussion

- *Epidemiology*: Subarachnoid hemorrhage, or bleeding into the subarachnoid space, is rare in children.[1,2] The incidence of subarachnoid hemorrhage in the general population is about 6 cases per 100,000 patient-years, but only 1–2 percent of those occur in pediatric patients.[1,3] The most common cause of pediatric subarachnoid hemorrhage is trauma (with non-accidental trauma being more common than accidental trauma), followed by aneurysmal bleeding, arteriovenous malformation bleeding, and mass.[1,2,4,5] Aneurysms in children are less common than arteriovenous malformations, but arteriovenous malformations are less likely to present as isolated subarachnoid hemorrhage.[1,4] Comorbid disease, such as sickle cell anemia, coarctation of the aorta, or connective tissue disorder, is common in patients with aneurysmal disease, and family history is a risk factor for this.[2]

- *Pathophysiology*: Subarachnoid hemorrhage occurs when blood vessels become disrupted and leak blood into the subarachnoid space. Disruption can be due to trauma, or may be due to blood vessel invasion from a tumor, increased wall stress as occurs with aneurysm, increase intravascular pressure as occurs with coarctation of the aorta, abnormal anatomy as with arteriovenous malformations, or abnormal vessel integrity as with connective tissue disorders. Regardless of the cause, blood in the subarachnoid space can cause mass effect, hydrocephalus, focal deficits, meningeal irritation, herniation, and death. In cases of subarachnoid hemorrhage from non-accidental trauma, the child may have multiple injuries.

- *Presentation*: Children with subarachnoid hemorrhage can present in a variety of ways. In non-verbal children, lethargy, seizures, poor tone, altered level of consciousness, vomiting, apnea, feeding difficulties, and breathing difficulties may be the predominant features.[1] Older, verbal children may present with altered mental status, vomiting, seizure, focal deficits, or complaint of severe headache.[1,2] It should be noted that the severity of clinical presentation is the strongest prognostic indicator in aneurysmal subarachnoid hemorrhage. The initial clinical severity can be reliably categorized by use of simple validated scales, such as that from Hunt and Hess, although it is important to note that this scale has been criticized for its inter-observer variability. Higher grades, which are reflective of progressively higher hemorrhage severity and neurologic dysfunction, are associated with higher overall mortality. The Hunt and Hess scale is as follows: grade 1 – asymptomatic or mild headache; grade 2 – cranial nerve palsy or moderate to severe headache/nuchal rigidity; grade 3 – mild focal deficit, lethargy, or confusion; grade 4 – stupor and/or hemiparesis; grade 5 – deep coma, decerebrate posturing, moribund appearance.

- *Diagnosis*: Diagnosis of subarachnoid hemorrhage is most commonly made on non-contrasted CT scan of the head.[6] Although the traditional standard for diagnosis has been CT followed by LP looking for xanthochromia and elevated red blood cells in the CSF if the CT is negative, with newer CT scan technology, this practice has been called into question, since the likelihood of a subarachnoid hemorrhage in the setting of a negative CT is very low, and is only about 5 percent even in the setting of a relatively high pre-test probability.[6] That said, in children with altered mental status, headache, or both, the differential includes numerous items besides hemorrhage, such as infectious processes, and many of these children require LP for exclusion of other dangerous diagnoses, independent of their CT status. Unfortunately, if xanthochromia is not present but the RBC are elevated, it can be difficult to distinguish traumatic LP from subarachnoid hemorrhage, and there are no definitive thresholds.

  In children with concern for intracranial bleeding or a symptomatic expanding aneurysm or dissection, CT angiography can be helpful to identify aneurysmal disease.[2,6] MRI can also help elucidate intracranial pathology in children with CNS symptoms.

- *Treatment*: Emergency physicians are not neurosurgeons, and do not provide definitive care for children with subarachnoid hemorrhage. The focus for care of these children needs to be reducing the secondary injury and getting the child to definitive care. The provider should start with the ABC algorithm. Many of these children will require airway management. Like other brain-injured patients, these patients should not be allowed to become hypoxic, as this can worsen their underlying injury. When intubating these children, care should also be taken to not hyperventilate them excessively. Although hyperventilation decreases intracranial pressure, it can also cause cerebral vasospasm, and, therefore, children should be ventilated to keep their end-tidal carbon dioxide at about 35.

  Optimal blood pressure management has not been studied in children with subarachnoid hemorrhage. In children with aneurysmal disease and concern for vasospasm, it is often appropriate to maintain higher blood pressures, to adequately perfuse the brain, and antispasmodics (nimodipine) are generally considered the standard of care.[2] Decisions regarding target blood pressures in these exceedingly ill children should be made in consultation with a pediatric neurosurgeon.

Definitive therapy is not well studied in a controlled fashion due to the rarity of this process and its multifactorial etiology, but in aneurysms, clipping as well as endovascular techniques are often performed.[2] Ventriculostomy for hydrocephalus and even craniectomy may be necessary in children with significant hydrocephalus. Arteriovenous malformations may require surgery, endovascular procedures, or radiation therapy. Regardless of specialist treatment, these children require management by a multidisciplinary team of neurologists and neurosurgeons, and consultation should be made to such specialists when a diagnosis of subarachnoid hemorrhage is made.

- *Disposition*: A child diagnosed with a subarachnoid hemorrhage should be transferred to a center with pediatric neurosurgical capability. The child should be closely monitored in a PICU regardless of interventions performed. Frequent neurologic assessments and blood pressure monitoring (and sometimes cerebrovascular pressure monitoring) are important to prevent and/or detect vasospasm and secondary ischemic insult. Subsequent to being discharged from the hospital the child should begin physical therapy to improve functionality as soon as possible and follow up with their neurologist regularly.

Historical clues	Physical findings	Ancillary studies
• Sudden headache • Vomiting • Slurred speech	• Altered mental status • Sluggish pupils • Hypertension	• CT with subarachnoid hemorrhage, CT angiography with aneurysm

Follow-Up

The child was diagnosed with subarachnoid hemorrhage from ruptured aneurysm based on her CT findings. She was transferred to a pediatric center and underwent endovascular coiling of the aneurysm. She ultimately had a good neurologic outcome after a several month rehabilitation stay.

References

1. Westra DL, Colohan ART. Pediatric subarachnoid haemorrhage. *Acta Neurochir Suppl* 2008; 104: 401–5.

2. Beez T, Steiger H-J, Hanggi D. Evolution and management of intracranial aneurysms in children: A systematic review of the modern literature. *J Child Neurol* 2016; 31: 773–83.

3. van Gijn J, Rinkel GJE. Subarachnoid haemorrhage: Diagnosis, causes and management. *Brain* 2001; 124: 249–78.

4. Stapf C, Mohr JP, Pile-Spellman J, et al. Epidemiology and natural history of arteriovenous malformations. *Neurosurg Focus* 2001; 11: article 1.

5. Wong G, Knuckey NW, Gubbay SS. Subarachnoid haemorrhage in children caused by cerebral tumour. *J Neurol Neurosurg Psychiatry* 1983; 46: 449–50.

6. Carpenter CR, Hussain AM, Ward MJ, et al. Spontaneous subarachnoid hemorrhage: A systematic review and meta-analysis describing the diagnostic accuracy of history, physical examination, imaging, and lumbar puncture with an exploration of test thresholds. *Acad Emerg Med* 2016; 23: 963–1003.

Genitourinary Complaints

Case 1

Contributing Author: Shellie Asher

History

The patient is a 12-month-old female who presents with one episode of blood in her diaper. Per mom the patient otherwise has been well. The child has not had a fever, and has been eating and drinking without difficulty. The patient was exclusively breast fed through 4 months, with the addition of table foods up until this week, at which time the parents introduced whole cow's milk. The patient normally has bowel movements every day, which are well formed. Today's bowel movement was softer and the parents noted blood in the diaper, which was bright red.

Past Medical History

- UTD on immunizations.
- Full-term spontaneous vaginal delivery without complications.

Medications

- None.

Allergies

- NKDA.

Physical Examination and Ancillary Studies

- *Vital signs*: T 98.4 °F, HR 105, RR 22, BP 98/56, O$_2$ sat 100% on room air.
- *General*: The patient is awake, alert, and appears comfortable.
- *HEENT*: PERRL. Extraocular movements intact. Moist mucous membranes. Tympanic membranes normal.
- *Neck*: Supple, with no adenopathy.
- *Cardiovascular*: Regular rate and rhythm, with no M/R/G.
- *Lungs*: Normal work of breathing, with clear and equal breath sounds. No W/R/R.
- *Abdomen*: Soft, non-tender, and non-distended, with normoactive bowel sounds throughout. There are no palpable masses. No apparent tenderness.
- *Genitourinary*: Normal genitalia, with no signs of trauma and no blood at the introitus.
- *Extremities and skin*: No rashes or skin changes. No signs of trauma.
- *Neurologic*: Appropriate for age, alert and interactive, no focal deficits.

Questions for Thought

- What is the differential diagnosis for blood in the diaper?
- What is the appropriate testing, should that bleeding be determined to be GI in origin?
- What is the ED management of this condition?

Diagnosis

- Blood in the stool due to milk protein allergy.

Discussion

- *Epidemiology:* GI bleeding in infants is rare, accounting for approximately 0.3 percent of chief complaints to a pediatric ED. Upper GI bleeding is less common than lower GI bleeding, occurring in 1 in 10,000 children each year.[1] GI bleeding in children increases in incidence with older age.
- *Pathophysiology:* The pathophysiology of GI bleeding is multifactorial and depends on age and

Table 11.1 Causes of GI bleeding by age. Bold type indicates more common reasons, regular font indicates less frequent etiologies.[1–3]

Neonate	1 month to 1 year	> 1 year
• **Anal fissures**	• **Esophagitis/GERD**	• **Peptic ulcer disease**
• **Milk protein allergy**	• **Gastritis**	• **Juvenile polyp**
• **Bacterial enteritis**	• **Anal fissures**	• **Meckel's diverticulum**
• **Intussusception**	• **Intussusception**	• **Infectious diarrhea**
• **Swallowed maternal blood**	• **Allergy**	• **Arteriovenous malformations**
• Infantile peptic ulcers	• **Enteritis**	• Variceal bleeding
• Adverse drug reaction	• Volvulus	• Duodenal ulcer
• Stress gastritis	• Foreign body	• Esophagitis
• Arteriovenous malformations	• Variceal bleeding	• Gastritis
• Volvulus	• Meckel's diverticulum	• Mallory–Weiss tears
• Coagulopathies	• Arteriovenous malformation	• Inflammatory bowel disease
• Meckel's diverticulum		• Henoch–Schönlein purpura

presentation. Bleeding may be essentially asymptomatic or may cause chronic (iron deficiency) anemia or acute blood loss anemia (Table 11.1). There is more information on anemia and blood loss in Chapter 3, Case 8.

- *Presentation*: The history and clinical course of pediatric GI bleeding varies with the patient's age and specific diagnosis. Pertinent historical elements include the nature of the bleeding (blood in the vomitus, blood in the stool, melena, acute vs. chronic bleeding), associated symptoms such as fever or abdominal pain, medication history, birth history, diet history, and family history.

  On physical examination, close attention should be paid to signs of shock, vital signs, any obvious sources of bleeding, abdominal examination including tenderness, mass, or organomegaly, and rectal/anal examination for gross blood and evidence of anal fissure.

- *Diagnosis*: The first step to the complaint of "blood in the diaper" is to determine if it is in fact blood. Parents have brought their children in to the ED for bloody diapers that were later discovered to be markers, crayons, beets, sports drinks, food coloring, and clothing dyes. This can be assessed using hemoccult. Once it is determined that there is in fact blood in the diaper, the next step is to determine the source. Blood may be urinary in origin, secondary to a UTI, or can be vaginal in origin. Vaginal bleeding may be from vaginal foreign body, sexual abuse, trauma, or, in the first weeks of life, from normal physiologic withdrawal from maternal

estrogens. A rectal examination may be necessary to determine the source of bleeding.

The keys to diagnosis are a thorough history and physical examination, as described above, directed toward the common etiologies of GI bleeding for the patient's age and chief complaint (i.e. bloody vomiting or blood in the stool). Ancillary studies in the ED may include CBC, serum chemistries, fecal occult blood, and coagulation studies. In addition, the Apt test can be used to determine the presence of fetal hemoglobin in a stool sample, to distinguish from the possibility of swallowed maternal blood in neonates or breastfeeding infants.[1,2] If an infectious etiology is suspected, fecal leukocytes, ova/parasites, and cultures can be obtained. Abdominal U/S is indicated if intussusception is suspected. Although often recommended, nasogastric irrigation and/or aspiration has very poor sensitivity for upper GI bleeding, incurs a significant amount of discomfort to the patient, and should not routinely be used as a diagnostic maneuver. For significant blood loss or recurrent bleeding, esophagogastroduodenoscopy or colonoscopy can be performed by a pediatric gastroenterologist for a definitive diagnosis.

- *Treatment*: Most children with a first episode of a small amount of blood in vomitus or stool, normal vital signs, and an unremarkable physical examination can be managed conservatively, with observation at home and primary care follow-up. If anal fissures are noted on examination, stool softeners should be prescribed. Children with larger amounts of bleeding or who appear ill or unstable require IV fluid resuscitation and, potentially, transfusion. Intussusception is often reduced with barium or air enema, but may require surgical intervention. Depending on the suspected cause of bleeding, medical management may include H_2 antihistamines, proton pump inhibitors, antacids, or hormone analogs such as octreotide or vasopressin. Significant GI bleeding of other etiologies may be treated endoscopically by a gastroenterologist, and surgical intervention may be indicated if the bleeding cannot be controlled.

- *Disposition*: The appropriate disposition of children with GI bleeding depends on the severity of the bleeding and associated symptoms. Children with a first episode of a small amount of bleeding in the setting of normal vital signs, benign physical examination, and no other associated symptoms can be discharged home with careful observation and primary care follow-up. Children who have more than a scant amount of bleeding, have abnormal vital signs, or appear ill require admission to a pediatric intensive care setting. Children presenting to a facility without these resources should be stabilized and transferred in an expeditious manner.

Historical clues	Physical findings
• Blood in diaper • Change in diet	• Normal vital signs • Benign abdominal examination

Follow-Up

The baby was found to have heme-positive stools. This patient was diagnosed with milk protein allergy. The patient's parents were instructed to stop cow's milk, and the patient was referred back to her pediatrician and an allergist for further dietary and allergy testing and counseling. The patient did well without any recurrence of GI bleeding.

References

1. Owensby S, Taylor K, Wilkins T. Diagnosis and management of upper gastrointestinal bleeding in children. *J Am Board Fam Med* 2015; 28: 134–45.

2. Hillemeier C, Gryboski JD. Gastrointestinal bleeding in the pediatric patient. *Yale J Biol Med* 1984; 57: 135–47.

3. Padilla BE, Moses W. Lower gastrointestinal bleeding and intussusception. *Surg Clin N Am* 2017; 97: 173–88.

Case 2

Contributing Author: Shellie Asher

History

The patient is a 4-month-old male who presents with parents who report a bulge in the baby's diaper area. The patient's mother noticed this when changing his diaper earlier today. She states that he has been feeding well, with no vomiting and normal stools. He has not had any fevers or other systemic symptoms. The patient is bottle-fed and has been taking his usual amounts of formula.

Past Medical History

- Full-term delivery with no complications.
- UTD on immunizations.

Medications

- None.

Allergies

- NKDA.

Physical Examination and Ancillary Studies

- *Vital signs*: T 98.4 °F, HR 105, RR 22, BP 100/65, O_2 sat 100% on room air.
- *General*: The patient is awake, alert, and appears comfortable.
- *HEENT*: PERRL. Red reflex intact. Moist oral mucosa. Tympanic membranes normal.
- *Neck*: Supple, with midline trachea and no adenopathy.
- *Cardiovascular*: Regular rate and rhythm. No M/R/G.
- *Lungs:* Clear, with normal respiratory effort. No W/R/R.
- *Abdomen*: Soft, non-tender, and non-distended, with normoactive bowel sounds throughout. No apparent tenderness.
- *Genitourinary*: There is a bulge in the right inguinal area, with fullness in the right scrotum. There is no erythema. No obvious tenderness.
- *Extremities and skin*: No rashes, deformity, or signs of trauma.
- *Neurologic*: Normal mental status, interactive and consoleable, symmetric strength, intact reflexes.
- *Pertinent laboratory values*: CBC and chemistry studies are normal.

- *Pertinent imaging*: U/S demonstrates a right indirect inguinal hernia containing a small loop of bowel.

Questions for Thought

- What are typical causes of this condition?
- What is the ED management for this condition?
- What signs and symptoms associated with this condition would be a cause for concern?

Diagnosis

- Inguinal hernia.

Discussion

- *Epidemiology*: The incidence of indirect inguinal hernia in the USA is between 1 percent and 5 percent, with highest rates in premature infants and males.[1,2] Inguinal hernias demonstrate the same predilection for children of all races, as opposed to umbilical hernias, which are more common in African American infants. Most hernias are detected in the first year of life, although asymptomatic hernias may present later.[2]
- *Pathophysiology*: Abdominal hernia is a defect in the ventral wall of the abdomen, which results in an opportunity for intra-abdominal structures such as omentum or bowel to protrude into extra-abdominal space. Indirect inguinal hernias are the most common type in children, and are the result of failure of the processus vaginalis to close (after the descent of the testis through the inguinal canal in males).[2] Other hernias of the ventral wall include direct inguinal hernias and femoral hernias (both of which are acquired rather than congenital, and are rare in children), umbilical hernias, epigastric hernias, and incisional hernias. Failure of the processus vaginalis to close may also result in hydrocele, when peritoneal fluid enters the scrotal sac.[1-3]
- *Presentation*: Infants or children with hernia typically present with an apparent bulge at the inguinal canal or in the scrotum. The majority of hernias occur on the right side, and a small number are bilateral. Bilateral hernias are more common in females.[1] This bulge may be constant or intermittent, often occurs with crying or straining, and may be associated with irritability

reflecting associated pain. If the hernia is incarcerated (abdominal contents are trapped in the defect), the patient may present with irritability or poor feeding. If strangulation (loss of blood flow to entrapped bowel) has occurred, the patient may additionally present with vomiting, decreased stool output, firm abdomen, or fever.[1-3]

- *Diagnosis*: The keys to diagnosis are a thorough history and physical examination. Other differential considerations include testicular torsion, epididymal appendage torsion, epididymitis, orchitis, hydrocele, skin infection, or tumor. Torsions, inflammatory syndromes, and incarcerated hernias are painful, while hydrocele, tumor, and most uncomplicated hernias are not. In situations where the diagnosis is in question, U/S can help differentiate among these possibilities, and is often diagnostic for torsion, tumor, or hernia.

  A history of previous episodes of bulging, birth history, changes in feeding, vomiting, fever, irritability/crying, and a family history should be obtained. On physical examination, a palpable smooth mass can often be felt in the inguinal region. If there is no mass felt with the child lying supine, reassess in the setting of increased abdominal pressure (crying or straining, or bearing down if the child is old enough to cooperate) or in an upright position. Girls should be assessed for palpable herniated ovary (often confused with an enlarged lymph node in the inguinal canal) and boys should be assessed for the presence of both testes in the scrotum. Signs of an incarcerated hernia on examination include signs of pain such as crying/irritability, a tender, firm mass in the area of the hernia, which is unable to be reduced, and discoloration of the overlying skin. If strangulation occurs, the bowel is at risk for necrosis and perforation. In this setting, the abdomen may be firm and diffusely tender. Ancillary studies in the ED may include CBC, serum chemistries, and U/S to evaluate for hernia and/or incarceration or strangulation. In boys, hernia and hydrocele often cannot be differentiated on clinical examination and U/S may be helpful to delineate between these diagnoses.
- *Treatment*: Well-appearing children who present with inguinal hernia should have reduction

attempted in the ED. Children with signs of an incarcerated hernia should have reduction attempted as long as there are no signs of systemic toxicity such as unstable vital signs, peritoneal abdominal examination, fever/leukocytosis, or severe discoloration of the hernia contents. If these signs are present, urgent surgical consultation is indicated. Definitive therapy is surgical repair of the hernia. Early repair is warranted in young children, as the risk of incarceration is high with delay in repair.[1,2]

- *Disposition*: Reducible simple inguinal hernias without incarceration or strangulation can be referred to a pediatric surgeon for close outpatient follow-up and repair. Surgical referral is always indicated, as the hernia defect will not spontaneously close and there is a 7–17 percent risk of incarceration if it is left untreated.[1,2] Parents should be counseled regarding the signs and symptoms of incarceration or strangulation which should prompt immediate return to the ED for urgent evaluation and management. Children with an unreducible hernia or signs of systemic toxicity should have urgent surgical consultation or be transferred to a facility where such consultation is available.

Historical clues	Physical findings	Ancillary studies
• Bulge found during diaper change • Normal feeding/stools • Lack of other symptoms	• Palpable inguinal hernia • Benign abdominal examination	• U/S showing indirect inguinal hernia • Normal laboratory tests

Follow-Up

This patient was diagnosed with a simple, reducible, indirect inguinal hernia. He was discharged home with next-day surgical follow-up, and the parents were instructed regarding signs and symptoms of incarceration and strangulation. The patient had an uncomplicated laparoscopic hernia repair and recovered without sequelae.

References

1. Chang SJ, Chen JY, Hsu CK, et al. The incidence of inguinal hernia and associated risk factors of incarceration in pediatric inguinal hernia: A nation-wide longitudinal population-based study. *Hernia* 2016; 20: 559–63.

2. Wang KS. Assessment and management of inguinal hernia in infants. *Pediatrics* 2012; 130: 768.

3. Davis JE, Silverman M. Scrotal emergencies. *Emerg Med Clin N Am* 2011; 29: 469–84.

Case 3

Contributing Author: Abhishek Chaturvedi

History

The patient is a 4-year-old boy who was brought to the ED by his caretaker for a 5-hour history of swelling and redness of the penis. The caretaker stated that the child became restless and started crying about 4 hours ago and did not stop, even after giving him his favorite candies and toys. On further questioning, the caretaker stated that about 5–6 hours ago, while giving a bath, she retracted the foreskin over the penis to clean it but subsequently could not move it back. She thought that it would go back on its own. When she saw that the child's penis was swollen and red, she immediately came to the ED to seek medical help. Review of systems is otherwise negative.

Past Medical History

- Healthy, immunizations UTD.

Medications

- None.

Allergies

- NKDA.

Physical Examination and Ancillary Studies

- *Vital signs*: T 98.8 °F, HR 112, BP 100/70, RR 28, O_2 sat 99% on room air.
- *General*: Crying, irritable, appears well-nourished, well-developed.
- *HEENT*: PERRL, mucous membranes moist.
- *Neck*: Supple and non-tender, with no adenopathy.
- *Cardiovascular*: Tachycardia, with regular rhythm. No M/R/G.
- *Lungs*: Clear, with normal work of breathing. No W/R/R.
- *Abdomen*: Soft, with no distension, masses, or tenderness. No organomegaly.
- *Genitourinary*: Irritable with examination of the genital area. Uncircumcised, the glans penis is edematous, erythematous, and congested, with a

collar of edematous foreskin (like a "doughnut" around the shaft near the glans). The remainder of the penile shaft is unremarkable. Testes are descended bilaterally, with normal cremasteric reflex. No discharge from the urethral meatus. No evidence of foreign-body insertion.

- *Extremities and skin*: No deformities noted. No swelling, redness, tenderness, rashes. Full range of motion at all the joints with 5/5 muscle strength in all four extremities.
- *Neurologic*: Interactive, age appropriate, normal reflexes.

Questions for Thought

- What are the typical causes of this condition?
- What is the ED management for this condition?
- What signs and symptoms associated with this condition would be a cause for concern?

Diagnosis

- Paraphimosis.

Discussion

- *Epidemiology*: According to the National Hospital Discharge Survey, circumcision rates in the USA declined from an all-time high of 78–80 percent in the mid to late 1960s to 55–60 percent in 2003.[1] While paraphimosis can occur at any age, its distribution is bimodal, occurring in uncircumcised young boys and adolescents and then again in older adult males.[2]
- *Pathophysiology:* Paraphimosis is the inability to completely reduce the penile foreskin distally back to its natural position overlying the glans penis after retraction. The entrapped foreskin forms a constricting band on the penile shaft. Compression inhibits venous drainage of the glans and results in a vicious cycle of progressive glans edema, which further prevents reduction of the foreskin. Glans edema may become so severe that arterial inflow is compromised and may result in necrosis and gangrene of the glans, which rarely may be complicated by the development of necrotizing fasciitis.
- *Presentation*: More common in young children and infants, paraphimosis is often discovered at a diaper change, but may be seen after the foreskin is forcibly retracted in an attempt to facilitate

cleaning, or following urinary catheter insertion.[3] Adolescents may have a delayed presentation because of embarrassment, and in this age group, paraphimosis has been reported in association with activities including sexual intercourse, genital piercing, or prolonged erotic dancing.[2,3] Poor hygiene and balanitis at any age are also associated with increased risk, as the inflammation can result in contracture of the distal foreskin. Ischemia can occur within hours, although some children will have minimal vascular compromise even in the setting of several days of symptoms.[3] Patients may complain of pain, or they may be agitated or fussy. Children may also present with urinary retention or abdominal distension.

- *Diagnosis*: Diagnosis is based upon physical examination. As such, it is critically important to completely examine all patients, particularly the pre-verbal child who cannot tell you what hurts. Other items to consider include hair tourniquet and phimosis. In cases of hair tourniquet, it may be very difficult to visualize the embedded hair. Phimosis, which is the inability to retract the distal foreskin over the glans penis, is physiologically normal in infants and children up to age 5–7, and considered pathologic only if it occurs after the foreskin was previously retractable, or after puberty. Parents should be counseled to never forcibly retract the foreskin of a young child, as this increases the risk of injury, infection, and both phimosis and paraphimosis. Young patients with phimosis can be followed by their PCP, and older patients can be referred to urology for outpatient follow-up and management.

  Once paraphimosis has been diagnosed, it is important to consider the underlying predisposing contributor to the paraphimosis. Although most cases are spontaneous or secondary to poor hygiene, paraphimosis may be secondary to *Plasmodium falciparum*, chancroid, lichen sclerosis, or contact dermatitis (application of celandine juice on the prepuce).[2] Paraphimosis may also be secondary to iatrogenic injury or neglect in disabled children who require assistance for activities of daily living.[2,3]
- *Treatment*: Paraphimosis is a urologic emergency that must be treated promptly to prevent glans necrosis. The treatment approach depends on the

presence of glans ischemia and the duration of the symptoms. In patients with no evidence of acute ischemia and symptoms less than 12 hours, the EM physician may attempt reduction of edema with osmotic agents and a single attempt to reduce the paraphimosis with adequate sedation/analgesia.[2-4] Patients with evidence of possible ischemia or symptoms for more than 12 hours should receive urgent urologic consultation and management.

The first step in reduction is adequate analgesia. Topical local anesthetic options include EML® (2.5% lidocaine and 2.5% prilocaine) cream or lidocaine gel. Regional anesthesia (with anxiolysis, as well) is accomplished with dorsal penile nerve block using 1% lidocaine (or 0.5% bupivacaine if a longer-lasting analgesia is preferred after reduction).[2-5] Calculate the maximum safe dose according to the child's body weight prior to injection. The total volume should not exceed 2 mL (1 mL on each side) – this will reduce the risk of any additional tourniquet effect from the local anesthetic. Local anesthetic should be infiltrated from the dorsal surface, as close to the base of the penis as possible. Insert the needle at the 2 o'clock and 10 o'clock positions, and wait for a "give" as it passes through the fascia. Discomfort can be minimized by using a small (i.e. 29-gauge) needle and injecting slowly. Procedural sedation may also be necessary.

Non-manipulative methods of reduction are considered first-line measures in the absence of any signs of ischemia in patients with symptoms less than 12 hours' duration.

- EMLA® glove technique: An appropriately sized surgical glove is cut at the base of the thumb. A single tube of EMLA® is emptied into the sleeve, which is advanced over the penis and left for approximately 30 minutes. The sleeve provides sufficiently prolonged local anesthesia and also allows it to soften the foreskin. Manual reduction can then be attempted.[5]
- Compression bandage (Colorado CoFlex® technique): After topical anesthesia or sedation, the penis is wrapped in three layers of flexible self-adherent bandage, beginning at the edematous area, then the entire penile shaft.

The first layer is applied loosely, with the following two layers progressively tighter.[4]
- Iced glove: After topical anesthesia, a glove is half-filled with ice and water, and then tied off like a balloon. The penis is placed into the invaginated thumb of the glove for 5 minutes. The glove is then compressed against the pubis.[4]
- Osmotic agents: Glucose, granulated sugar, or mannitol-soaked gauze may be wrapped around the paraphimosis for 30–45 minutes, to draw out edema fluid.[4]

NOTE: Ice and osmotic agents may take 1–2 hours to have an effect and should not be used when arterial compromise is suspected.

Regardless of initial methods to reduce edema, when the preputial swelling and edema have subsided, correct the paraphimosis by gentle manual reduction. To reposition the prepuce, place both thumbs on the glans penis and wrap the fingers behind the prepuce. Apply gentle steady pressure to the prepuce with counter-pressure to the glans penis as the prepuce is pulled down.

If there is any concern for ischemia of the glans penis or after an initial failed attempt at manual reduction under adequate sedation/analgesia, a urologic surgical consultation should be obtained emergently. If surgical intervention is not immediately available and an attempt at non-surgical intervention has failed, the following invasive techniques can be attempted (by an experienced provider or in consultation with a surgical expert):

- Hyaluronidase method: Injection of 1-mL aliquots of hyaluronidase (using a tuberculin syringe) into one or more sites of the edematous prepuce. Hyaluronidase disperses extracellular edema by modifying the permeability of intercellular substance in connective tissue.
- Aspiration is a method using a tourniquet applied to the shaft of the penis, and then inserting a 20-gauge needle parallel to the urethra to aspirate 3–12 mL of blood from the glans. This reduces the volume of the glans sufficiently to facilitate manual reduction.
- The Dundee technique involves multiple needle punctures to drain out the collected

fluid, thereby leading to manual reduction of the foreskin.

· Dorsal slit procedure and emergent circumcision are the last resorts for reducing paraphimosis. For the dorsal slit procedure, a vertical incision is placed in the 12 o'clock position to incise the constricting band of the foreskin. This frees the constricting ring and allows for reduction of the paraphimosis. The incised margins can then be approximated using 4/0 nylon sutures.

• *Disposition*: Patients with reduction of paraphimosis in the ED should be observed after reduction to assure adequate pain control and the ability to urinate. Patients meeting criteria for discharge should be instructed not to retract the foreskin for at least 2 weeks and counseled regarding signs and symptoms of recurrence, phimosis, and infection. They should be referred to urology for outpatient follow-up. Patients requiring surgical intervention should be managed per the post-operative instructions of the surgical team.

Historical clues	Physical findings
• Penis pain • History of retraction during cleaning • Penile erythema	• Paraphimosis on examination • No evidence of ischemia

Follow-Up

The paraphimosis was reduced after application of ice packs, followed by a compression bandage and manual reduction of the prepuce over the glans. Following reduction, it was ensured that the child could pass urine. On discharge, the parents and caretaker were instructed not to retract the foreskin for at least 2 weeks and informed to expect dysuria and/or hematuria and the need to continue simple analgesia for 24–48 hours. They were also instructed to place triple antibiotic ointment on the prepuce and follow up with urology or their PCP for evaluation in 3–4 weeks, to review clinical progress and to assess indications for circumcision.

References

1. Centers for Disease Control and Prevention. National Hospital Discharge Survey. See www.cdc.gov/nchs/nhds/ (accessed February 2017).

2. Dubin J, Davis JE. Penile emergencies. *Emerg Med Clin N Am* 2011; 29: 485–99.

3. Clifford ID, Craig SS, Nataraja RM, et al. Paediatric paraphimosis. *Emerg Med Australasia* 2016; 28: 96–9.

4. Pohlman GD, Phillips JM, Wilcox DT. Simple method of paraphimosis reduction revisited: Point of technique and review of the literature. *J Pediatr Urol* 2013; 9: 104–7.

5. Khan A, Riaz A, Rogawski KM. Reduction of paraphimosis in children: The EMLA® glove technique. *Ann R Coll Surg Engl* 2014; 96: 168.

Case 4

Contributing Author: Jennifer Pelesz

History

The patient is a 15-year-old female who comes in with her mom to the ED with a complaint of pelvic and abdominal pain. She states the pain is across her lower abdomen and began a day or so ago. It has been intermittent but has become worse over the last day. She describes it as "pressure" and it is becoming more severe. She also has pain across her lower back. She denies fever or chills, any nausea or vomiting, and has been eating and drinking normally. She denies urinary symptoms. She states her periods have been "irregular" and the last menstruation was "last month," but doesn't recall the exact date. She denies any vaginal discharge. She denies being sexually active. She is a high school student and lives at home with her mother, father, and a younger sister. She denies use of tobacco, alcohol, or recreational drugs.

Past Medical History

• Asthma.

• Myringotomy tubes as an infant.

• Immunizations UTD.

• Menarche at age 12, last menstrual period about a month ago.

Medications

• Albuterol as needed.

Allergies

• NKDA.

Physical Examination and Ancillary Studies

• *Vital signs*: T 98.7 °F, HR 108, RR 16, BP 143/72, O_2 sat 100% on room air.

- *General*: Patient is obese, appears uncomfortable, and is holding her abdomen as she walks into the room.
- *HEENT*: PERRL. Extraocular movements intact. Moist oral mucosa.
- *Neck*: Supple and non-tender, with no adenopathy.
- *Cardiovascular*: Regularly tachycardic, with no M/R/G.
- *Lungs*: Clear bilaterally, with no W/R/R.
- *Abdomen/genitourinary*: Obese, diffusely tender, firm mass palpable from pelvis to above the umbilicus. Small amount of clear, thin discharge on vaginal examination.
- *Extremities and skin*: Warm and well-perfused, with no signs of trauma and no rashes.
- *Neurologic*: Awake and appropriate, non-focal neurologic examination.
- *Pertinent laboratory values*: Urine positive for pregnancy, 1+ leukocyte esterase, trace protein.

Questions for Thought

- What is the differential diagnosis for this patient?
- What are the potential complications?
- What social ramifications and issues are involved with this patient?
- What other tests/studies should be performed?

Diagnosis

- Third-trimester pregnancy, in active labor.

Discussion

- *Epidemiology*: Early and unplanned pregnancy and childbirth are significant consequences of adolescent sexual activity. The vast majority of pregnancies in this age group are unplanned. Pregnant adolescents are more likely to delay seeking prenatal care, some not getting any care at all until childbirth. Therefore, there are higher rates of unfavorable outcomes, such as prematurity, infant mortality, and poor health and developmental outcomes in this group.[1] Additionally, adolescent mothers are more likely to drop out of school and rely on public assistance for support.[2]
- *Pathophysiology*: The complications of pregnancy are among the life-threatening gynecologic causes of pelvic pain in adolescents. While pelvic pain is an uncommon primary complaint for intrauterine pregnancy, lower abdominal or pelvic pain is often the presenting complaint in ectopic pregnancy, which is discussed in detail in Chapter 8, Case 8. Placental abruption is the premature separation of the placenta from the uterus, and often presents with lower abdominal pain and/or vaginal bleeding. The peak incidence of abruption is between the 24th and 26th week, although it may occur at any time. Uterine rupture is rare in first pregnancies, and generally occurs in laboring women who have had previous uterine surgeries. Both abruption and rupture are associated with high maternal and fetal mortality. Pregnancy may spontaneously miscarry, but if not all products of conception are passed, the patient may become septic from superinfection. Domestic violence during pregnancy is frequently directed at the gravid uterus, and adolescents in violent relationships may also present with abdominal pain or pelvic complaints.
- *Presentation*: Because of denial in this age group and the reluctance to seek care, adolescents may present with any number of complaints at any time during the pregnancy. Vague complaints such as dizziness, nausea and vomiting, or fatigue are common in the first trimester. Also, pelvic pain, cramping, and vaginal bleeding can occur. Later, weight gain or amenorrhea may prompt a visit to the PCP, urgent care, or ED. Often, adolescent females have irregular and sporadic menstrual cycles and missed menses go unnoticed, prompting presentation later in the pregnancy. It is important to separate the adolescent from adult caregivers and ask about menstrual history and sexual activity in all females of this age group. A routine pregnancy test should be considered in all females who have reached sexual maturity.

  Pregnant adolescents may also present with miscarriage. Spontaneous abortion or miscarriage occurs in about 20 percent of all pregnancies. Presenting symptoms commonly include crampy pelvic pain and vaginal bleeding, sometimes with the passage of clots and/or visible products of conception. Young women with irregular or sporadic menstrual cycles may mistake these symptoms for their normal period. If not all tissue is passed, the patient may become septic from bacterial superinfection and may present with fever, diffuse abdominal and pelvic pain, and malodorous vaginal discharge.

- *Diagnosis*: The key to diagnosis is a careful history, physical examination, and urine or serum β-hCG testing. Once pregnancy is confirmed in an adolescent female, there are several important studies/tests that should be performed. First, a complete physical examination in these patients includes a speculum and bimanual pelvic examination. This may be the patient's first pelvic examination and it is important to take the time to explain the details of the examination and obtain informed consent. Important findings on pelvic examination include vulvar, anal, or vaginal trauma; cervical motion tenderness; vaginal bleeding or discharge; uterine tenderness; and adnexal tenderness or masses. Bimanual examination should *not* be performed in girls with vaginal bleeding who are believed to be in the second trimester or later until it can be ascertained that they do not have placenta previa (placenta overlying the cervical os).

  Pregnancy in a minor may be a presentation of sexual abuse or assault. Care should be taken to evaluate for signs of trauma or injury during the physical examination, and to interview the patient in a safe and private environment.

  Socially, the pregnant adolescent faces many challenges. Many feel stigmatized and socially isolated. The reported rates of postpartum depression range from 7 to 37 percent in adolescents, and teenagers are at greater risk to complete suicide. A history of mental illness or a prior suicide attempt places a patient at an increased risk for a repeat attempt. The provider should assess the patient's mental health as well as her physical health.

  Clinicians should be aware of the state laws governing adolescent confidentiality and privacy, as well as those involving mandatory reporting and notification of the legal guardians. A minor's ability to consent for healthcare and/or treatment varies from state to state.

  In addition, laboratory testing should be performed to include:

  - Serum quantitative β-hCG: In the absence of a defined intrauterine pregnancy, serum β-hCG can be performed serially to assist in the diagnosis of ectopic pregnancy or fetal demise. β-hCG should double about every 48–72 hours in a normal pregnancy and should decrease in a spontaneous abortion. Abnormal increases can point to an ectopic pregnancy.
  - CBC to assess for possible infection as well as anemia.
  - Blood typing, including determination of rhesus status. In the rhesus-negative patient, administration of rhesus immunoglobulin is indicated in the setting of ectopic pregnancy or vaginal bleeding to prevent alloimmunization.
  - Testing for sexually transmitted infections: Early treatment during pregnancy is important to reduce the risk of complications and potential for fetal transmission in certain cases.[1-3]

  Imaging studies should be performed in the pregnant adolescent with abdominal or pelvic pain to determine the location of the pregnancy. In the absence of assisted fertility treatments, the identification of an intrauterine pregnancy effectively rules out ectopic pregnancy, as spontaneous heterotopic pregnancy (one embryo in the uterus and additional embryo[s] in an ectopic location) is very rare.

- *Treatment*: The appropriate treatment of pregnant adolescents varies depending on the stage of pregnancy. Most early-pregnancy complaints other than ectopic pregnancy can be effectively managed as an outpatient and do not require any specific treatment other than hydration, prenatal vitamins, and treatment of pregnancy-associated nausea and vomiting as needed. Adolescents presenting in late pregnancy (later than 20 weeks) should be assessed for active labor and treated accordingly.

- *Disposition*: Patients with an intrauterine pregnancy earlier than 20 weeks' gestation should be referred to obstetrics for outpatient prenatal care and follow-up. Patients presenting with abdominal complaints after 20 weeks' gestation should have urgent obstetrics consultation in the ED or be transferred for urgent evaluation if they are not in active labor. If an intrauterine pregnancy cannot be identified in the ED, the disposition should be determined in conjunction with obstetrics and gynecology, based on the β-hCG levels and U/S findings.

  In addition to the medical concerns, there are many social and legal issues that surround adolescent pregnancy. Currently, two-thirds of the states in the USA explicitly allow minors to consent for prenatal care. Some require the minor to be of a certain age or be classified legally as a "mature minor." The remaining states have no relevant policy or laws. In some states, a legal guardian may need to be informed for certain examinations, tests, or procedures. It is important to be familiar with local statutes when evaluating the pregnant adolescent in the ED.

For various reasons, the ED provider, rather than the pediatrician or family physician, may be the one to diagnose an adolescent's pregnancy. Depending on how far along the pregnancy is at diagnosis, there are many medical, legal, and social issues to consider. In a busy department this can be challenging. Medical emergencies must be promptly addressed and treated immediately, but the social and legal implications should not be ignored. It is important to ensure access to proper follow-up care and adequate support for the adolescent who is found to be pregnant in the ED prior to discharge.

Historical clues	Physical findings	Ancillary studies
• Crampy abdominal and back pain	• Gravid uterus (above umbilicus corresponds to > 20 weeks' gestation)	• Positive urine pregnancy test

Follow-Up

The patient initially denied the possibility of pregnancy, even after being told of the positive urine test. She was then interviewed after mom stepped out of the room and admitted to the provider that she was sexually active and was not using any birth control. Her pain continued to increase in intensity and it was determined she was in active labor. She was transferred to the labor and delivery department and later that evening gave birth to a healthy male child.

References

1. Fernandes de Azevedo W, Baffi Diniz M, Borges da Fonseca ES, et al. Complications in adolescent pregnancy: Systematic review of the literature. *Einsten (Sao Paulo)* 2015; 13: 618–26.

2. Centers for Disease Control and Prevention. Reproductive health: Teen pregnancy. www.cdc.gov/teenpregnancy/ (accessed February 2017).

3. McCracken KA, Loveless M. Teen pregnancy: An update. *Curr Opin Obstet Gynecol* 2014; 26: 355–9.

Case 5

Contributing Author: Pamela Young

History

The patient is a 15-year-old female who presents with complaints of foul-smelling, yellow, vaginal discharge. She states that this has been going on for about 3 days. She complains of mild lower abdominal pain. She is unsure of her last menstrual period. She is currently sexually active with one long-term boyfriend. She states that she was taking birth control pills a few months ago but forgot to take them for a while. She is currently waiting for her next period to begin so that she can resume the medication. She is not currently using any contraception. The patient denies any fever or chills. She denies any previous history of sexually transmitted infections (STIs). She denies any vomiting or diarrhea, but has felt nauseous at times.

Past Medical History

• Attention deficit–hyperactivity disorder.
• Allergic rhinitis.
• UTD on immunizations.

Medications

• Oral contraception (non-compliant).

Allergies

• NKDA.

Physical Examination and Ancillary Studies

• *Vital signs*: T 98.2 °F, HR 72, RR 14, BP 98/62, O$_2$ sat 98% on room air.
• *General*: Normal body habitus. Awake and alert, in no acute distress.
• *HEENT*: PERRL, moist mucous membranes, unremarkable examination.
• *Neck*: Supple and non-tender, with no adenopathy.
• *Cardiovascular*: Regular rate and rhythm, normal S1 and S2, no M/R/G.
• *Lungs*: Clear and equal, with no W/R/R. Normal respiratory effort.
• *Abdomen*: Bowel sounds in all four quadrants normal; mild, diffuse abdominal tenderness, increased in suprapubic region. No organomegaly,

no guarding or rebound. No costovertebral angle percussion tenderness.

- *Genitourinary*: External genitalia is normal, without any lesions noted. Cervix is non-friable. Large amount of thick, yellow discharge noted at cervical os as well as brownish bleeding noted. Bimanual examination notes normal uterus, cervical os closed, adnexa not palpable, no cervical motion tenderness. Mild bilateral inguinal lymphadenopathy.
- *Extremities and skin*: Warm and well-perfused, with normal capillary refill and no signs of trauma.
- *Neurologic*: Awake and alert, grossly non-focal.
- *Pertinent laboratory values*: U/A negative for leukocytes, 3+ blood. Urine hCG negative, rapid HIV antibody negative.

Questions for Thought

- What are the most common STIs in teenagers?
- What is the role for empiric treatment of STIs in a patient with this presentation?
- Is there any indication for imaging in this patient?
- What is the definitive treatment of this patient?
- Are their special concerns for STIs in sexually active teenagers?

Diagnosis

- Chlamydial cervicitis and bacterial vaginosis.

Discussion

- *Epidemiology*: The average age of first coitus is approximately 16 years among American adolescents, but the age is lower in certain populations, such as inner-city youth.[1] Adolescents have barriers affecting access to STI prevention and management, including transportation, conflict between clinic hours and school or work, and the inability to pay for the examination and treatment. Embarrassment, risk-taking behavior, peer norms, and concerns about confidentiality and parent involvement also factor into adolescent sexual activity and the reluctance to seek medical care. As a result, adolescents are at very high risk for STIs. The CDC estimates that nearly 20 million new sexually transmitted infections occur every year in the USA, approximately half of which occur

among young people aged 15–24.[2] Recent epidemiologic data suggest that one in four sexually active adolescent females has an STI such as chlamydial disease or human papilloma virus, and 10 percent of asymptomatic adolescents screened in a pediatric ED were positive for *Chlamydia trachomatis* or *Neisseria gonorrhoeae*.[3] During 2013–2014, the rate of reported primary and secondary syphilis cases increased by 11.6 percent among persons aged 15–19 years and by 13.1 percent among persons aged 20–24 years.[1]

In addition to a high rate of primary infection, repeated acquisition of STIs is common, with as many as 40 percent of the annual incidence of chlamydial or gonococcal disease occurring in adolescents previously infected with the causative organisms. Many adolescents are re-infected within a few months of an index infection. Repeated acquisition of STIs is a risk factor for subsequent development of HIV infection.

Certain groups have been identified as higher risk of HIV infection and co-infection with other STIs. In a recent study of very young men who have sex with men, urban and non-white status indicated a higher incidence of infection as well as co-infection.[4] Other risk factors included the use of alcohol or drugs during sexual activity.[2,4] In very young pediatric populations, care must be taken to screen for sexual abuse or assault. An STI may be the first hint of sexual assault in a victim who has not reported the abuse.

- *Pathophysiology*: STIs are typically transmitted via contact by an infected individual to the oropharyngeal area or genitourinary tract of another individual, where thin mucous membranes are susceptible to microbial passage. Causative agents include bacteria such as *C. trachomatis*, *N. gonorrhoeae*, and *Treponema pallidum*, viruses such as herpes, human papilloma virus, and HIV, and parasites such as *Trichomonas vaginalis*, pubic lice, and scabies.
- *Presentation*: STIs may present with localized complaints of discharge, drainage, or dysuria, cutaneous complaints, or abdominal pain and systemic complaints.

  · *Urethral or vaginal discharge and dysuria* are the hallmarks of gonorrhea and chlamydia, as well as trichomoniasis, bacterial vaginosis, and candidiasis. Classically, chlamydial and gonorrheal cervicitis cause purulent drainage, trichomoniasis causes malodorous gray to green discharge with vulvar irritation, bacterial vaginosis causes a watery, foul-smelling discharge with minimal irritation, and candida vaginitis causes vulvar irritation with scant white discharge. Vaginitis and vulvitis are discussed in more detail later in this chapter, Case 7. Genital herpes is sometimes associated with dysuria and a scant, mucoid urethral discharge; however, these infections usually have associated skin findings.

- *Skin findings* are typical of genital warts (condyloma acuminata), caused by human papilloma virus, herpes infections, syphilis, and disseminated gonococcal infection. The skin lesions of genital warts are typically not painful and are soft and fleshy, and located on the perineal area. Herpes infections nearly always present with painful genital ulcers, which may be confused with "hair bumps," particularly in adolescents who shave the genital region. These are sometimes accompanied by systemic complaints in primary infection, as opposed to recurrences. They can appear very similar to Behçet's disease. The rash of disseminated *N. gonorrhoeae* is erythematous and papular to pustular. It is painful, and is usually accompanied by joint pain. The rash of syphilis is typically genital in location and is painless. It is associated with a high rate of HIV co-infection.

- *Abdominal pain and systemic complaints* are common in adolescents presenting with pelvic inflammatory disease, and any adolescent with abdominal pain or tenderness should be queried privately regarding sexual activity. Pelvic inflammatory disease is a common sequela of untreated gonorrhea or chlamydia and should be suspected in the female patient presenting with severe lower abdominal pain, with or without associated fever. Pain with intercourse is another common presenting symptom.

- *Diagnosis*: Screening of sexually active female adolescents for gonorrhea and chlamydia should be performed at least annually and as indicated by complaint or presentation.[5] Screening of adolescent males should be performed dependent upon risk factors, i.e. anal intercourse, reported unprotected sexual activity, and symptoms upon presentation. The CDC recommended in 2006 that "opt-out" HIV testing be routinely offered to all patients aged 13 to 64 years.[2] This involves informing the patient, orally or in writing, that HIV testing will be performed unless he or she declines. The AAP recommends that routine HIV screening be offered at least once to all adolescents by 16 to 18 years.[5] Annual HIV testing should be offered to high-risk adolescents who use IV drugs or have sex with multiple partners, or men who have sex with men. If a patient is being tested for other STIs, then HIV testing should be included.

For symptomatic patients, diagnoses of gonorrhea and chlamydia are most commonly made by a DNA probe or nucleic acid amplification from either a genitourinary swab specimen or from urine testing. Gram's stain is both sensitive and specific for the diagnosis of gonococcal urethritis in symptomatic males. Although cultures are not routinely indicated, they may be warranted in the instance of suspected sexual abuse or assault. Herpes is typically diagnosed on clinical examination, although wound culture of active lesions provides a definitive diagnosis.

Serologic testing for HIV is performed via ELISA screening for HIV-1 and -2. Positive results are confirmed via HIV-1/HIV-2 differentiation assay or Western blot.

- *Treatment*: The CDC routinely publishes updated treatment guidelines for STIs, most recently in 2015, reflecting developing resistance patterns. It has been estimated that upwards of 30 percent of adolescents are non-compliant with STI treatment.[6] Therefore, single-dose therapy or treatment at the time of examination, if there is a high index of suspicion, is preferable. Expedited partner therapy allows for the provision of appropriate single-dose antibiotics to patients with chlamydia or gonorrhea for delivery to partners. This measure may help to reduce the incidence of re-infection by repeat exposure to an untreated partner. Current recommendations also endorse a test of cure within 3 to 12 months, particularly if there is a question regarding compliance or treatment of the partner.

Briefly, the CDC recommends that chlamydia infection be treated with azithromycin 1 g orally or doxycycline 100 mg twice daily for 7 days. *N. gonorrhoeae* infections should be treated with ceftriaxone 250 mg IM plus azithromycin 1 g orally. First-line treatment of initial presentation of genital herpes is a 7–10-day course of acyclovir, though there may be increased compliance with the once daily dosing of valacyclovir. The complete recommendations may be found on the CDC website.

- *Disposition*: Patients presenting with signs and symptoms of sexually transmitted infections should be screened for co-infections, with close follow-up arranged for test results and ongoing care, including a test of cure to assure eradication of the current infection. Providers should be watchful for signs of sexual abuse/assault and offer forensic examination and notification of law enforcement as per local law and practice.

Historical clues	Physical findings	Ancillary studies
• Vaginal discharge • Sexually active • Abdominal pain	• Mucopurulent cervical discharge • Inguinal adenopathy	• Negative pregnancy test

Follow-Up

This patient's presentation of foul-smelling discharge with mild lower abdominal pain is typical for chlamydia infections, for which her nucleic acid amplification test was positive. The patient was notified of her positive test and prescriptions for doxycycline were provided to the patient and her partner. The patient returned 1 month later with concerns for a STI as her partner may not have been compliant with the treatment regimen, and she tested positive for both *N. gonorrhoeae* and *C. trachomatis*. She was treated with IM ceftriaxone and oral azithromycin. The patient denied any concerns for sexual assault/abuse or human trafficking and stated that she had a safe living environment. Her partner was notified to seek treatment at the Department of Health. The patient was subsequently lost to follow-up.

References

1. Kann L, Kinchen S, Shankin SL, et al. Youth risk behavior surveillance United States, 2013. *MMR Suppl* 2014; 63: 1–168.
2. Centers for Disease Control and Prevention (CDC). Reproductive health: Teen pregnancy. See www.cdc.gov/teenpregnancy/ (accessed February 2017).
3. Schneider K, FitzGerald M, Bychzkowski T, et al. Screening for asymptomatic gonorrhea and chlamydia in the pediatric emergency department. *Sex Transm Dis* 2016; 43: 209–15.
4. Garofalo R, Hotton AL, Kuhns LM, et al. Incidence of HIV infection and sexually transmitted infections and related risk factors among very young men who have sex with men. *J AIDS* 2016; 72: 79–86.
5. American Academy of Pediatrics. Recommendations for preventive pediatric health care. See www.aap.org/en-us/Documents/periodicity_schedule.pdf (accessed February 2017).
6. Schneider K, Byckowski T, Reed J. Treatment compliance among asymptomatic adolescents with sexually transmitted infections. *JAMA Pediatr* 2015; 169: 1065-6.

Case 6

Contributing Author: Leah A. Perez

History

The patient is a 4-year-old female who presents with a 24-hour history of urinary frequency and dysuria. Per mom the patient started complaining of pain when voiding yesterday after she came home from preschool which the patient attends all day. The mother reports the patient has had decreased appetite with nausea, but mom denies vomiting, diarrhea, abdominal pain, or fever. The patient is toilet trained and per mom she had an accident last night and woke up wet this morning which is unusual for her. The patient's mother is also concerned as the patient appears more uncomfortable when voiding this morning and is crying intermittently, which is causing her to stop mid-stream when voiding. The patient is voiding more frequently as well. She has no previous history of UTIs.

Past Medical History

- Tonsillectomy and adenoidectomy.
- UTD on immunizations.

Medications

- Loratidine daily.

Allergies

- NKDA.

Physical Examination and Ancillary Studies

- *Vital signs*: T 98.4 °F, HR 95, BP 118/69, RR 18, O_2 sat 99% on room air.
- *General*: The patient is awake, alert, and appears comfortable.
- *HEENT*: PERRL. Oropharynx clear, with moist mucous membranes.
- *Neck*: Supple, with no adenopathy.
- *Cardiovascular*: Regular rate and rhythm, with no M/R/G.
- *Lungs*: Clear and equal, with normal work of breathing and no W/R/R.
- *Abdomen*: Soft, not distended. Normal bowel sounds throughout. There are no palpable masses. There is suprapubic tenderness on palpation.
- *Extremities and skin*: No rashes, deformity, or evidence of trauma.
- *Neurologic*: Appropriate for age, non-focal.
- *Pertinent laboratory values*: Urine dipstick with specific gravity 1.020, pH 6.0, glucose negative, ketones negative, leukocyte esterase moderate, nitrite positive, protein trace, hemoglobin trace, bilirubin negative, and urobilirubin negative.

Questions for Thought

- What are typical laboratory findings in this condition?
- What further laboratory testing should be initiated in the ED?
- What items on the differential diagnosis are important not to miss?

Diagnosis

- Lower UTI/cystitis.

Discussion

- *Epidemiology*: UTI is one of the most common pediatric infections, second only to otitis media, and accounts for 1.5 million office visits a year.[1,2] These infections distress the child, concern the parents, and may cause permanent kidney damage and hypertension.[2] UTIs occur with equal frequency in boys and girls under 1 year of age, but are more common in girls after that age.[1,2] Circumcision offers some protection from UTI in boys.[1,2]

- *Pathophysiology*: Urine in the proximal urethra and urinary bladder is normally sterile. UTIs develop when pathogens ascend to the bladder (cystitis, or lower tract disease) or to the kidneys (pyelonephritis, or upper tract disease) via the urethra. Pathogens may then enter the blood stream and cause systemic illness (bacteremia). Poor containment of infection, including bacteremia, is most common in infants less than 2 months old. Pathogens may enter the urinary tract secondary to turbulent urinary flow during normal voiding, voiding dysfunction, or catheterization.[1] In addition, sexual intercourse or genital manipulation may foster the entry of bacteria into the urinary bladder.[1] More rarely, the urinary tract may be colonized during systemic bacteremia (sepsis); this is more common in infants than in older children. Pathogens can also infect the urinary tract through direct spread via the fecal–perineal–urethral route.

  The majority of UTIs are caused by *Escherichia coli*, which accounts for 75–90 percent of UTIs.[2] Most of the remainder are also caused by bowel flora such as *Enterococcus* or *Klebsiella* species or other Gram-negative rods, but fungi such as *Candida albicans* and even viruses may cause UTI. *Staphylococcus* and *Streptococcus* species also cause UTIs, particularly in neonates and adolescent females.

- *Presentation*: The history and clinical course of a UTI vary with the patient's age and specific diagnosis. No one specific sign or symptom can be used to identify UTI in infants and children. Contributing factors to making a decision to pursue UTI testing includes a prior history of a UTI, circumcision history in very young boys, and, in older children, typical symptoms such as increased urinary frequency, abdominal or suprapubic discomfort, loss of urinary continence, or dysuria. Typical presentations for children of various age groups are as follows:

  - Children aged 0–2 months: Neonates and infants up to age 2 months generally present with upper tract disease, and the UTI is discovered as part of an evaluation for neonatal sepsis. They may present with jaundice, fever, poor feeding, vomiting, or irritability.[1,2]
  - Infants and children aged 2 months to 2 years: Infants with UTIs may present with poor

feeding, fever, vomiting, strong-smelling urine, abdominal pain, or irritability.[2] They often lack local symptoms or are unable to communicate those symptoms, although parents may note crying with urination or increasing frequency.

· Children aged 2–6 years: Preschoolers with lower tract disease usually have voiding symptoms such as urgency, frequency, hesitancy, dysuria, or incontinence, with no fever. They may have suprapubic pain or tenderness. Upper tract disease may present with vomiting, abdominal pain, fever, strong-smelling urine, enuresis, or regression with milestones in terms of toilet training, as well.[1]

· Older children and adolescents with lower tract disease usually present with dysuria, urgency, and frequency with or without abdominal pain.[1] Fever is usually absent. With upper tract disease, children may have fever, flank pain, abdominal pain, and vomiting. It is important to remember that adolescent girls with sexually transmitted infections or vaginitis may present with similar symptoms, and the history and physical examination should consider these possibilities.

• *Diagnosis*: The AAP recommends that all children with fever with no source under the age of 2 years be evaluated for UTIs.[3] Although peripheral blood collection may risk-stratify individuals from a sepsis standpoint and assess renal function, the diagnosis of a UTI is made by urine studies. Although the AAP does allow for non-invasive collection of urine for analysis, bagged urine samples should not be used for culture, as they have a very high false positive rate.[1,3,4] A negative bag urine culture is strong evidence that there is no UTI present. However, given the limitations to this mode of collection, consideration for catheterization should be given for children with a high suspicion of UTI who are unable to provide a clean-catch specimen.[4]

U/A is insufficient to make a diagnosis of UTI, and lacks the sensitivity to rule it out.[4] The data obtained may change the clinical suspicion of the disease, however, and therefore it is not an unreasonable test to obtain along with the gold standard, which is urine culture and microscopy. For instance, with a 10 percent pre-test probability, a positive nitrite on U/A increases the probability of UTI to 75 percent (as the specificity of nitrite is 98 percent).[4] This may change the provider's threshold for antibiotic administration. Likewise, the visualization of bacteria on microscopy increases the probability of UTI to 35 percent, which may bring the likelihood of the disease sufficiently high for an individual provider to choose to treat.[4] If a child does not have sufficient urine for U/A and culture, culture is the diagnostic test of choice, and U/A should not be performed.[4]

Urine should be cultured within 4 hours or the urine should be refrigerated to prevent bacterial overgrowth. Culture positivity is defined at different thresholds depending upon the method of obtaining the specimen. Current established thresholds are 10,000 colony forming units (cfus) of a single pathogen per milliliter in a catheter-obtained specimen and 100,000 cfus/mL in a clean-catch specimen.[4] Some advocate for treating at lower counts in patients who have symptomatic disease.[4]

When a UTI has been diagnosed, the medical provider should consider the underlying associated risk factors to optimize management. Constipation is a common risk factor, as is diabetes.[4] Voiding dysfunction and anatomic anomalies should be considered in patients with recurrent disease.[3,4] A recent history of broad-spectrum antibiotic use may alter antibiotic choice, and should be specifically questioned.

• *Treatment*: Symptomatic relief in children is generally supportive, with anti-inflammatory medications and increased fluid intake to enhance urine dilution. Antiemetics may also be used. Urinary anesthetics, such as phenazopyridine, are not recommended for children under 12 years of age.

Children with cystitis typically respond well to appropriate antibiotic therapy and symptomatic treatment. Antibiotic therapy is started on the basis of clinical history, physical examination, and U/A results before the culture provides a definitive diagnosis, in most cases. Certainly, all ill children should receive antibiotics. In older children with an unclear etiology of symptoms, observation alone pending urine culture is not unreasonable as many will clear their bacteriuria spontaneously and there are no untoward affects from delaying therapy for a day.[4] In patients who are not toxic, a 4-day course of an oral antibiotic agent is recommended for the treatment of cystitis.[4] A systematic review of treatments for cystitis in children showed no difference in efficacy with 7–14 days of therapy compared with 2–4 days.[4] Empiric antibiotic therapy should be based on resistance patterns for typical uropathogens in the patient's community, with an appropriate first-line agent such as sulfamethoxazole–trimethoprim, amoxicillin–clavulanic acid, cephalexin, cefixime, cefpodoxime, or nitrofurantoin. Of note, the limited tissue penetration of nitrofurantoin limits its use to cystitis and excludes its use for pyelonephritis. If the clinical response is not satisfactory after an initial course of empiric therapy, antibiotic choice should be altered on the basis of antibiotic susceptibility. Children with upper tract disease (systemic symptoms or WBC casts on urine microscopy diagnostic for pyelonephritis) should be treated for longer, typically 10–14 days.[4] Ill children, children less than 2 months old, and children unable to take fluids by mouth should be admitted for IV antibiotics.

Former recommendations included a voiding cystourethrogram in the follow-up for all first febrile UTIs, but newer guidelines from the AAP state that U/S should be performed in young children with first UTIs, particularly all boys and girls under 3 years, and febrile girls with UTIs, under age 7.[3,4] The risk–benefit on more detailed imaging, using modalities requiring radiation exposure, are best deferred to the primary care team. Likewise, decisions for antibiotic prophylaxis for recurrent UTIs should be made in concert with the primary care team.

- *Disposition*: Neonates (birth to 6 weeks) with fever and a UTI should be admitted and started on parenteral antibiotics pending culture results and clinical response to therapy. The majority of older infants and children with simple cystitis or pyelonephritis can be discharged home with oral antibiotics if they are well-appearing and can take oral fluids and medication. Patients who have signs of sepsis and/or cannot take oral fluids/medications should be admitted to the hospital for fluid resuscitation and parenteral antibiotic therapy.

Historical clues	Physical findings	Ancillary studies
• Frequency • Dysuria • Enuresis	• Suprapubic tenderness	• U/A suggestive of a UTI, with positive nitrites and leukocyte esterase

Follow-Up

This patient was diagnosed with an uncomplicated cystitis and discharged to home with ibuprofen and trimethoprim–sulfamethoxazole based on clinical history, examination, U/A results, and local patterns of antibiotic resistance. The patient and her mom were encouraged to increase PO intake and take warm baths for comfort and return to the ED with any new or worsening symptoms.

References

1. Becknell B, Schober M, Korbel L, et al. The diagnosis, evaluation, and treatment of acute and recurrent pediatric urinary tract infections. *Expert Rev Anti Infect Ther* 2015; 13: 81–90.

2. Copp HL, Schmidt B. Work up of pediatric urinary tract infection. *Urol Clin North Am* 2015; 42: 519–26.

3. Newman TB. The new American Academy of Pediatrics urinary tract infection guidelines. *Pediatrics* 2011; 128: 572–5.

4. White B. Diagnosis and treatment of urinary tract infections in children. *Am Fam Phys* 2011; 83: 409–15.

Case 7

Contributing Authors: Shellie Asher and Rebecca Jeanmonod

History

The patient is a 4-year-old female, who is brought in by mom for vaginal discharge. The patient's mother states that she was giving the child a bath this evening when she noted a foul-smelling vaginal discharge and a yellow stain in the patient's underwear. There have been no recent fevers, vomiting, abdominal pain, or other illnesses. The patient complains that it "feels itchy down there" but denies other complaints. The patient's mother notes that the child recently completed toilet training and has been independently managing her toileting and associated hygiene.

Past Medical History

- None.

Medications

- None.

Allergies

- NKDA.

Physical Examination and Ancillary Studies

- *Vital signs*: T 98.4 °F, HR 110, RR 22, BP 95/60, O_2 sat 98% on room air.
- *General*: Well-nourished and well-appearing child, in no acute distress.
- *HEENT*: PERRL. Mucous membranes moist with no lesions.
- *Neck*: Supple, with no tenderness or adenopathy.
- *Cardiovascular*: Regular, normal S1/S2, without M/R/G. Good capillary refill.
- *Lungs*: Clear bilaterally, with no W/R/R.
- *Abdomen*: Soft and non-tender with no masses, rebound, or guarding.
- *Genitourinary*: Tanner 1. Slightly erythematous vulva with a small amount of foul-smelling discharge. There is a small foreign body at the vaginal introitus, which appears to be retained toilet tissue. There is no bleeding or other evidence of injury on external examination.
- *Extremities and skin*: Warm and well-perfused, with no rashes or signs of trauma.
- *Neurologic*: Normal mentation for age. Non-focal examination.
- *Pertinent laboratory values*: Wet mount with 3+ WBC, Gram's stain negative, culture with normal vaginal flora.

Questions for Thought

- What is the differential diagnosis for this presentation?
- What are the possible causes of this diagnosis?
- What social or safety concerns should you consider for this child?

Diagnosis

- Non-specific vulvovaginitis.

Discussion

- *Epidemiology*: Symptoms referable to the vulva and vagina are common in girls of all ages. The exact incidence is difficult to determine, as the underlying diagnoses are numerous. The cause of vulvovaginitis differs as a factor of the patient's age, with post-menarcheal girls having pathogens similar to adult women of reproductive age, and pre-menarcheal girls having non-specific vulvovaginitis or infections with respiratory flora.
- *Pathophysiology*: In prepubertal girls, most cases of vulvovaginitis begin with irritation of the vulva, followed by involvement of the vagina. The anatomy and physiology of the pediatric vagina and vulva is predisposed to irritation because of the relatively small labia minora, the absence of labial fat pads and pubic hair, low levels of estrogen with a resulting thin vaginal epithelium, and alkaline pH.[1,2] Behavioral factors such as poor hygiene (particularly related to toilet training), self-exploration, foreign-body insertion, tight-fitting clothing, and chemical exposures such as bubble baths and damp swim suits also play a role.[1,2] While most cases are non-specific, infectious agents such as respiratory pathogens (typically *Streptococcus* or *Haemophilus* species), enteric pathogens, STIs, viral infections (such as EBV), and parasitic infections may be associated with vulvovaginitis.[1–4] Autoimmune and idiopathic causes also occur, such as lichen sclerosis, vasculitis, psoriasis, or Behçet's disease.[1] Candidal vulvovaginitis is uncommon in prepubertal girls, although it occurs in association with diaper rash in children who are not toilet trained.

  In girls who have reached puberty, the vaginal mucosa is thicker, fat pads have developed, and pubic hair is present. The pH of the vaginal secretions is more acidic. All of these items offer protection from the causes of vaginitis that plague the smaller child. Rather, the vast majority of all cases of vaginitis in post-menarcheal young women are caused by candidal species, *Gardnerella vaginalis*, and *Trichomonas vaginalis*.[5,6] These pathogens cause varying degrees of inflammation and discharge and displace normal vaginal flora.
- *Presentation*: Patients who are in diapers will typically present with irritation, noted by the

caregiver, or with discharge. Older children or adolescents may present with complaints of irritation or itching, or parents may note staining or discharge in their underwear. Children may also complain of burning, vaginal pain, and dysuria.

It is important to remember that vulvovaginitis exists on a spectrum. In post-menarcheal girls with vulvovaginitis, candidal infections most commonly present with significant irritation but a paucity of discharge, although patients may complain of a thick plaque or discharge present at the introitus. Those with bacterial vaginosis typically have copious discharge, which is thin and malodorous, but very little true inflammation. Those with trichomoniasis have both inflammation and discharge. The provider should have a high index of suspicion for vaginal and vulvar pathology in girls of all ages who complain of itching, dysuria, drainage, irritation, or lower abdominal pain.

- *Diagnosis*: The diagnosis of vulvovaginitis depends on a careful history and physical examination. While the diagnosis is typically derived clinically, there are many potential causes of vulvovaginitis that may need to be investigated, including infection, chemical irritation, foreign bodies, allergy, systemic diseases, and sexual abuse. Important historical elements include hygiene habits, recent illnesses (particularly respiratory and GI), chemical irritant exposure, history of foreign body or masturbation, and sexual abuse. The provider should interview verbal children privately to query regarding inappropriate touching and abuse. The provider should do this in a way that is not frightening to the child.

  The provider should perform a complete physical examination, paying attention to other signs of injury, abuse, or neglect. When performing a vaginal examination on an infant, the easiest method is to perform an external examination in frog-legged position. As children become older, they may be very resistent to being examined. Other ways to examine a child that are sometimes more acceptable to the child is to have the child on knees and elbows on the bed, or to have the child in frog-legged position while seated on the caregiver's lap. In extreme cases, such as suspected abuse or irretrievable foreign body, the child may require an examination under anesthesia. Older, post-menarcheal girls may require a speculum examination, particularly if sexually active and the diagnosis of vaginitis versus cervicitis is unclear. Remember that cervicitis does not typically cause vaginal irritation, although it does cause discharge.

  The provider should carefully inspect the vulva and vaginal introitus, with attention to color, signs of injury, foreign body, or discharge. Vulvovaginitis should be distinguished from other common vulvar disorders including lichen sclerosis (which presents with intense pruritus and sharply demarcated, white, finely wrinkled skin around the vagina and anus), trauma, and labial adhesions (inability to separate the labia minora, which may be associated with concomitant vulvovaginitis). If inflammation and discharge are significant, diagnostic studies including wet mount, Gram's stain, and culture may be performed.

  Wet mount, pH, and a whiff test are by far the best immediate diagnostic tools at the disposal of the clinician in the setting of post-menarcheal girls, as candida species, *G. vaginalis*, and *T. vaginalis* are all identifiable with sensitivities in the mid 80s for these pathogens.[5] Candidal species will demonstrate budding yeast and a pH <5, with no significant odor to the discharge in the clinical setting of intense vulvar/vaginal irritation.[5] Bacterial vaginosis will present with pH >5, clue cells on microscopy, and a positive whiff test in the clinical setting of copious malodorous discharge.[5] Trichomoniasis will present with a pH >5.4 and a positive whiff test in the setting of discharge and irritation with a strawberry cervix.[5] A DNA probe for *T. vaginalis* is appropriate in this patient population, as well. Testing for specific pathogens (such as sexually transmitted infections and pinworms) may also be performed as indicated by the history and examination.

- *Treatment*: Mainstays of treatment for non-specific vaginitis are good hygiene and local care of inflamed tissues. The area should be cleaned gently with a mild fragrance- and dye-free soap and gently dried. Clothes similarly should be washed with mild fragrance- and dye-free detergents, and the child should be dressed in loose, breathable clothing. Small amounts of non-medicated ointment or barrier cream may be applied to protect tissues during the healing process. Cases refractory to these measures may be treated with short courses of topical low-potency corticosteroid creams. Antimicrobials may be administered if history, examination, and testing suggest a specific microbiologic cause or for cases that do not respond to the previously discussed measures. In post-menarcheal girls in whom wet mount does not provide a diagnosis, treatment for all three common causes of vaginitis is appropriate, as this covers more than 90 percent of all cases of vulvovaginitis in this age group. It is important to determine pregnancy status prior to initiation of treatent, as treatment regimens differ in pregnant and non-pregnant patients.

- *Disposition*: Most patients can be discharged home with supportive care as noted above. Arrangements should be made for outpatient follow-up with the patient's PCP.

Historical clues	Physical findings	Ancillary studies
• Vaginal discharge • Recent toilet training	• Vaginal discharge • Retained foreign body	• WBC on wet mount • Normal flora on culture

Follow-Up

The patient and mother were queried separately about the possibility of child abuse, and no concerns were identified. Symptoms were attributed to the retained foreign body secondary to inadequate hygiene. The foreign body was removed and the vulva cleaned gently with warm water and mild soap. The patient's mother was counseled regarding supervision of hygiene at this age, and the patient's pediatrician was contacted to assure close follow-up.

References

1. Van Eyk N, Allen L, Giesbrecht E, et al. Pediatric vulvovaginal disorders: A diagnostic approach and review of the literature. *J Obstet Gynaecol Can* 2009; 31: 650–62.

2. Yilmaz AE, Celik N, Soylu G, et al. Comparison of clinical and microbiological features of vulvovaginitis in prepubertal and pubertal girls. *J Formosan Med Assoc* 2012; 111: 392–6.

3. Beyitler I, Kavukcu S. Clinical presentation, diagnosis, and treatment of vulvovaginitis in girls: A current approach and review of the literature. *World J Pediatr* 2017; 13: 101–5.

4. Kim H, Chai SM, Ahn EH, et al. Clinical and microbiologic characteristics of vulvovaginitis in Korean prepubertal girls, 2009–2014: A single center experience. *Obstet Gynecol Sci* 2016; 59: 130–6.

5. Hainer BL, Gibson MV. Vaginitis: Diagnosis and treatment. *Am Fam Phys* 2011; 83: 807–15.

6. Zeger W, Holt K. Gynecologic infections. *Emerg Med Clin N Am* 2003; 21: 631–48.

Chapter 12

Skin Complaints

Case 1

Contributing Author: Efrat Rosenthal

History

The patient is a 6-year-old female, who presents with a painful lesion on her right buttocks. The lesion has been present for the last week, mildly red and elevated, and tender to touch. The patient has been seen by her pediatrician, who had started her on trimethoprim–sulfamethoxazole, which she has taken for 5 days, with no improvement or change in symptoms. She has not had any fevers and denies any discharge from the lesion. Her pediatrician saw her in the office again today and gave a prescription for cephalexin, and then sent her to the ED for possible incision and drainage. She has otherwise been in her usual health. Of note, the patient was on vacation about two weeks ago and was playing on a wooden structure. She did incur a splinter in the same area at the time; however, mom was able to pull it out (approximately 1 cm in length).

Past Medical History

- Healthy with no medical problems.
- UTD on immunizations.

Medications

- Currently taking trimethoprim–sulfamethoxazole.
- Has prescription for cephalexin, but has not started it yet.

Allergies

- NKDA.

Physical Examination and Ancillary Studies

- *Vital signs*: T 98.8 °F, HR 88, RR 18, BP 105/68, O$_2$ sat 100% on room air.

- *General*: The patient is a well-appearing, playful girl in no distress.
- *HEENT*: The patient's extraocular eye movements are intact, she has moist mucous membranes and a clear oropharynx. No overt trauma.
- *Neck*: No obvious trauma. Her neck is supple with no lymphadenopathy.
- *Cardiovascular*: The heart rate and rhythm are regular and there are no murmurs. The distal pulses are normal.
- *Lungs*: There are clear breath sounds bilaterally, with comfortable work of breathing.
- *Abdomen*: The abdomen is soft, non-tender, non-distended, with no masses or hepatosplenomegaly.
- *Extremities and skin*: The patient has an approximately 1-cm erythematous lesion on her right buttock that is mildly swollen, with no induration or fluctuance appreciated. The lesion is tender to palpation and has a punctate center with an overlying scab. Extremities are normal.
- *Neurologic*: Normal mental status and non-focal examination.
- *Pertinent imaging*: Bedside U/S performed and shown in Figures 12.1 and 12.2.

Questions for Thought

- What is the difference between inert and organic cutaneous foreign bodies?
- What are some complications that may stem from retained foreign bodies?
- What is the best diagnostic imaging to visualize an organic foreign body?
- Is antibiotic therapy necessary?

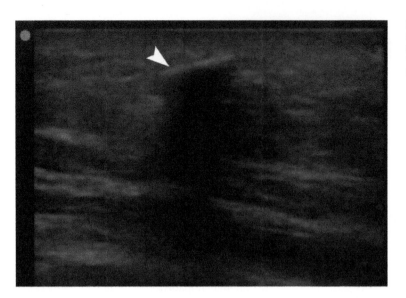

Figure 12.1 Bedside U/S (long-axis view) demonstrating a thin, elongated, approximately 1-cm foreign body about 1.5 cm deep in the tissue. No fluid collection or abscess visualized.

Diagnosis

- Foreign-body granuloma.

Discussion

- *Epidemiology*: There are millions of ED visits annually in the USA due to open wounds.[1] There is more information on uncomplicated soft-tissue wounds in Chapter 6, Case 4. Puncture wounds account for 3–5 percent of traumatic injuries presenting to the pediatric ED.[2] They are more frequent in the summer months, and penetrating wounds of the lower extremities are common, with more than half occuring in the foot.[1,2] Most puncture wounds occur as isolated minor events and medical care is generally not sought or required. Any object becomes a foreign body when it penetrates the skin and lodges in the soft tissue. It is estimated that 38 percent of foreign

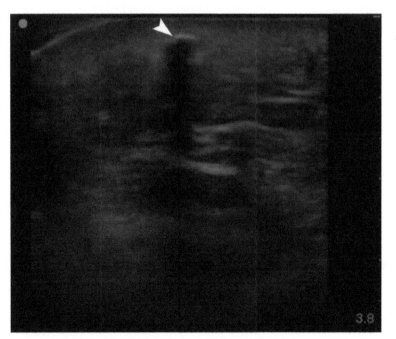

Figure 12.2 U/S Short-axis view of the foreign body, with the probe rotated by 90 degrees.

bodies are overlooked on initial examination, although history and imaging increase the diagnostic yield and make discharge of patients with an acute wound with a retained foreign body relatively uncommon. The majority of the injuries are caused by wood, metal, and glass; many are caused by thorns or fragments of wood that are retained in the limb, creating a foreign-body granuloma.[1-4]

- *Pathophysiology*: A retained foreign body may result in allergic, inflammatory, and infectious complications. The inflammatory response varies in intensity based on the composition of the object: inert materials (glass, plastic, metal) are non-reactive and generate less response than organic materials (bones, wood, rubber, soil, stones, or vegetative materials).[1,2,5] Inert materials are relatively low risk for infection and can be left in place if they are inaccessible and will not cause tissue damage or function deficit, while organic materials pose a higher risk.[1,5] Organic objects can cause a variety of bacterial and fungal infections, including synovitis from joint penetration, periosteal reactions, foreign-body granulomas, draining fistulas, and pseudotumors of the soft tissue. Wood is notorious for splintering and fragmenting, which is part of the reason it is high risk for being left as a foreign body and why extraction is so difficult.[1-3,5] Missed foreign bodies are a frequent cause of wound infections that are resistant to antibiotic therapy. Foreign-body granuloma, a chronic inflammatory process, may occur with foreign bodies left in place over time. Tissue becomes inflamed, and histolytic and macrophage reactions occur, forming multinucleated giant cell infiltration.[5] The foreign body may then become encapsulated with fibrous tissue and form a granuloma. The patient may present with chronic pain or inflammation at the skin site.
- *Presentation*: In acute foreign body, most patients will relate a history (such as breaking glass or stepping on an object) that suggests the possibility of a foreign body. In most cases of a retained foreign body, there is no clear history and patients cannot reliably report its presence, but a high index of suspicion is needed. Patients may present for evaluation several months or even years after the initial injury. Any injury with glass should raise the suspicion of a retained fragment, as these

are most commonly missed. Erythema, swelling, or persistent pain in the area of the puncture site suggests a retained foreign body. Chronic or recurrent infections at a specific site are also very suspicious for a retained foreign body. Foreign-body granulomas can also present as pseudotumors of both bone and soft tissue years after the initial injury. Depending on the time since the initial injury, a puncture wound overlying the lesion may or may not be visible.

- *Diagnosis*: A thorough history, exploring the possibility of a foreign body, is an important first step. Superficial foreign bodies can sometimes be palpated or visualized; however, relying solely on a clinical examination may lead to many missed foreign bodies on the initial examination.[1,3] Gently running a gloved finger over the suspected foreign-body site can elicit a characteristic foreign-body sensation in the patient.[2,3,5] Deeper foreign bodies may require imaging or surgical exploration to localize. Radiographs have traditionally been the first images obtained as they can detect approximately 80 percent of all foreign bodies, even the size of a pinpoint, if the foreign body is radiodense. Almost all types of glass (95 percent) 2 mm in size can be seen by X-ray, although smaller fragments are often missed.[1,3] Wooden foreign bodies have been reported to be visible by radiography in only about 10–15 percent of all cases, however, these may become invisible after 48 hours due to fluid absorption. U/S is a non-radiation modality that has been shown to accurately demonstrate the size, shape, and location of soft-tissue foreign bodies that are 2 mm or larger and it is superior to CT in the ability to detect objects.[6,7] Wood has a distinct signature on U/S; hyperechoic foci, often with acoustic shadowing and a hypoechoic halo; which is helpful in the identification of these otherwise difficult-to-find foreign bodies.[1,6] Though it has its limitations, U/S is portable, can be used real time, and does not utilize ionizing radiation, making it the preferred modality for the initial investigation of foreign bodies.[1,6,7]
- *Treatment*: The first step in treatment is to decide whether a removal attempt should be made in the ED. Removal is more likely to be successful if the object has been under the skin for less than 1 week, the entry wound is fresh, the object is visible, the object can be localized with imaging,

or the object can be felt during probing. Foreign bodies within or proximal to joints, flexor tendons, or blood vessels may require surgical consultation and removal within the OR.[7] Local anesthesia should be limited to minimize swelling near the foreign body, which can make localization more difficult. Using a number 15 scalpel blade, an incision over the entry point should be made and a small curved clamp can be used to explore the incision site for the foreign body.[5] Raking through the site to feel for the foreign body may assist localization. Raking is not recommended over delicate structures (i.e. nerves, flexor tendons) such as in the palm.[5] Once localized, the foreign body is grasped and removed. If the foreign body is wood, a small incision parallel to the course and angle of the object should be made so the splinter can be removed without leaving behind smaller splinters. After removal, the wound should be irrigated. Suturing of small incisions is not recommended as the site should be left open to drain, if necessary. Antibiotics should only be prescribed if there is evidence of an infection and tetanus prophylaxis should be given as necessary.[1] If a foreign body cannot be removed within 5 to 10 minutes, surgery should be consulted.

- *Disposition*: Most patients with foreign bodies are discharged from the ED after successful removal.[3] Patients with objects that cannot be extracted require outpatient surgical follow-up. Complications of foreign bodies can also dictate the patient disposition, such as infections requiring IV antibiotics and, therefore, admission.

Historical clues	Physical findings	Ancillary studies
• History of recent splinter removal • Persistent pain	• Normal vital signs • Tender erythematous lesion • Punctate center (entry site)	• U/S with foreign body

Follow-Up

The ED provider felt the foreign body was amenable to attempt at removal. A small incision was made and prior to probing, a splinter was easily extracted with external pressure. The wound was then irrigated and dressed. The patient was UTD with her vaccinations and did not require a tetanus booster. Her antibiotics were discontinued.

References

1. Wagstrom Halaas G. Management of foreign bodies in the skin. *Am Fam Phys* 2007; 76: 683–90.
2. Baldwin G, Colbourn M. Puncture wounds. *Pediatr Rev* 1999; 20: 21–3.
3. Levine MR, Gorman SM, Young CF, et al. Clinical characteristics and management of wound foreign bodies in the ED. *Am J Emerg Med* 2008; 26: 918–22.
4. Strecker-McGraw MK, Jones TR, Baer DG. Soft tissue wounds and principles of healing. *Emerg Med Clin N Am* 2007; 25: 1–22.
5. Trott AT. Common wound care problems. In *Wound and Lacerations: Emergency Care and Closure*, 4th edition. Philadelphia, PA: Saunders, 2012, pp. 220–35.
6. Graham DD. Ultrasound in the emergency department: Detection of wooden foreign bodies in the soft tissues. *J Emerg Med* 2002; 22: 75–9.
7. Boyse TD, Fessell DP, Jacobson JA, et al. Ultrasound of soft-tissue foreign bodies and associated complications with surgical correlation. *Radiographics* 2001; 21: 1251–6.

Case 2

Contributing Author: Efrat Rosenthal

History

The patient is a 12-year-old boy with history of autism, presenting with a rash on his lower legs bilaterally for 2 days. The patient has otherwise been in his usual state of health, afebrile, with no cold symptoms, cough, vomiting, diarrhea, fatigue, or weakness. The rash is not itchy or painful. It is located mostly on his lower legs, with some spots on his upper legs and trunk. Of note, the patient presented about 1 week ago to the ED with a chief complaint of left knee pain. The pain was thought to be secondary to a possible trauma at school because the patient does occasionally fall, though this injury was unwitnessed. At that visit the patient had an X-ray that was normal, and, given the history and normal physical examination, he was discharged home with acetaminophen and ibuprofen.

Past Medical History

- Autism.
- UTD on immunizations.

Medications

- Acetaminophen for knee pain.

Allergies

- NKDA.

Physical Examination and Ancillary Studies

- *Vital signs*: T 98.9 °F, HR 96, RR 18, BP 115/70, O_2 sat 99% on room air.
- *General*: The patient is alert, well-appearing, and interactive.
- *HEENT*: No signs of trauma. The patient has moist mucous membranes with no pharyngeal erythema. He has a few petechial spots in his posterior soft palate, with no vesicular or ulcerative lesions. The extraocular muscles are intact and PERRL.
- *Neck*: Supple and non-tender, with shotty cervical lymph nodes.
- *Cardiovascular*: Regular rate and rhythm. Intact and normal distal pulses.
- *Lungs*: Clear breath sounds bilaterally, with easy work of breathing.
- *Abdomen*: The patient's abdomen is soft, non-tender, non-distended, and there is no hepatosplenomegaly.
- *Extremities and skin*: The patient's skin shows a non-blanching petechial rash on both his lower extremities, with a few isolated lesions appreciated on his trunk. He has no signs of limb deformity or trauma.
- *Neurologic*: Awake and interactive, with a grossly normal neurologic examination.
- *Pertinent laboratory values*: WBC 42,000, Hb 7.9, Plt 37,000. On his peripheral blood differential, there are 31 percent blast forms. Electrolytes, phosphate, and uric acid normal.
- *Pertinent imaging*: Right knee radiograph from prior visit is normal.

Questions for Thought

- What are the typical laboratory findings in this type of patient?
- What other imaging would you like to get in the ED?
- What are two complications from this illness with which a patient can present to the ED?

Diagnosis

- Acute lymphoblastic leukemia (ALL).

Discussion

- *Epidemiology*: Childhood cancer is rare, with a reported incidence in the USA of approximately 1 case per 7,000 among children aged 15 years and younger.[1,2] Almost 40 percent of childhood cancers are hematologic malignancies. Acute leukemia is the most common form of childhood malignancy, comprising approximately 30 percent of all childhood cancers, with ALL being four to five times more common than acute myeloid leukemia (AML).[1,2] The incidence of ALL is approximately 3.4 cases per 100,000, with a peak incidence occurring between 2 and 5 years of age, and more commonly among boys than girls.[1,2] Several genetic disorders are associated with an increased risk of leukemia, including but not limited to Down's syndrome (trisomy 21), ataxia–telangiectasia, Wiskott–Aldrich syndrome, Bloom syndrome, Fanconi anemia, Kostmann disease, Klinefelter syndrome, Blackfan–Diamond anemia, and neurofibromatosis.[1]
- *Pathophysiology*: There is strong evidence that acquired genetic changes from environmental or genetic predisposition are central to the development of leukemia.[1–3] The exact causal factor is usually unknown, but the changes result in unregulated monoclonal cellular proliferation of hematopoietic or lymphoid cells, which then cause symptoms through bone-marrow replacement or proliferation of the malignant cells in other organs.
- *Presentation*: Leukemia proliferation within the bone marrow results in decreased production of normal white blood cells, red blood cells, and platelets. This decreased production of normal blood cells is often related to the initial signs and symptoms of leukemia, including fatigue, pallor, petechiae (as in this case), ecchymoses, mucosal bleeding, and a higher risk of infection.[1–4] The leukemic expansion within the bone marrow may also cause severe bone pain, limp, or refusal to walk; this presentation occurs in approximately 25 percent of children with newly diagnosed leukemia.[4] The extramedullary organs that are most frequently involved with leukemic infiltration are the liver, spleen, and lymph nodes.[1,2] Many affected children initially present with an enlargement of these organs on physical examination. Any body organ can be potentially

involved in leukemia, including the CNS, testes, skin, kidneys, lungs, pleura, pericardium, eyes, breasts, ovaries, and GI tract.

- *Diagnosis*: Hematologic malignancy should be considered in children with longstanding, unexplained fevers, longstanding, unresolved adenopathy, organomegaly, petechial rash, atraumatic bone pain, or recurrent infection. Initial blood work with a CBC and manual differential will detect circulating leukemic blast cells in most patients. There are other conditions, such as infectious mononucleosis, that can result in atypical white cells in the blood. A bone marrow examination, therefore, is essential for conclusive diagnosis of leukemia, as well as an adjunct in identifying specific subtypes of leukemia, which may require different approaches in management.[3] Once the suspicion of leukemia is high on the differential, a CXR should be performed to evaluate for the presence of a mediastinal mass, which may be present in the setting of a lymphoma.

- *Treatment*: Initial management includes initiation of IV fluids, blood work (including CBC with manual differentiation, electrolytes, uric acid, renal and liver function tests, coagulation studies), and admission to a pediatric cancer center. Patients then commonly receive transfusion support, treatment of suspected or proven infections with broad-spectrum antibiotics, and correction of any metabolic imbalances that may be present in patients with high tumor burden secondary to tumor lysis syndrome. Rarely, a patient may require leukophoresis or exchange transfusion to control extreme leukocytosis.[1] Patients are scheduled for urgent bone-marrow aspiration and biopsy for diagnostic accuracy and cytogenetics, as well as LP to assess CNS involvement.[3] These results are used for a risk-group stratification of the patient in order to reduce toxicity in low-risk patients while ensuring appropriate, more aggressive therapy for those with high-risk disease or relapse.[3] Successful treatment of children with ALL involves the administration of a multidrug regimen, which is divided into several phases: induction, consolidation, and maintenance.

- *Disposition*: Children diagnosed with leukemia should be referred to a pediatric cancer center for admission and to undergo the above treatment.

Historical clues	Physical findings	Ancillary studies
• Atraumatic leg pain • New rash	• Petechial rash • Lymphadenopathy	• CBC with elevated WBC and blast forms • Negative knee X-ray

Follow-Up

The likely diagnosis of leukemia was recognized in this patient presenting with a petechial rash in the setting of left knee pain. Given the clinical finding of petechiae and associated differential diagnoses, the patient quickly had a CBC that revealed lymphoblastic cells, consistent with a leukemic process. The patient subsequently had a CXR to rule out a mediastinal mass. Hematology–oncology was consulted, and he had further blood tests to assess for possible tumor lysis syndrome, the results of which were within normal range. He was started on IV fluids and admitted for further evaluation, including LP and bone-marrow aspiration, followed by the initiation of chemotherapeutic treatment.

References

1. Campana D, Pui CH. Childhood leukemia. In Niederhuber JE, Armitage JO, Dorshow JH, Kastan MB, Tepper JE, eds., *Abeloff's Clinical Oncology*, 5th edition. Philadelphia, PA: Elsevier, 2014, pp. 1849–72.
2. Hunger SP, Mulligan CG. Acute lymphoblastic leukemia in children. *N Engl J Med* 2015; 373: 1541–52.
3. Hutter JJ. Childhood leukemia. *Pediatr Rev* 2010; 31: 234–40.
4. Simone JV, Verzosa MS, Rudy JA. Initial features and prognosis in 363 children with acute lymphocytic leukemia. *Cancer* 1975; 36: 2099–108.

Case 3

Contributing Authors: Sundeep M. Shukla and Rebecca Jeanmonod

History

The patient is a 3-year-old male who presents to the ED after pulling hot water onto himself. While the patient's mother was boiling a pot of water to make rice, the child used a stepstool and pulled down the pot of water. His mother ran in from the pantry closet to find him lying on the ground with hot water over his trunk and hands. The patient did not have any loss of consciousness and cried immediately.

The mother applied calamine lotion to the effected regions and then brought the child in for evaluation.

Past Medical History

- Asthma.
- Prior clavicle fracture.

Medications

- Albuterol as needed.

Allergies

- NKDA.

Physical Examination and Ancillary Studies

- *Vital signs*: T 98.6 °F, HR 121, RR 27, BP 92/68, O$_2$ sat 100% on room air.
- *General*: The child looks underweight and has tattered clothes. The patient is crying but without cyanosis or stridor.
- *HEENT*: PERRL. Mucous membranes moist. Oropharynx clear.
- *Neck*: Supple and non-tender, with no adenopathy.
- *Cardiovascular*: Regular tachycardia, with no M/R/G.
- *Lungs*: Normal work of breathing, with clear and equal breath sounds.
- *Abdomen*: Soft and non-distended. No masses or organomegaly.
- *Extremities and skin*: There is erythema over the head, face, and neck, with blisters containing serous fluid present on the anterior surface of the neck. There is also erythema and blisters on the anterior chest, epigastric region, and on the right hand. The patient has 14 percent total burns on the body. There is no extremity deformity.
- *Neurologic*: All wounded skin has intact sensation to light touch.
- *Pertinent laboratory values*: WBC 8,000, Hb 12, HCT 38, CPK 190, BUN 10, Cr 0.9, K 3.6, all other laboratory values are normal.

Questions for Thought

- Is the mother's description of the injury consistent with the patient's physical findings?
- What management should be initiated in the ED?
- How does management of this patient differ from that of patients who are victims of electrical burns?

- How does management of this patient differ from that of patients with staphylococcal scalded skin syndrome, Stevens–Johnson syndrome, toxic epidermal necrolysis, or other desquamating rashes?

Diagnosis

- Superficial and superficial partial-thickness burns.

Discussion

- *Epidemiology*: Burns are a common problem in children, and scald burns are the most common cause of burns in children younger than 5 years of age.[1] Hot-tap-water burns cause more hospitalizations than any other hot liquid. Burns are discussed in more detail in Chapter 2, Case 5. Electrical burns are less common than scald burns, but can have significant morbidity and mortality.
- *Pathophysiology*: Burns disrupt the integrity of the skin, causing a local and systemic inflammatory reaction, which ultimately results in fluid shifts from the vascular space into the interstitial space. This occurs as a consequence of changes in vascular permeability due to the presence of mediators including histamine, serotonin, prostaglandins, platelet products, complement components, and kinin.[2,3] There is more information on the pathophysiology of cutaneous burns in Chapter 2, Case 5.

  Electrical burns are caused by electrical current passing through the body to the ground, closing a circuit. Like cutaneous burns, electrical burns disrupt tissue, increase capillary permeability, and result in fluid shifts and intravascular volume depletion. Unlike cutaneous burns, however, the extent of the tissue damage from electrical burns is difficult to assess based on physical examination alone. This is because electricity travels along the course of least resistance (neurovascular bundles) and creates heat in areas of high resistance (bone), and therefore the tissue damage and destruction are not evident on skin examination. The provider may only be able to appreciate an entrance wound/eschar and an exit wound/eschar. Furthermore, an electrical current may cause involuntary muscle contraction (resulting in musculoskeletal injury, blunt/blast injury, or rhabdomyolysis), seizure, or cardiac arrest.

Staphylococcal scalded skin syndrome is caused by infection with *Staphylococcus aureus*, which releases an exfoliative toxin.[4] It occurs predominantly in young children and neonates, with almost all cases presenting before age 6.[4] The disease is typically contracted from asymptomatic carriers of the bacteria.

Toxic epidermal necrolysis (which involves greater than 30 percent of the skin surface) and Stevens–Johnson syndrome (which involves less than 10 percent of the skin's surface, but has mucosal involvement) occur most commonly due to pharmacologic agents, athough infections, radiation, sunlight exposure, connective-tissue disorders, and malignancies may also be involved.[5] Although the cleavage site within the skin differs in staphylococcus scalded skin syndrome as compared to toxic epidermal necrolysis and Stevens–Johnson syndrome, the end result is disruption of the barrier function of the skin, just like in a cutaneous burn. Thus, patients undergo the same fluid shifts and pathophysiologic consequences as burn patients.

- *Presentation*: Most patients with a burn will present with a consistent history for the injuries you see. Presentation depends upon the type of burn, the depth of the burn, and the burn location. There is more information on burn presentation in Chapter 2, Case 5. In cases of an electrical burn, patients may present with severe pain, seizure, renal failure, rhabdomyolysis, hypotension, or cardiac arrest. They may also present with isolated mouth burns from chewing on electrical wires.

- *Diagnosis*: It is critically important to assess the total surface area involved in cutaneous burns. All patients must be completely disrobed and examined. When available, the Lund and Browder chart is a reliable method to assess burn area in children. Otherwise, a modified rule of 9s may be used (Figure 2.7).

  In children with exfoliating rashes and no history of a burn, a history should be sought for new pharmacologic agents and infectious disease symptoms. The involved surface area should be calculated for these children, as well, and a note made of mucosal lesions.

- *Treatment*: Initial management should focus on the airway. Burn patients will need supplemental oxygen immediately on arrival and a quick examination of the airway, as singed facial hairs and carbonaceous sputum are important signs that an inhalational injury has occurred. The use of a nasopharyngoscope can help evaluate injury from the burns.

  IV access and fluid resuscitation are an important aspect of burn care management. Many resuscitation formulas are available, with the most prominent being the modified Parkland formula. The patient is to receive IV fluids at 4 mL/kg per percentage burn area, with half of the volume given in the first 8 hours (starting from when burn occurred) and the remaining half administered over the next 16 hours. In addition, adding maintenance fluids has also been vital to resuscitating tissues in children and is widely practiced in most burn centers.[6-8] Superficial or first-degree burns are not used in calculating the total body surface area involved when using the modified Parkland formula.

  Careful volume resuscitation is also important in children with other exfoliating conditions, following typical resuscitation endpoints, such as urine output. Children believed to have staphylococcus scalded skin syndrome should receive anti-staphylococcal antibiotics. There is no role for routine antibiotic use in other exfoliating dermatoses or in cutaneous burns.

  Care of cutaneous burns is outlined in detail in Chapter 2, Case 5.

- *Disposition*: Depending on what burns are encountered the patient can be managed at home, in the hospital, or may need to be transferred to a burn center. Transfer to a burn center should occur in the following circumstances, which are outlined in criteria established by the American Burn Association:[1]

  · Partial-thickness burns greater than 10 percent of the total body surface area.
  · Burns that involve the face, hands, feet, genitalia, perineum, or major joints.
  · Full-thickness burns in any age group.
  · Electrical burns, including lightning injury.
  · Chemical burns.
  · Inhalation injury.

- Burn injury in patients with preexisting medical disorders that could complicate management, prolong recovery, or affect mortality.
- Any patient with burns and concomitant trauma (such as fractures) in which the burn injury poses the greatest risk of morbidity or mortality. In such cases, if the trauma poses the greater immediate risk, the patient may be initially stabilized in a trauma center before being transferred to a burn unit. Physician judgment will be necessary in such situations and should be in concert with the regional medical control plan and triage protocols.
- Burned children in hospitals without qualified personnel or equipment for the care of children.
- Burn injury in patients who will require special social, emotional, or rehabilitative intervention.

Some patients may need to be admitted to a hospital, but not necessarily transferred to a burn center. Cases in which there is concern that the caretaker may not be able to provide appropriate wound care is one example. Inability to provide adequate pain management, poor access to follow-up care, and concern for child abuse are other indications for admission.

Patients who are discharged home must have adequate training on dressing changes. Methodical dressing changes are required to keep the burn sites clean. Adequate supplies of dry gauze and ointments should be arranged for home. Instructions should be given detailing the procedure for dressing changes and also providing recommendations for close follow-up. Patients may also benefit from a visiting nurse to help with dressing changes. As previously discussed, appropriate pain control is essential when administering dressing changes, and also ensuring adequate comfort of the burn patient at home.

Providers need to educate the patient and guardians about potential complications, such as infections. Variations such as discharge color, worsening appearance of the wound, and bleeding from the wound should promptly lead to notification of their provider. Photos taken during dressing changes can help evaluate the progress of wound healing. Another possible delayed complication is compartment syndrome, which could limit blood flow and cause irreversible tissue damage. Pain may intensify, necessitating narcotic medications, but return precautions should be given for severe pain as this could also indicate infection or compartment syndrome.

Historical clues	Physical findings	Ancillary studies
• History of pulling down boiling water	• Cutaneous blisters • Splash burns	• Unremarkable laboratory tests

Follow-Up

This patient had superficial partial-thickness burns greater than 10 percent of the body surface area and required transfer to a burn center. His injury was consistent with the mechanism described by his mother. He received appropriated pain medications and IV fluids per the modified Parkland formula. His care included several weeks of follow-up within a burn clinic after discharge from the inpatient burn center. The patient had a full recovery. The mother was also educated on using a back burner and other ways to prevent injury.

References

1. Kramer CB, Rivara FP, Klein MB. Variations in US pediatric burn injury hospitalizations using burn repository data. *J Burn Care Res* 2010; 31: 734–9.

2. Merz J, Schrand C, Mertens D, et al. Wound care of the pediatric burn patient. *AACN Clin Issues Adv Pract Acute Crit Care* 2003; 14: 429–41.

3. Reed J, Pomerantz W. Emergency management of pediatric burns. *Pediatr Emerg Care* 2005; 21: 118–29.

4. Mishra AK, Yadav P, Mishra A. A systematic review on staphylococcal scalded skin syndrome: A rare and critical disease of neonates. *Open Microbiol J* 2016; 10: 150–9.

5. Usatine RP, Sandy N. Dermatologic emergencies. *Am Fam Phys* 2010; 82: 773–80.

6. Alharbi Z, Piatkowski A, Dembinski R, et al. Treatment of burns in the first 24 hours: Simple and practical guide by answering 10 questions in a step-by-step form. *World J Emerg Surg* 2012; 7: 13.

7. Hettiaratchy S, Papini R. Initial management of a major burn: II – Assessment and resuscitation. *BMJ* 2004; 329: 101–3.

8. Sharma RK, Parashar A. Special considerations in paediatric burn patients. *Ind J Plast Surg* 2010; 43: S43–50.

Case 4

Contributing Author: Amanda Shorette

History

The patient is a 5-year-old female, who presented from an outside hospital after sustaining a dog bite to the face. She had been bitten by a pitbull, who was owned by a family friend, while visiting the child's home. The attack was witnessed by the patient's older sister and the dog's owner but neither were present in the ED to provide exact details. The dog's vaccination status was unknown but the animal was taken into custody by animal control. The child was evaluated at a community ED, where she was noted to have extensive injuries to the right side of her face, including several complex lacerations, with eyelid and intraoral involvement. IV antibiotics and analgesia were provided and she was subsequently transferred to a tertiary hospital.

Past Medical History

- UTD on immunizations.
- No significant medical problems.

Medications

- None.

Allergies

- NKDA.

Physical Examination and Ancillary Studies

- *Vital signs*: T 99.0 °F, HR 129, RR 24, BP 107/73, O_2 sat 98% on room air.
- *General*: The patient is awake, alert, sitting up in bed. She is anxious but responds appropriately.
- *HEENT*: The patient's globes are grossly intact bilaterally, with intact extraocular movements. PERRL. There is a 2-cm full-thickness laceration of the right lower lid. Her vision is grossly intact. She has a complex 8-cm laceration to the right fronto-temporal scalp and forehead, just lateral to the right orbit. There is a separate 2-cm laceration to her right cheek. In addition, there are multiple puncture wounds on her right cheek and along the angle of the mandible. There is a large intraoral laceration seen at the gum line at the right lateral jaw. There is mobility of the right lower jaw and right lower teeth. There are no lacerations or trauma noted to the tongue. The posterior oropharynx is patent. There is no nasal or ear involvement.
- *Neck*: There is no swelling or tenderness to the neck. She has full range of motion.
- *Cardiovascular*: Mildly tachycardic but regular, without M/R/G.
- *Lungs*: Respirations are non-labored, with no stridor or adventitious upper-airway noise. There are clear lung sounds bilaterally and no evidence of chest-wall trauma.
- *Abdomen*: Her abdomen is soft, non-tender, and non-distended, with normal bowel sounds.
- *Extremities and skin*: No evidence of extremity injury.
- *Neurologic*: The patient is alert and oriented. She has good postural tone. She has a GCS of 15. She is able to appreciate touch to the right side of her face but the examination is limited by pain and the extent of the injury. There is right upper lid weakness and limited smile on the right. The remainder of her cranial nerve examination is intact.
- *Pertinent laboratory values*: Hb 11.8, HCT 33.1.
- *Pertinent imaging*: CT reconstruction shown in Figure 12.3.

Questions for Thought

- Which animal bite wounds should be closed primarily?
- When should prophylactic antibiotics be used for animal bites?
- When is post-exposure prophylaxis (tetanus, rabies) indicated?
- When should you consider ancillary testing, such as imaging, in this kind of patient?
- When should you consider urgent/emergent specialty consultation?

Diagnosis

- Severe facial dog-bite injury, complicated by complex maxillofacial fractures.

Discussion

- *Epidemiology*: Animal and human bites represent a significant health issue in the USA with 3–6 million occurrences per year. Dogs cause 80–90 percent of these animal bite wounds, with 800,000 Americans seeking medical attention for

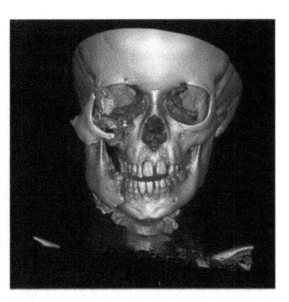

Figure 12.3 CT of head and face. There is no acute intracranial injury. There are numerous comminuted facial fractures, notably a comminuted orbital floor fracture, comminuted zygomaticomaxillary complex fracture, zygomatic arch fracture, fracture of the greater wing of the right sphenoid, and open comminuted mandible fracture–dislocation, with displacement of multiple primary teeth. The right orbit is also noted to be displaced inferiorly but without radiographic evidence of globe injury or optic nerve injury. For the color version, please refer to the plate section.

dog bites.[1-4] Dog attacks kill approximately 20–35 people each year, mainly infants and small children.[1] Most affected individuals know the dog that attacked them. Children are especially vulnerable to dog attacks because of their small size and proximity to the dog's mouth as well as their uninhibited behavior around dogs. Cat bites are the second most common type of animal bite with 400,000 annual cases, representing 5–15 percent of animal bite wounds. Feline attacks typically are underreported because they are perceived as less serious than other forms of animal bites; however, approximately 6 percent of patients inflicted with cat bites will require hospitalization.[2,3] Compared to dog bites, cat bites tend to affect older individuals, with females being predominantly affected.[2,3]

- *Pathophysiology*: Dog bites can lead to a range of injuries, but given their rounded teeth and powerful jaws they typically cause crush injuries.[3,5] Abrasions, lacerations, puncture wounds, and even avulsion injuries or amputation can be seen.[3,5] Cats inflict wounds with both their

teeth and their claws, with injuries typically presenting as abrasions or small, deep puncture wounds.[2,3] Bite wounds tend to colonize with the native oral flora of the animal that inflicted the injury, notably anaerobic (i.e. *Pasteurella*), *Staphylococcus*, and *Streptococcus* species. Dog bites are known to inoculate wounds with *Prevotella* species and *Capnocytophaga canimorsus*, which can rarely result in fulminant systemic infection characterized by a profound inflammatory response, leading to shock, disseminated intravascular coagulation, and multi-system organ failure.

- *Presentation*: In children less than 9 years, the head and neck are the most common sites of dog-bite injury, while in people older than 10 years, the extremities, particularly the hand, are mostly affected.[2,3] Dog-bite patients tend to present either within 8–12 hours after the injury for acute wound management and concern for rabies prophylaxis or much later after the development of signs of infection. Patients with infection tend to present around 35 hours after the bite. Dog bites have an infection rate ranging from 1.6 to 30 percent.[2,3,6] Cat bites typically present later than dog bites, often only after the patient has developed an infectious complication. Cat wound infection rates are high, with an incidence of 15–50 percent.[6] The penetrating nature of cat bites predisposes patients to deep abscess formation and osteomyelitis. Signs of infection can occur rapidly, often within 12–24 hours, which is typical of *Pasteurella* infections.[3] Animal-bite patients may also present with wounds infected after primary repair, which can manifest as fever, erythema, swelling, tenderness, purulent drainage, and lymphadenitis near the site. These patients typically present 24 hours or later after the time of injury.

- *Diagnosis*: A detailed history of the circumstances surrounding the injury is critical, including (1) time and location of the bite event, (2) type/breed of the animal, (3) vaccination history of the animal, (4) vaccination history of the victim, (5) behavior of the animal and its current whereabouts, (6) provoked versus unprovoked attack, (7) anatomic location of the wound(s), (8) any pre-hospital treatment, and (9) any underlying medical factors that may impair wound healing or increase the risk of infection (i.e. immunocompromised state, diabetes, asplenic patients).[2-4,6] These factors are important in determining the risk of wound infection and the need for rabies prophylaxis. The wound should be thoroughly inspected under local anesthesia to assess the extent and depth of the injury, to identify an injury to deeper structures, including neurovascular or tendon injuries, to visualize devitalized tissue, and to determine the presence of a foreign body.[6] The bottom of the wound should be visualized and examined under range of motion, if possible. Laboratory studies are indicated only in patients who present with infected bite wounds and signs of systemic infection; in such cases, the clinician should consider a CBC, CRP, and ESR but should know that normal values may still be seen in patients with cellulitis, joint infection, osteomyelitis, and even sepsis. Wound cultures should be obtained in infected bites when possible before initiating antibiotic therapy and the laboratory should be notified that the sample is an animal bite, since oral flora common in infected bite wounds (*Pasteurella multocida* in cats and dogs) tend to be fastidious and easily misidentified. Wound cultures are not indicated in clinically uninfected bites since they do not correlate with a risk of subsequent infection or pathologic organism in later-occurring infections. Consider radiography if there is concern for an underlying fracture, such as with deep bite wounds or bites near joints. Also obtain radiographs if there is concern for retained foreign bodies such as embedded teeth. Plain radiographs may be indicated in markedly infected wounds to assess for bony injury, subcutaneous gas, and a change associated with osteomyelitis. U/S is helpful when assessing for abscess formation or radiolucent foreign bodies. Dog bites to the head can result in penetration of the skull and even meningitis or brain abscess formation; head CT scans are warranted with deep dog bites and puncture wounds to the scalp or face to assess for fracture, especially in children less than 2 years of age.

- *Treatment*: All wounds should be assessed for active bleeding and a neurovascular assessment should be performed. Direct pressure should be applied to any active bleeding, and resuscitation should be promptly initiated when needed. If the patient is stable and no emergent intervention is needed, then the clinician can proceed with wound care. Meticulous wound care is central to treating animal bites. Copious pressurized irrigation with 5–8 psi (18–20-gauge blunt needle attached to a 30–60-mL syringe using 250–500 mL of solution) is the most important means of preventing infection by reducing bacteria counts in the wound.[2-4,6,7] This method may reduce infection rates fivefold, although it should be noted that this is less effective for puncture wounds. Any devitalized tissue should be debrided as this has been shown to be effective in preventing infection by removing a potential infection nidus.[2-4,6,7] Careful wound exploration and foreign-body removal should be done, with special attention to any fascial or joint capsule violation. Puncture wounds are more challenging to manage since no specific wound treatment method has been proven to reduce infection rates; however, the general consensus states that any superficial debridement of non-viable tissue should be performed. "Coring," or removal of deep tissue, is not recommended.

There is an abundance of literature addressing how to repair animal bites; however, the evidence is conflicting. The general consensus suggests that when considering whether or not to close a wound primarily, by delayed primary closure, or by secondary intention, the clinician should consider the location, the complexity, and the age of the wound.[2,3,7] Untreated bites more than 6–12 hours old are at higher risk of infection. Primary closure of wounds can be performed in simple lacerations, those that are clinically uninfected, face and scalp wounds, and bites less than 12 hours old on the extremities or body.[2,3] Wounds at higher risk for infection with primary closure include (1) crush injuries, (2) puncture wounds, (3) bites involving the hands and feet, (4) wounds more than 24 hours old on the face and more than 12 hours old elsewhere, (5) cat and human bites not located on the face, and (6) bite wounds in immunocompromised hosts.[2,3] Hand bites have an infection rate of 30–40 percent.[7] In contrast, scalp and facial bites demonstrate a low infection rate and it is therefore recommended to close all of these when presenting within 24 hours. Facial injuries presenting greater than 24 hours are more controversial, but the consensus shows that primary closure for uninfected wounds and delayed primary closure for contaminated-appearing wounds are acceptable approaches. Deep sutures and cyanoacrylate tissue adhesive (glue) should be avoided when possible as these repair methods can create an anaerobic environment and inhibit drainage of infected material, if wound infection should occur.[2,3] Wounds that cannot be closed primarily should be left open to drain, dressed with wet-to-dry dressings twice a day, and examined daily to assess for infection, with debridement as needed. If after 72 hours the wound does not appear clinically infected and it is in a cosmetically important area, then delayed primary closure can be performed. Secondary intention should be allowed for very-high-risk wounds and wounds complicated by infection.

Evidence is especially mixed on the use of antibiotic prophylaxis in animal-bite wounds. Cat bites as well as other deep puncture wounds should receive prophylaxis due to the high risk of infection.[2-7] Antibiotics should also be strongly considered in moderate to severe injuries with associated crush injury; wounds located on the hands, genitalia, or in close proximity to bones or joints; bites in compromised hosts; and human bites through the dermis.[2-7] Prophylaxis should be given for 3–5 days. When clinically infected, antibiotic courses should be for at least 10 days, and any suture material from a prior repair should be removed. Antibiotic choice should be directed toward coverage of anaerobes and *Staphylococcus*, *Streptococcus*, and *Pasteurella* species. First-line choice is amoxicillin–clavulanate. Alternative therapies include an agent with activity against *P. multicoda* (doxycycline, trimethoprim–sulfamethoxazole, penicillin VK, cefuroxime, moxifloxacin) plus an agent with anaerobic activity (metronidazole, clindamycin).

Animal bites are tetanus-prone wounds, therefore the immunization status of the patient should be addressed and tetanus toxoid vaccine administered when indicated. The need for tetanus immune globulin should also be assessed. Children with no immunizations require both tetanus immune globulin and tetanus immunization.

The patient's risk for rabies exposure should be evaluated especially in unprovoked animal bites, if the animal appears ill, or if the animal is wild or a stray. The rabies vaccination status of the dog or cat should be determined when possible. The CDC provides guidelines regarding the risk of contracting the rabies virus and when to administer post-exposure prophylaxis.[1] Previously unvaccinated individuals with potential rabies exposure should receive both the rabies vaccine and rabies immune globulin.

Surgical consultation should be considered for deep wounds that penetrate bone, tendons, and joints.[3] Complex facial lacerations, wounds associated with neurovascular compromise, and wounds with complex infections (abscess formation, osteomyelitis, and septic joint), especially of the hand, also warrant surgical consultation.

- *Disposition*: Patients with simple bite wounds can be treated in the ED and discharged home with good wound care instructions, close follow-up, and prophylactic antibiotic therapy, if warranted. Superficial wound infections can be managed with wound debridement as needed, oral antibiotic therapy, and close outpatient follow-up. Wounds complicated by abscess formation require surgical intervention. Wounds with either infection involving deep structures, associated signs of systemic infection, or persistent infection despite outpatient antibiotic therapy require admission for IV antibiotics and possible surgical management. Admission should also be considered for immunocompromised individuals and those with poor follow-up or history of medication non-adherence.

Historical clues	Physical findings	Ancillary studies
• Dog bite • Pitbull • UTD immunizations for both dog and child	• Obvious facial deformity and injury • Intact airway • Unstable facial and jaw bones	• Unremarkable laboratory tests • Head CT with orbital and mandibular fractures

Follow-Up

The patient was managed by an interdisciplinary team of surgical specialists and required multiple reconstructive surgeries. Post-operatively, she does have some facial scarring and ptosis of her right eyelid but has preserved vision and intact function of her face and jaw.

References

1. Centers for Disease Control and Prevention (CDC). Preventing dog bites. See www.cdc.gov/features/dog-bite-prevention/ (accessed February 2017).

2. Ellis R, Ellis C. Dog and cat bites. *Am Fam Phys* 2014; 90: 239–43.

3. Eilbert WP. Dog, cat and human bites. Providing safe and cost-effective treatment in the ED. *Emerg Med Pract* 2003; 5: 1–20.

4. Aziz H, Rhee P, Pandit V, et al. The current concepts in management of animal (dog, cat, snake, scorpion) and human bite wounds. *J Trauma Acute Care Surg* 2015; 78: 641–8.

5. Chhabra S, Chhabra N, Gaba S. Maxillofacial injuries due to animal bites. *J Maxillofac Oral Surg* 2015; 14: 142–53.

6. Nakamura Y, Daya M. Use of appropriate antimicrobials in wound management. *Emerg Med Clin N Am* 2007; 25: 159–76.

7. Kennedy SA, Stoll LE, Lauder AS. Human and other mammalian bite injuries to the hand: evaluation and management. *J Am Acad Orthop Surg* 2015; 23: 47–57.

Case 5

Contributing Author: Benjamin Kitt

History

The patient is a 24-month-old female accompanied by her mother, who presents to the ED with a complaint of a mark on her cheek that mom believes is secondary to some kind of trauma incurred while playing with her brother. The mother reports that she was in the kitchen when she heard her daughter start crying in the bedroom, where she was playing with her 4-year-old brother. When her mother entered the room, she found the patient crying and holding her face. The patient told her mother that her brother hit her in the face, but the brother denied this and reported that the patient hit her face on the door. The mother is now concerned about the bruise on her daughter's face and wants to make sure "everything is alright." Since the incident, the patient has been acting normally, has not vomited, and is not complaining of pain. The child lives with mom, mom's boyfriend, and her older brother.

Past Medical History

- UTD on immunizations.
- No medical problems or known bleeding diathesis.

Medications

- None.

Allergies

- NKDA.

Physical Examination and Ancillary Studies

- *Vital signs*: T 99.1 °F, HR 95, RR 24, BP 96/60, O$_2$ sat 100% on room air.
- *General*: The patient is alert, awake, and acting appropriately for her age. She is happy, smiling, and playful with staff.
- *HEENT*: PERRL. No subconjunctival or retinal hemorrhages. Mucous membranes are moist. There is a large bruise over the patient's left cheek, which has petechiae and purpura in parallel lines. There are no other regions of petechiae or ecchymoses. There are no obvious facial fractures, Battle's sign, raccoon eyes, or hemotympanum.
- *Neck*: Supple and non-tender, with midline trachea and no adenopathy.
- *Cardiovascular*: Regular rate and rhythm, with no M/R/G.
- *Lungs*: Clear and equal, with normal work of breathing. No W/R/R.
- *Abdomen*: The patient has normoactive bowel sounds. Her abdomen is soft and non-tender to palpation. No signs of trauma or noticeable bruising.
- *Extremities and skin*: There is no swelling or tenderness. Full range of motion with good capillary refill.
- *Neurologic*: Intact cranial nerves. Non-focal examination.

Questions for Thought

- What concerns do you have about the bruise?
- What reasons might the history be concerning?
- Would you order any laboratory or radiographic imaging?
- What is the patient's disposition?

Diagnosis

- Child abuse with facial hand-slap bruising.

Discussion

- *Epidemiology*: According to the US Department of Health and Human Services, a 2013 report estimated that 679,000 children were victims of abuse and neglect, which roughly translates to an incidence of 1 percent amongst the population.[1] Although the rate of child abuse has been declining, physicians need to be aware that roughly 1 out of 100 children they see will be a victim of neglect or abuse. Most victims of abuse or neglect are below the age of 5 (47 percent) with 27.3 percent below 3 years old and 19.7 percent between 3 and 5 years old.[1] Males and females are victims of abuse or neglect in similar percentages: 48.7 percent for males and 50.9 percent for females. According to the 2013 data, 82 percent of abusers are the biological parent and 18 percent are others, such as another relative, foster parent, daycare worker, etc.[1]

- *Pathophysiology*: According to the Child Abuse Prevention and Treatment Act the term "child abuse and neglect" means, at a minimum, any recent "act or failure to act on the part of a parent or caretaker, which results in death, serious physical or emotional harm, sexual abuse or exploitation, or an act or failure to act which presents an imminent risk of serious harm."[2] According to the act, "The term 'child' means a person who has not attained the lesser of the age of 18; or except in the case of sexual abuse, the age specified by the child protection law of the State in which the child resides."[2] The risk factors for abuse are hard to identify and track; however, a few have been described. The greatest risk factor for a patient is age. If the child is younger than 5 years old he or she falls into the age range with the highest percentage of abuse. Parental risk factors include but are not limited to lack of child care skills, substance abuse, and history of child maltreatment. Child abuse is divided into four types of abuse and includes neglect, physical abuse, emotional abuse, and sexual abuse.[1,2] Neglect is the most common type of maltreatment, followed by physical abuse, with emotional and sexual abuse having roughly similar percentages.
- *Presentation*: Child abuse and neglect can present in a variety of ways, and therefore physicians must be vigilant in performing a thorough history and physical examination on any patient where abuse or neglect is suspected. Obtaining a history from the patient is often difficult as over half of the children abused are under the age of 5. Initial

questioning should be open-ended.[3] Open-ended questions can be followed by more specific questions but yes or no questions should be avoided.[3,4] For patients who are non-verbal, the history will be based on the parent or family account of what happened. Clinical gestalt will be important when assessing the validity of the parent's story. Concerning factors for abuse include a vague history or the injury not matching the history. An account not matching the patient's developmental abilities and inconsistent histories are also more concerning for abuse. More information on presentation of child abuse is available in Chapter 2, Case 4.

A thorough physical examination must be performed if abuse is suspected, which includes a head-to-toe examination with the patient undressed. Examine the skin looking for bruising in different stages of healing or in centrally located areas. Children who are walking commonly have bruising on their anterior shins, but centrally located bruising such as to the abdomen, ears, and neck are concerning for abuse.

Look at the pattern on the bruise. Does it look like a hand slap, belt, or cord? In the case described above the slap was in the shape of a hand and contained multiple parallel lines, which occur when capillaries break between the fingers. When assessing burns, assess to see if the distribution of burned area matches with the story. If the story is a cup of hot tea pulled down from the table, is the burn consistent with a splash or is it uniform and suggestive of submersion in hot water? Look for signs of fractures and order appropriate imaging studies. A thorough ophthalmologic examination should be performed to assess for signs of "shaken baby syndrome," such as bilateral retinal hemorrhages. Assess the genitalia and perineum for signs of trauma or lesions.

- *Diagnosis*: If there are any red flags in the history or physical examination, a physician should pursue the appropriate investigation for child abuse. The diagnostic work-up is guided by your physical examination. The AAP recommends a skeletal survey for children under the age of 2 who are suspected victims of physical abuse.[5] The skeletal survey can assess for both acute and healing fractures. A typical skeletal survey has specific radiographic view requirements of the skull, spine, pelvis, femur, legs, feet, humerus, forearms, and hands. The diagnosis for child abuse becomes more likely if the patient has multiple fractures, multiple rib fractures, femoral, humeral, or skull fractures.[6] The AAP recommends neuroimaging in suspected child abuse patients with head trauma, altered mental status, or skull fracture seen on X-ray to assess for intracranial bleeding. Liver enzymes, specifically ALT and AST, can be useful in assessing for intra-abdominal trauma without external signs.[7] CPS must be contacted and their investigation can also help make the diagnosis.

- *Treatment*: Any life-threatening injuries should be treated according to the ATLS protocols, and appropriate consultations should be made according to the child's injuries. Once medical management is addressed, social workers, CPS, and physicians who specialize in child abuse should be consulted. Chapter 2, Case 4 has more information about this.

- *Disposition*: Hospitalization is necessary for all patients with serious medical conditions secondary to their abuse; however, consider hospitalization if you are concerned that the child will be returning to an unsafe environment or CPS is unavailable to assess the patient until a later time. Hospitalization will allow for close monitoring of the patient while providing a safe environment for the child until an appropriate investigation can be undertaken. The physician's primary responsibilities are to help in the identification of possible child abuse, provide medical treatment, ensure detailed documentation, and contact CPS, who will ultimately determine the social disposition of the child.

Historical clues	Physical findings
• Story inconsistent with examination findings • Trauma being attributed to a small sibling • Patient in high-risk age group for abuse	• Parallel bruising pattern consistent with hand slap

Follow-Up

Social work and CPS were consulted and felt that the patient was unsafe to return home until a representative could assess the home. The patient was admitted to the hospital and a physician specially trained in child abuse was consulted. It was determined that the mother's boyfriend was responsible for the bruise. The child was discharged in the care of her mother, with appropriate social services follow-up.

References

1. Heisler K. US Department of Health and Human Services. Child maltreatment 2013. See www.acf.hhs.gov/sites/default/files/cb/cm2013.pdf (accessed February 2017).

2. Child Abuse Prevention and Treatment Act (CAPTA). United States Code title 42, chapter 67, reenacted 2010.

3. Lamb ME, Sternberg KJ, Orbach Y, et al. Age differences in young children's response to open-ended invitations in the course of forensic interviews. *J Consult Clin Psychol* 2003; 71: 926–34.

4. Lamb ME, Orbach Y, Hershkowitz I, et al. Structured forensic interview protocols improve the quality and informativeness of investigative interviews with children: A review of research using the NICHD investigative interview protocol. *Child Abuse Negl* 2007; 31: 1201–31.

5. American Academy of Pediatrics. Diagnostic imaging of child abuse. See http://pediatrics.aappublications.org/content/123/5/1430 (accessed February 2017).

6. Kemp AM, Dunstan F, Harrison S, et al. Patterns of skeletal fractures in child abuse: a systematic review. *BMJ* 2008; 337: a1518.

7. Lane WG, Dubowitz H, Langenberg P. Screening for occult abdominal trauma in children with suspected physical abuse. *Pediatrics* 2009; 124: 1595–602.

Case 6

Contributing Author: Rebecca Jeanmonod

History

A 14-month-old girl presents to the ED accompanied by her grandfather for a rash. Grandpa states that he babysits the child most weekends, and when she was dropped off today he had noted red bumps on her arms and ankles. When he changed the child's diaper, he realized the bumps actually involved most of the child's bilateral legs as well, and he saw a lesion or two on the back of her neck. He did not see anything in the diaper area. The child has seemed bothered by the rash, scratching at it and saying "boo-boo." She has otherwise been acting like herself. She has been playful with Grandpa, and he states she ate her breakfast and her lunch with usual appetite. She has not had fever, vomiting, cough, runny nose, or diarrhea. She has been making a usual number of wet diapers, and has not had any recent dietary changes.

Past Medical History

- Eczema.
- Seasonal allergies.
- UTD on immunizations.

Medications

- Topical steroids as needed, although no recent use.
- Loratidine.

Allergies

- Amoxicillin – rash.

Physical Examination and Ancillary Studies

- *Vital signs*: 98.7 °F, HR 110, RR 25, BP 97/61, O$_2$ sat 100% on room air.
- *General*: Awake, alert, interactive, and well-appearing.
- *HEENT*: PERRL. Oropharynx without lesions. Mucous membranes moist.
- *Neck*: Supple and non-tender, with no adenopathy. Midline trachea.
- *Cardiovascular*: Regular rhythm, with no M/R/G. Capillary refill < 2 seconds.
- *Lungs*: Normal work of breathing, clear lung sounds, with no W/R/R.
- *Abdomen*: Soft, without tenderness, masses, or guarding. Normal bowel sounds.
- *Extremities and skin*: Warm and well-perfused. There are several scattered erythematous blanching papules of about 7–10 mm in diameter, which are located on the patient's extremities. They are not confluent. The child has no lesions on the palms or soles. There are several lesions on the child's posterior neck. The child does not have lesions on the trunk. The lesions are not pustular or vesicular. The child is scratching at the lesions.
- *Neurologic*: Non-focal neurologic examination.

Questions for Thought

- What findings in rashes are worrisome?
- What is the differential diagnosis for generalized rash?
- How should this child be treated?

Diagnosis

- Insect bites.

Discussion

- *Epidemiology*: Rashes are a common presenting complaint in primary care and EDs. They can be seen in any age group, and can be localized or generalized, painful, pruritic, or essentially asymptomatic. They can be evidence of an isolated skin process or secondary to a systemic process, arising from infectious, inflammatory, immune, or toxicologic causes. Most importantly, they can be dangerous or benign, and although the clinical diagnosis of the exact etiology of a rash may be challenging, the provider should be able to recognize the rash that suggests severe disease. A full discussion of every specific rash is outside the scope of this book.
- *Pathophysiology*: Rashes are caused in a number of ways. Wheals and hives are a result of increased capillary permeability, leading to extravasation of fluid into the skin, often secondary to a type I hypersensitivity reaction (acute allergy/anaphylaxis). Fluid-filled papules/vesicles and bullae may also be secondary to a hypersensitivity reaction (topical dermatitis, such as with poison ivy exposure) when localized, or secondary to viral infection (varicella, disseminated herpes) when generalized. Diffuse, non-descript maculopapular rashes may be secondary to drug eruptions or viral infections. Exfoliating rashes may be caused by erythema multiforme, toxic shock syndrome, staphylococcal scalded skin syndrome, or immune-mediated disease. Petechiae may be caused by malignancy, vasculitis, meningococcemia, or Rocky Mountain spotted fever. The rash of Lyme disease is pathognomonic for the disease and is discussed elsewhere. Finally, scaling rashes may be from underlying chronic conditions, such as psoriasis or eczema, or can be from fungal infections.
- *Presentation*: Small children may present when parents notice a rash in an otherwise asymptomatic child, or they may present for a complex of symptoms of which the rash is only a small part. It is important to do a thorough physical examination in all pediatric patients so as not to miss serious pathology. It is also important to obtain the relevant history that contributes to

the rash: recent travel, time of year, outdoor activity (for insect, arthropod, and allergen exposure), medications, immunization history, progression and migration of the lesions, sick contacts or others with lesions, joint symptoms or fever, and involvement of palms, soles, and mucosae.

- *Diagnosis*: The differential diagnosis for a rash is large, and not one that can be easily committed to memory. However, in the ED, it is important to narrow down the differential diagnosis to exclude dangerous items. One way to begin is to divide rashes into "localized" rashes and "systemic" rashes.

  Localized rashes do not involve the entire body by definition. Contact dermatitis from exposure to poison ivy as well as insect bites often present in this way, and have a paucity of other symptoms beyond rash and pruritis, as in our patient. It is important to note the pattern of the rash. Is it on exposed areas that are likely to be susceptible to insect bites? Is the rash localized to intertriginous areas (more common in streptococcal or candidal infections) or between fingers and toes (common in scabies)? A single lesion may also be evidence of cellulitis or, in the right clinical setting, primary Lyme disease. In all these scenarios, there is generally no further testing needed for diagnosis and treatment – the child may be treated based on the clinical diagnosis alone.

  Generalized rashes are more challenging, as the differential diagnosis is larger and contains many concerning items. When facing these rashes, the provider should begin by assessing the overall status of the patient, and whether or not the patient appears ill. Ill children with benign-appearing rashes are ill children nonetheless and require resuscitation, treatment, and diagnostic testing. Likewise, well-appearing children with dangerous-appearing rashes also typically require evaluation beyond examination. It is only the well-appearing child with a benign-appearing generalized rash who requires nothing more than symptomatic care.

  What makes a rash "dangerous-appearing?"

  - Although there are exceptions to every rule, *rashes that do not blanch* when pressed are worrisome. Non-blanching rashes (e.g. petechiae and purpura) occur from the presence of blood in the tissue. This occurs because of injury to blood vessels or disease to platelets. In other words, these rashes are evidence of underlying vasculitis or coagulopathy, such as occurs with autoimmune or idiopathic vasculitis, leukemic crises, meningococcemia, or Rocky Mountain spotted fever. Although children may have localized petechiae to the face from forceful vomiting, petechiae elsewhere are concerning for dangerous disease processes. It is important to note that the rash of Rocky Mountain spotted fever or meningococcemia may initially appear benign, so if there is any concern at all for these diagnoses, the child should be observed for several hours to assess for evolution of lesions, and a low threshold should be maintained for initiation of treatment.

  - *Rashes that involve the palms and soles* are also concerning. Although the clinician should be aware of benign common causes of palm and sole rashes (such as hand–foot–mouth disease, a self-limited, highly contagious disease of early childhood – see Figure 12.4), rashes in these regions can be evidence of erythema multiforme, Kawasaki disease, Rocky Mountain spotted fever, staphylococcal scalded skin syndrome, Stevens–Johnson syndrome, toxic epidermal necrolysis, and toxic shock syndrome, all of which may present with hand and foot involvement.

  - *Rashes with blistering, exfoliation, or skin sloughing* are generally "bad" rashes. Blisters/vesicles suggest viral disease, such as disseminated herpes or varicella. Rashes with skin loss not only imply a significant underlying disease (such as toxic shock syndrome, staphylococcal scalded skin syndrome, or toxic epidermal necrolysis) but the rash causes breakdown of the skin's barrier function to further infection and fluid loss. Therefore, these children are at risk for dehydration and electrolyte imbalances, and should be treated similarly to burn patients. Further discussion of this can be found in this chapter, Case 3.

  - *Rashes with significant systemic symptoms*, such as diffuse urticaria, with shortness of breath or vomiting/diarrhea should always be taken

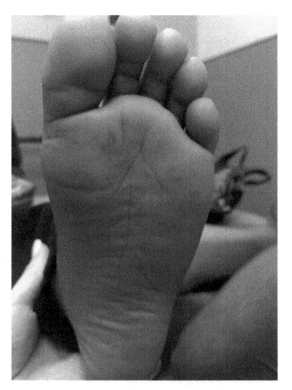

Figure 12.4 Rash on sole caused by hand–foot–mouth disease. For the color version, please refer to the plate section.

seriously. The rash may be the presenting complaint for anaphylaxis, sepsis, malignancy, or significant infectious disease, such as measles, chickenpox, or rubella.

· *Rashes involving the mucosa* should raise consideration for Kawasaki disease and Stevens–Johnson disease.

   Most rashes are benign. Most are non-specific, blanching, non-exfoliating, and resolve spontaneously. To distinguish among dangerous rashes, CBC, blood cultures, pathogen assays, and biopsy may be required, but the vast majority of rashes require no further diagnostic work-up beyond a good history and physical examination.

• *Treatment*: If the inciting process is known and treatable (for example, a child with a rash secondary to an antibiotic), the child should be treated for the underlying cause. Children with concern for significant infectious disease should receive antibiotics and admission to the hospital. The vast majority of non-specific rashes require only symptomatic care, which is typically topical or systemic steroids for allergic rashes (systemic steroids are often needed for extensive contact dermatitis) and antihistamine for pruritis.

• *Disposition*: Most cases of rash can be discharged home with follow-up with pediatrics. Careful return precautions should address worrisome rash findings, which should prompt a repeat ED visit.

Historical clues	Physical findings
• Itchy rash on exposed areas • No other complaints	• Papules consistent with insect bites located on areas not covered by clothing • Otherwise well child

Follow-Up

Grandpa was encouraged to use symptomatic care for the child's insect bites and was counseled regarding the use of insect sprays to prevent further bites. The child was discharged home.

Case 7

Contributing Author: Dorka M. Jiménez Almonte

History

A 10-month-old boy presents with fever, irritability, and a rash of 8 hours duration. The parents report that the baby was doing well until approximately 8 hours ago when he woke up from his nap with a high fever. The patient has been very fussy and crying inconsolably ever since. The parents gave acetaminophen by mouth at home, which lowered the temperature but did not alleviate the fussiness. The infant has been refusing to drink fluids or eat solids. He has had only one barely wet diaper in the last 8 hours. A couple of hours ago, the parents noticed a reddish rash on his chest, abdomen, and legs. The child had two episodes of non-bilious vomiting at home, prompting the parents to bring him in. En route to the ED, his rash darkened in color. He has not had diarrhea or URI symptoms. He has no known sick contacts.

Past Medical History

• Term normal spontaneous vaginal delivery.
• UTD on immunizations.
• Meeting developmental milestones with no issues.

Medications

- Vitamin D supplement daily.

Allergies

- NKDA.

Physical Examination and Ancillary Studies

- *Vital signs*: T 103.2 °F, HR 180, RR 45, BP 85/45, O_2 sat 99% on room air.
- *General*: The patient's size and weight appears appropriate for age. He is ill-appearing, crying inconsolably, sitting on his mother's lap. He is not producing tears despite crying.
- *HEENT*: No signs of trauma. Anterior fontanelle is bulging. PERRL. Clear conjunctivae. Dry mucous membranes. No oral lesions.
- *Neck*: Supple, with no tenderness to palpation. The range of motion appears intact as the patient moves his head in all directions without restrictions. There is no evident nuchal rigidity.
- *Cardiovascular*: Regular tachycardia, with no M/R/G. Femoral pulses are equal bilaterally. Capillary refill > 4 seconds.
- *Lungs*: Clear and equal bilaterally, with no W/R/R.
- *Abdomen*: The abdomen is not distended. It is soft and depressible and is not tender to palpation. There is no organomegaly.
- *Extremities and skin*: Extremities intact, with no signs of trauma. There are red macules and some slightly raised maculopapular lesions on the trunk and extremities. There are a few non-blanching petechial lesions on the trunk and lower extremities. There are approximately 3-mm purpuric, slightly elevated lesions on the dorsal aspect of the feet. These purpuric lesions are tender to palpation.
- *Neurologic*: Awake and crying, inconsolable. No focal abnormalities.
- *Pertinent laboratory values*: WBC 27,500 with 30% bands, Plt 100,000, ESR 100.

Questions for Thought

- How would you describe this patient's condition?
- What would be your initial steps to manage the patient?
- What diagnostic tests would you obtain?
- What medications if any do you consider in this patient?

- What measures would you take to protect other patients and the medical staff?

Diagnosis

- Meningococcemia.

Discussion

- *Epidemiology*: Meningococcal disease is endemic to North America and the annual incidence varies from 0.5 to 1.5 cases per 100,000 in multiyear cycles.[1,2] Globally, epidemics occur at irregular year intervals, every 7–10 years, mostly in sub-Saharan Africa, known as the "meningitis belt," with rates as high as 1 case per 1,000 during these epidemics.[2] *Neisseria meningitidis*, an encapsulated Gram-negative diplococcus, is an obligate human pathogen. Humans are reservoirs for *N. meningitidis* via asymptomatic nasopharyngeal carriage. Carrier rates increase progressively with age from 0.7 percent of children less than 4 years old to 10–20 percent in adolescence and up to 30 percent in 25-year-olds.[1,2] This increase is thought to be secondary to changes in social behavior that occur with age (kissing, intimate contact) and overcrowding (e.g. poverty, military barracks). Transmission occurs via close contact with infected respiratory droplets or secretions, and there is a 2–10-day incubation period.[2] Rates of disease are significantly higher in children younger than 2 years of age, with a second peak during adolescence through young adulthood.[1,2] Higher disease rates in less developed countries are likely to be partially due to poverty, crowding, poor sanitation, and malnutrition. The overall mortality rate is 8–14 percent and the morbidity rate is 11–19 percent for those who survive.[1-3] Long-term sequelae are typically devastating and include hearing loss, neurodevelopmental delays, and amputations.[2,3]
- *Pathophysiology*: *N. meningitidis* exclusively infects humans.[1] Nasopharyngeal colonization by *N. meningitidis* is a prerequisite for the development of systemic infection. Invasive meningococcal disease is only caused by six serogroups, classified by the polysaccharide capsule surrounding the bacterium; serogroups A, B, C, W-135, X, and Y.[2] The bacterium adheres to

and invades the human epithelial and endothelial cells. The polysaccharide capsule inhibits phagocytosis and uses numerous virulence factors to escape the human immune response, such as phase variation, antigenic variation, and molecular mimicry of human antigens. Nasopharyngeal carrier state, exposure to *N. meningitidis*, and certain immune defects such as asplenia and complement deficiencies are known risk factors for invasive meningococcal disease.[2,3] Damage to the nasopharyngeal epithelium (changes in temperature, URIs, low humidity, and sand particles) combined with host susceptibility leads to invasive disease.[2,3] Vascular collapse and shock are caused by damage to the microvasculature, resulting in increased vascular permeability (capillary leak), pathologic vasoconstriction and vasodilation, and intravascular coagulation. Microvascular thrombosis is responsible for serious complications such as purpura fulminans.

- *Presentation*: Patients may present with one of three syndromes: meningitis (30–50 percent), meningitis with bacteremia (40 percent), or bacteremia alone (10 percent).[1-3] Meningitis is the most common presentation. Clinical presentation varies according to the age of the patient. Presentation in infants and young children is less specific and can present a diagnostic challenge. Fever is typically the first symptom in infants and young children.[2,3] Headaches are more common in children older than 5 years of age.[2,3] Many children initially present with upper respiratory symptoms such as cough, sore throat, coryza, and otalgia.[2,3] Most children are irritable and develop loss of appetite, nausea, and vomiting. Symptoms rapidly evolve (over a few hours) to a more serious presentation with neck stiffness, altered mental status, and seizures.[2,3] Bacteremia (acute meningococcemia) presents with non-specific symptoms, such as fever, lethargy, reduced oral intake, headache, nausea, and vomiting, with or without clinical signs of sepsis, such as tachycardia, tachypnea, and fever.[2,3] Myalgias can be present in older children and are typically more painful than those seen with viral illnesses such as influenza. The cardinal presentation is a non-blanching, hemorrhagic (petechial or purpuric) rash.[1-6] The lesions are commonly seen on the trunk and extremities but they can be present in any location. Purpura are initially small, irregular, and painful. Multiple large hemorrhagic lesions are associated with a worse prognosis. The hemorrhagic rash may progress to purpura fulminans, a cutaneous manifestation of disseminated intravascular coagulation, which presents as a purpuric rash, shock, and gangrene, often requiring amputation.[2-5] Patients can also present a mixture of both meningitis and meningococcemia. An initially mild condition may progress to a fulminant disease, multi-organ failure, and death within hours.[2,3] Ill appearance, petechial rash below the nipple line, and purpura measuring more than 2 mm have been identified in the literature as predictors of meningococcal disease or serious bacteremia.[2-5] In children, 95 percent of cases of non-blanching petechial rash and fever are caused by viral pathogens such as enterovirus or adenovirus and not meningococcal disease.[4] Early in meningococcemia the rash can have a maculopapular appearance. Given that it can be very difficult to distinguish early meningococcal disease from a viral exanthem, a period of observation is recommended for a well-appearing child with an acute, non-blanching rash, to safely distinguish between the two.

- *Diagnosis*: In children presenting with petechial rash and fever, laboratory studies including CBC, blood culture, ESR, and CRP are usually warranted. Infants should also undergo age-appropriate fever work-up per current guidelines. The diagnosis of *N. meningitidis* invasive disease is confirmed by positive cultures of the blood, CSF, or joint fluid. The CBC typically shows leukocytosis with left shifting (predominance of granulocytes). The platelet count may be decreased. The inflammatory markers such ESR and CRP are usually elevated. If the patient has meningitis the CSF analysis will show pleocytosis (increased white blood cells), decreased glucose, and increased protein. In the Gram's stain, Gram-negative diplococci can be seen. In advanced disease, coagulation studies can be used to evaluate for a consumptive coagulopathy. BUN and Cr should also be obtained to evaluate renal function and electrolytes. Electrolyte disturbances are common in patients who have shock. Other etiologies that present with fever and a hemorrhagic rash should be considered, such as vasculitis (Henoch–Schönlein purpura), Rocky Mountain spotted fever, toxic shock syndrome, enteroviral infection, leptospirosis, and bacteremia that is caused by other pathogens such as *Streptococcus pneumoniae*.[4,5]

- *Treatment*: This is an infectious emergency and treatment must not be delayed. If the diagnosis is seriously considered, blood cultures must be drawn and antibiotics administered within 30 minutes. It is of utmost importance that antibiotic therapy is not delayed for diagnostic procedures such as LP. The drug of choice to treat suspected or culture-proven meningococcal infection is a third-generation cephalosporin, such as cefotaxime or ceftriaxone. If susceptible, the treatment could later be switched to penicillin G. Serious complications, such as shock, disseminated intravascular coagulation, and purpura fulminans should be treated early and aggressively. The patient should be placed on droplet precautions until 24 hours after the initiation of effective antimicrobial therapy. Chemoprophylaxis is warranted to intimate contacts who have been exposed to the patient's oral secretions (kissing, eating utensils, toothbrushes), such as household, daycare, nursery, and school contacts. People who frequently slept in the same dwelling as the patient should also receive prophylaxis. For healthcare staff, chemoprophylaxis is not routinely recommended except when involved in orotracheal intubation, suctioning of secretions, and examination of the eye area. Meningococcal quadrivalent vaccine is an adjunct to chemoprophylaxis when an outbreak is caused by a serogroup covered by the vaccine (A, C, Y, and W-135).

- *Disposition*: Patients with a concern of meningococcal infection should be admitted to the hospital. If the child is ill-appearing or if there are signs concerning for meningitis (neck stiffness) or septic shock (poor perfusion, hypotension), the child should be treated for meningococcal disease immediately and admitted to the PICU for further monitoring and management.

Historical clues	Physical findings	Ancillary studies
• Age • Fever • Rapid symptom progression • Rash	• Fever • Bulging fontanelle • Irritability • Clinical findings of dehydration • Purpuric lesions	• Leukocytosis with left shift (elevated bands) • Thrombocytopenia • Elevated ESR

Follow-Up

A petechial and purpuric rash developed within an hour of presentation to the ED. The patient was promptly identified as requiring resuscitation and was placed on contact precautions. IV access was immediately obtained and fluid resuscitation was initiated expeditiously. Laboratory tests were drawn including CBC, ESR, CRP, electrolytes, glucose, BUN/Cr, and blood culture. Additionally, coagulation studies were obtained, given the presence of purpuric lesions. Antibiotic treatment was started with ceftriaxone within 15 minutes. The patient was admitted to the PICU. One hour later an LP was performed. All household and daycare contacts were treated prophylactically. The next day the blood culture confirmed the diagnosis of invasive *N. meningitidis* infection.

References

1. Centers for Disease Control and Prevention (CDC). Meningococcal disease incidence, United States, 1970–2015. See www.cdc.gov/meningococcal/images/meningococcal-disease-incidence-lg.jpg (accessed February 2017).

2. Sabatini C, Bosis S, Semino L, et al. Clinical presentation of meningococcus in childhood. *J Prev Med Hyg* 2012; 53: 116–19.

3. Pace D, Pollard AJ. Meningococcal disease: Clinical presentation and sequelae. *Vaccine* 2012; 30 Suppl 2: B3–9.

4. Aber C, Alvarez Connelly E, Schachner LA. Fever and rash in a child: When to worry? *Pediatr Ann* 2007; 36: 30–8.

5. Ramos-e-Silva M, Pereira AL. Life-threatening eruptions due to infectious agents. *Clin Dermatol* 2005; 23: 148–56.

6. Klinkhammer MD, Colletti JE. Pediatric myth: Fever and petechiae. *CJEM* 2008; 10: 479–82.

Case Key

Chapter	Case	Diagnosis
2	1	Multiple trauma
2	2	Head trauma
2	3	Cervical spine injury
2	4	Non-accidental trauma
2	5	Burns
2	6	Drowning
2	7	Hypovolemic shock
2	8	Cardiogenic shock
2	9	Respiratory failure
2	10	Septic shock
2	11	Anaphylaxis
3	1	Foreign-body airway
3	2	Periodic breathing
3	3	Gastroesophageal reflux disease (GERD)
3	4	Bronchiolitis
3	5	Acute asthma exacerbation
3	6	Brief resolved unexplained event (BRUE)
3	7	Congestive heart failure, congenital heart disease (CHF, CHD)
3	8	Symptomatic anemia
4	1	Febrile seizure
4	2	Neonatal fever
4	3	Neutropenic fever
4	4	Neuroleptic malignant syndrome (NMS)
4	5	Fever with sickle cell disease
4	6	Fever with transplant
4	7	Aspirin overdose
4	8	Environmental hyperthermia
4	9	Acute viral perimyocarditis
5	1	Foreign body ENT
5	2	Anterior epistaxis
5	3	Globe rupture
5	4	Acute mastoiditis
5	5	Orbital fracture
5	6	Lemierre syndrome
5	7	Peritonsillar abscess
5	8	Otitis media
5	9	Retropharyngeal abscess
6	1	Nursemaid's elbow
6	2	Ankle sprain
6	3	Septic arthritis
6	4	Lacerations
6	5	Lyme arthritis
6	6	Osteomyelitis
6	7	Supracondylar fracture
6	8	Shoulder dislocation
6	9	Fractures

Chapter	Case	Diagnosis
7	1	Inborn error of metabolism
7	2	Acute gastroenteritis
7	3	Iron toxicity
7	4	Intussusception
7	5	Seizure
7	6	Intracranial mass
7	7	Bulimia nervosa
7	8	Malrotation
7	9	Strep throat
7	10	Overfeeding
8	1	Appendicitis
8	2	Urinary retention, constipation
8	3	Diabetic ketoacidosis
8	4	Ingested foreign body
8	5	Sexually transmitted disease
8	6	Pneumonia
8	7	Torsion
8	8	Ectopic pregnancy
9	1	Idiopathic ketotic hypoglycemia
9	2	Infant botulism
9	3	Congenital heart disease
9	4	Hypernatremia
9	5	Congenital heart disease
9	6	Intoxication
9	7	Intussusception
9	8	Acute psychosis
10	1	Carbon monoxide poisoning
10	2	Hypertensive emergency
10	3	Epidural hematoma
10	4	Medulloblastoma
10	5	Meningitis
10	6	Migraine
10	7	Lyme disease
10	8	Retropharyngeal abscess
10	9	Subarachnoid hemorrhage
11	1	Milk protein allergy
11	2	Inguinal hernia
11	3	Paraphimosis
11	4	Pregnancy
11	5	Sexually transmitted disease
11	6	Urinary tract infection (UTI)
11	7	Vaginitis
12	1	Retained foreign body
12	2	Acute lymphoblastic leukemia (ALL)
12	3	Burns
12	4	Animal bite
12	5	Child abuse
12	6	General rash
12	7	Meningococcemia

Index

AAP guidelines
  bronchiolitis, 51
  BRUE, 56, 57
  child abuse, 287
  febrile seizure, 69
  HIV screening, 265
  infant botulism, 204
  infant feeding, 172
  iron supplements, 65
  otitis media, 115, 116
  over-the-counter preparations,
    216
  UTIs, 268, 269
ABCDE algorithm, 5
abdominal pain, 173–200
  appendicitis, 173–5
  constipation. See constipation
  diabetic ketoacidosis, 180–3
  ectopic pregnancy. See ectopic
    pregnancy
  foreign-body ingestion, 183–6
  intussusception, 220
  pelvic inflammatory disease, 265
  pneumonia. See pneumonia
  pregnancy, 260, 261
  referred, 190
  STIs. See sexually transmitted
    infections (STIs)
  gonadal torsion, 192–5
  urinary retention, 176–80
abscess
  drainage, 113
  peritonsillar. See peritonsillar abscess
  retropharyngeal. See retropharyngeal
    abscess
absolute neutrophil count (ANC),
  75
abusive head trauma, 17
acetaminophen, 218
activated charcoal, 87
acute asthma exacerbation, 52–5
  diagnosis, 54
  disposition, 55
  pathophysiology, 53
  presentation, 53
  treatment, 54–5
acute gastroenteritis, 150–2
  diagnosis, 151
  epidemiology, 151

pathophysiology, 151
presentation, 151
treatment, 151–2
acute lymphoblastic leukemia (ALL),
  35, 73, 276–8
  diagnosis, 278
  epidemiology, 277
  pathophysiology, 277
  presentation, 277
  treatment, 278
acute myeloid leukemia (AML),
  277
acute psychosis, 221–3
  diagnosis, 222
  epidemiology, 222
  pathophysiology, 222
  presentation, 222
  treatment, 223
acute respiratory distress syndrome
  (ARDS)
  burns and, 21
  drowning and, 25
acute viral perimyocarditis, 91–4
altered mental status, 201–23
  acute psychosis, 221–3
  brain tumors, 162
  coarctation of the aorta, 211–15
  coronary artery anomaly, 206–8
  hypernatremia, 209–11
  idiopathic ketotic hypoglycemia,
    201–3
  infant botulism, 203–6
  intoxication, 215–18
  intussusception. See intussusception
American Academy of Pediatrics
  (AAP). See AAP guidelines
American Burn Association, criteria,
  280
anaphylaxis, 38–41
  diagnosis, 40
  disposition, 40
  epidemiology, 39
  pathophysiology, 39
  presentation, 40
  red flags, 40
  treatment, 40
anemia, 64–7, 254
  diagnosis, 65–6
  epidemiology, 65

pathophysiology, 65
presentation, 65
treatment, 66
anesthesia
  lacerations, 131
  paraphimosis, 259
  shoulder dislocation, 143
aneurysms, subarachnoid hemorrhage,
  250, 251, 252
animal bites, 282–5
  diagnosis, 283–4
  disposition, 285
  epidemiology, 282
  pathophysiology, 283
  presentation, 283
  treatment, 284–5
anion gap, elevated, 217
ankle fracture, 144–6
ankle sprain, 123–6
  diagnosis, 125
  disposition, 126
  epidemiology, 123
  grading, 124, 125
  pathophysiology, 123–4
  presentation, 123, 124
  treatment, 125
anorexia nervosa, 164–5
anosmia, 161
anticoagulants, 111
antidotes, and poisons, 218
antiemetics, 242
aorta, coarctation of, 211–15
apnea, 46
  bronchiolitis and, 51, 52
  definition, 46
apparent life-threatening event
  (ALTE). See also brief resolved
  unexplained event (BRUE)
  GERD and, 48
  periodic breathing vs., 46
appendectomy, 175
appendicitis, 173–5
  diagnosis, 175
  epidemiology, 174
  pathophysiology, 174
  presentation, 175
  treatment, 175
Apt test, 254
arterial blood gas (ABG)

drowning, 25
reference values, xvi
respiratory failure, 34
arteriovenous malformations, 250, 252
arthritis
Lyme. *See* Lyme arthritis
septic. *See* septic arthritis
arthrocentesis, 128, 129, 134, 135
aseptic meningitis, 237, 245
aspiration method, 259
aspirin overdose, 85–8
diagnosis, 86
epidemiology, 85
pathophysiology, 86
presentation, 86
treatment, 87
asthma
acute exacerbation. *See* acute asthma
exacerbation
anaphylaxis and, 39
epidemiology, 53
ataxia, 161
atrial septal defect (ASD), 61, 63
autism spectrum disorder, 76, 183
axillary nerve, 142

bacteremia, 267, 293
bacterial meningitis
epidemiology, 237
pathophysiology, 238
Bacterial Meningitis Score, 238
balloon catheter, 97, 101
Bankart lesion, 142
basilar skull fracture, 8
bee allergy, 38–41
benzodiazepines, 70, 159
beta-agonists, 54, 55
beta-hCG levels, 197, 198, 199, 262
beta-hydroxybutyrate, 181
bicycle accidents
head trauma, 7–10
multiple trauma, 3–6
botulism immunoglobulin, 205
biphasic reaction, 41
bipolar disorder, 222
bladder-bowel dysfunction, 176–80
BLEEP examination, 214
blood typing, 262
blowout fractures, 107, 108
blue CHD, 60, 61
blunt trauma, 5, 21
bone conduction theory, 107
bone marrow examination, 278
Borrelia burgdorferi, 134, 244
Borrelia mayonii, 244
botulinum neurotoxin (BoNT), 205
botulism, infant, 203–6
bougienage method, 186
bowel perforation, 183–6

brain tumors. *See* medulloblastoma,
intracranial mass
breastfeeding, 172, 204, 210
breathing difficulties, 42–67
acute asthma exacerbation, 52–5
anemia. *See* anemia
bronchiolitis, 49–52
congestive heart failure, 59–63
foreign-body aspiration, 42–4
GERD. *See* gastroesophageal reflux
disease (GERD)
periodic breathing, 45–6
respiratory failure, 32–5
brief psychotic disorder, 222
brief resolved unexplained event
(BRUE), 55–8
diagnosis, 57
epidemiology, 56
pathophysiology, 56
presentation, 56
treatment, 57–8
bronchiolitis, 48, 49–52
diagnosis, 51
disposition, 52
epidemiology, 50
pathophysiology, 50
presentation, 51
treatment, 51–2
bronchoscopy, 43, 44
bruising
BRUE and, 58
child abuse, 286–8
B-type natriuretic peptide (BNP), 31
buckle fracture, 145
bulimia nervosa, 163–5
diagnosis, 164
epidemiology, 164
pathophysiology, 164
presentation, 164
treatment, 164
burn center, transfer to, 22, 280, 281
burn shock, 20
burns, 19–23, 278–81
classification, 20
diagnosis, 280
disposition, 22, 280–1
epidemiology, 20, 279
pathophysiology, 20, 279–80
presentation, 20, 280
treatment, 21–2, 280
burr hole, 233
button batteries, ingestion, 186

Canadian C-spine Rule, 12
cancer. *See also specific cancers*
neutropenic fever and, 73–6
Candida albicans, 188
carbon monoxide poisoning, 21, 224–6
diagnosis, 225

epidemiology, 225
pathophysiology, 225
presentation, 225
treatment, 226
carboxyhemoglobin levels, 225, 226
cardiac arrest, 211
cardiogenic shock, 29–32
diagnosis, 31
epidemiology, 30
pathophysiology, 30
presentation, 30
septic shock and, 36, 213, 214
treatment, 31
cardiopulmonary resuscitation (CPR)
BRUE patient, 57, 58
drowning patient, 23, 25
carditis
endocarditis, 30, 31
Lyme, 245
myocarditis, 30
pericarditis. *See* pericarditis
cat bites, 283, 285
CATCH criteria, 232
catheterization, 97, 101, 179, 186
c-collar immobilization, 11
Centers for Disease Control and
Prevention (CDC), 264, 265
Centor score, 170
cerebral edema, 181, 182
cerebral palsy, 178
cerebral perfusion pressure, 232
cerebrospinal fluid (CSF)
meningitis, 238
pleocytosis, 238
reference values, xvi
CHALICE criteria, 232
chest pain, pericarditis, 93
chest X-ray (CXR)
acute asthma exacerbation, 54
bronchiolitis, 51
CHD, 62
CHF, 59
coarctation of the aorta, 213
foreign-body aspiration, 44
foreign-body ingestion, 185
pneumonia, 190, 191
child abuse, 1, 286–8. *See also*
non-accidental trauma
diagnosis, 287
disposition, 288
epidemiology, 286
pathophysiology, 287
presentation, 287
risk factors, 287
sexual, 189, 262, 264, 271
treatment, 288
Child Abuse Prevention and
Treatment Act, 287
chlamydial infection, 187–9, 263–6

choking episode, 43
circumcision, 258, 260, 267
clinical decision rules
    head trauma, 232
    neutropenic fever, 75
Clostridium botulinum, 204
Clostridium difficile, 82
coagulation reference values, xvi
coarctation of the aorta, 211–15
    diagnosis, 213–14
    disposition, 214
    epidemiology, 212
    pathophysiology, 212–13
    presentation, 213
    treatment, 214
cognitive behavioral therapy, 165
colic, 206–8
    definition, 207
    diagnosis, 208
    epidemiology, 207
    presentation, 207
colloid therapy, 28
Colorado CoFlex® technique, 259
community-acquired pneumonia,
    189–91
compartment syndrome, 281
compensated shock, 27
complete blood count (CBC), xv
compression bandage, 259, 260
congenital heart disease (CHD), 59–63
    coarctation of the aorta. *See*
        coarctation of the aorta
    coronary artery anomaly, 206–8
    cyanotic, 60, 61
    diagnosis, 61
    epidemiology, 60, 212
    pathophysiology, 60
    pink, 60, 61, 62
congestive heart failure (CHF), 59–63
    definition, 61
    diagnosis, 61
    pathophysiology, 61
    presentation, 61
    treatment, 62–3
constipation, 176–80
    diagnosis, 178–9
    epidemiology, 176
    foreign-body ingestion and, 184, 185
    infant botulism and, 204, 205
    pathophysiology, 177–8
    presentation, 178
    treatment, 179
convulsions, seizures and, 158
corn syrup, contaminated, 204
coronary artery anomaly, 206–8
    red flags, 208
cow milk protein intolerance, 48
cranial nerve palsies, 205
cricothyroidotomy, 5

crying, persistent, 206, 207–8
c-spine injury, 10–14
    diagnosis, 12–14
    epidemiology, 11
    imaging, 232
    pathophysiology, 11
    presentation, 11–12
    treatment, 15
CT scanning, 1
    animal bite, 283
    appendicitis, 175
    brain tumors, 162
    epidural hematoma, 230, 232
    foreign-body ingestion, 185, 186
    globe rupture, 103
    head trauma, 8
    intussusception, 221
    Lemierre syndrome, 111
    mastoiditis, 105, 106
    multiple trauma, 6
    non-accidental trauma, 18
    orbital fracture, 108, 109
    peritonsillar abscess, 113
    retropharyngeal abscess, 118, 119,
        248, 249
    subarachnoid hemorrhage, 250, 251
cyanide, 21
cyanotic CHD, 60, 61
cystitis, 266–9
cytomegalovirus (CMV),
    transplant-associated, 81–4

deep partial-thickness burns, 20
deferoxamine, 154
dehydration
    acute gastroenteritis, 151
    diabetic ketoacidosis, 181, 182
    epidemiology, 209
    hypernatremic, 209–11
depression, 222
    postpartum, 262
dextromethorphan overdose, 215–18
diabetes, types, 181
diabetic ketoacidosis, 180–3
    diagnosis, 182
    epidemiology, 181
    pathophysiology, 181
    presentation, 181
    treatment, 182
diarrhea, 210
    hypovolemic shock from, 27
digital rectal exam, 178
diplopia, 161
disseminated intravascular
    coagulation, 293, 294
distributive shock, 36
dog bites, 282–5
dorsal slit procedure, 260
double-bubble sign, 167

Down's syndrome, 166
drainage
    abscess, 113
    joint, 128
    mastoiditis, 106
dressing changes, burns, 281
drowning, 23–6
    disposition, 25
    epidemiology, 24
    pathophysiology, 24
    presentation and diagnosis, 25
    prevention, 25
    resuscitative measures, 23
    treatment, 25
ductal-dependent lesions, 211–15
Dundee technique, 259
duodenal atresia, 166
dysentery, acute gastroenteritis and,
    151
dysuria, 264

ear complaints. *See* eye, ear, nose, and
    throat
ear pain, 115, 116
early disseminated Lyme disease, 244,
    245, 246
early localized Lyme disease, 244
echocardiography
    cardiogenic shock, 31, 32
    CHD, 62, 63
    coarctation of the aorta, 214
ectopic pregnancy, 195–9
    diagnosis, 196–7
    epidemiology, 196, 197, 284
    pathophysiology, 196
    presentation, 196
    treatment, 197–8
elbow, supracondylar fracture, 138–40
electrical burns, 279
electrocardiogram (EKG)
    acute viral perimyocarditis, 92, 94
    cardiogenic shock, 31
    CHD, 62
    CHF, 60
    coronary artery anomaly, 208
electroencephalography (EEG),
    seizures, 159, 160
ELISA, 134
EMLA® glove technique, 259
endocarditis, 30, 31
endoscopy, 185
enema, 156, 157, 220
enteroviral meningitis, 236–9
environmental hyperthermia, 88–91
    diagnosis, 90
    epidemiology, 88
    pathophysiology, 89
    presentation, 89–90
    treatment, 90

enzyme immunoassay, 245
epididymitis, 188
epidural hematoma, 230–3
    diagnosis, 231
    epidemiology, 230
    pathophysiology, 231
    presentation, 231
    treatment, 232–3
epilepsy
    febrile seizure and, 69, 70
    seizures and, 158, 159
epinephrine, 38, 40, 41
epistaxis, 98–101
    diagnosis, 99–100
    epidemiology, 99
    pathophysiology, 99
    posterior, 101
    presentation, 99
    treatment, 100–1
Epstein–Barr virus (EBV), 82, 84
erythema migrans, 134, 244, 245
Escherichia coli, 267
esophageal foreign body, 96
    diagnosis, 96
    presentation, 96
    treatment, 97
extravaginal torsion, 193
eye, ear, nose, and throat, 95–120
    epistaxis, 98–101
    foreign body in, 95–8
    globe rupture, 102–4
    Lemierre syndrome, 109–11
    mastoiditis, 104–6
    orbital fracture, 106–9
    otitis media, 104, 105, 114–16
    peritonsillar abscess, 112–14
    retropharyngeal abscess, 117–20

facial nerve palsy, 243–6
FAST examination, 4, 5
febrile seizure, 68–70
    diagnosis, 69–70
    epidemiology, 69
    pathophysiology, 69
    presentation, 69
    treatment, 70
fever, 68–94
    acute viral perimyocarditis, 91–4
    aspirin overdose, 85–8
    environmental hyperthermia, 88–91
    febrile seizure, 68–70
    neonatal, 71–3
    neuroleptic malignant syndrome, 76–8
    neutropenic, 73–6
    with sickle cell disease, 78–80
    with transplant, 81–4

fluid resuscitation
    aspirin overdose, 87
    burns, 21, 23, 280
    cardiogenic shock, 31
    hypovolemic shock, 28–9
    septic shock, 37
fluorescein staining, 103
Foley catheter, 101, 186
forced expiratory volume in one
    second (FEV1), 54
forced vital capacity (FVC), 54
foreign body
    esophageal. See esophageal foreign
    body
    eye, 102, 103
    lacerations, 131
    nasal. See nasal foreign body
    vaginitis, 272
foreign-body aspiration, 42–4
    diagnosis, 43–4
    epidemiology, 43
    pathophysiology, 43
    presentation, 43
    treatment, 44
foreign-body granuloma, 273–6
    diagnosis, 275
    epidemiology, 274
    pathophysiology, 275
    presentation, 275
    treatment, 275
foreign body in the ear, 95–8
    diagnosis, 96
    epidemiology, 95
    pathophysiology, 96
    presentation, 96
    treatment, 97–8
foreign-body ingestion, 183–6
    diagnosis, 185
    disposition, 186
    epidemiology, 184
    pathophysiology, 184
    presentation, 185
    treatment, 185–6
formula feeding, 171, 172, 204
    overconcentration, 210
four-extremity pulse oximetry, 213
fractures, 144–6
    diagnosis, 145–6
    epidemiology, 144
    maxillofacial, 282–5
    pathophysiology, 144–5
    presentation, 145
    rib, 16, 17
    supracondylar, 138–40
    treatment, 146
free radicals, 153
full-thickness burns, 20
Fusobacterium necrophorum, 110, 111

gait problems, 127
Gardnerella vaginalis, 188, 263–6
Gartland classification, 139
gastric decontamination, 206
gastric outlet obstruction, 153
gastroenteritis, 48
    acute. See acute gastroenteritis
    viral, 26–9
gastroesophageal reflux, 47
gastroesophageal reflux disease
    (GERD), 48–9
    diagnosis, 48
    differential diagnosis, 48
    epidemiology, 47
    overfeeding and, 172
    pathophysiology, 48
    presentation, 48
    red flags, 48
    treatment, 49
gastrointestinal bleeding, 253–5
    diagnosis, 254
    disposition, 255
    epidemiology, 253
    iron toxicity, 154
    pathophysiology, 253
    presentation, 254
    treatment, 254
gastrointestinal irritation, 153
generalized rashes, 290
genital warts, 265
genitourinary complaints, 253–72
    inguinal hernia, 255–7
    milk protein allergy, 253–5
    paraphimosis, 257–60
    pregnancy. See pregnancy
    STIs. See sexually transmitted
    infections (STIs)
    UTIs. See urinary tract infection
    (UTI)
    vaginitis, 269–72
Glasgow Coma Scale (GCS), 3, 6
globe rupture, 102–4
    diagnosis, 103
    epidemiology, 102
    pathophysiology, 102
    presentation, 103
    treatment, 103
globe to wall theory, 107
glucocorticoids, 54
glycerin suppositories, 179
gonococcus, 265
gonorrhea, 127, 188, 264, 265
greenstick fracture, 145
growth centers, elbow, 139
G-tube, feeding through, 209, 210

Haemophilus influenzae, 115, 237, 239
hair tourniquet, 258
hallucinations, 217, 218, 222

head and neck pain, 224–52
  carbon monoxide poisoning, 224–6
  epidural hematoma, 230–3
  hypertensive emergency, 226–9
  Lyme disease, 243–6
  medulloblastoma, 234–6
  meningitis. See meningitis
  migraine, 240–2
  retropharyngeal abscess, 247–9
  subarachnoid hemorrhage, 249–52
head trauma, 5, 7–10. See also epidural
    hematoma, traumatic brain injury
    (TBI)
  abusive, 17
  diagnosis, 8–9
  disposition, 9
  epidemiology, 8
  globe rupture in, 103
  pathophysiology, 8
  presentation, 8
  treatment, 9
headache
  brain tumors, 161
  epidemiology, 241
  episodic, 226
  migraine, 240–2
  red flags, 241
heart failure, 30–1. See also congestive
    heart failure (CHF)
heat cramps, 89
heat exhaustion, 89
heat stroke, 88, 89. See also
    environmental hyperthermia
  classic, 89
  exertional, 89
Heimlich maneuver, 42, 44
hematogenous seeding, 136
hemodialysis, 87
hemorrhagic shock, 27, 28
  treatment, 29
hepatotoxicity, 153
herpes infections, 188, 265, 266
heterotaxy, 166
high ankle sprain, 124, 126
high-flow nasal cannula (HFNC), 52
hip, septic arthritis, 126–9
Hirschsprung's disease, 178
HIV infection, 188, 264, 265
HIV testing, 265
homonymous hemianopsia, 161
honey, contaminated, 204
human papilloma virus, 264, 265
Hunt and Hess scale, 251
hyaluronidase method, 259
hydraulic theory, 107
hydrocele, hernia and, 256
hydrocephalus, GERD and, 48
Hymenoptera anaphylaxis, 39
hyperbaric oxygen, 226

hypercarbia, 33
  bronchiolitis and, 51, 52
hypernatremia, 209–11
  diagnosis, 210
  disposition, 210
  pathophysiology, 210
  treatment, 210
hypertonic saline solution, 233
hypertensive emergency, 226–9
  diagnosis, 228
  epidemiology, 227
  pathophysiology, 227–8
  presentation, 228
  treatment, 228–9
hypertensive encephalopathy, 227,
    228
hyperthermia. See environmental
    hyperthermia
hypoglycemia
  idiopathic ketotic. See idiopathic
    ketotic hypoglycemia
  inborn error of metabolism and, 148,
    149
hyponatremia, 182
hypotension
  septic shock and, 37
hypotensive shock, 27
hypothermia, induced, 25
hypovolemic shock, 26–9
  cardiogenic shock and, 30
  diagnosis, 28
  epidemiology, 27
  pathophysiology, 27
  presentation, 27
  septic shock and, 36
  treatment, 28–9
hypoxia, 33, 225

iced glove, 259, 260
idiopathic ketotic hypoglycemia,
    201–3
  diagnosis, 202
  epidemiology, 202
  pathophysiology, 202
  presentation, 202
  treatment, 202
immune system, chemotherapy and,
    74
immunofluorescence assay, 245
inborn error of metabolism, 147–50
  diagnosis, 149
  epidemiology, 148
  idiopathic ketotic hypoglycemia and,
    202
  pathophysiology, 148
  presentation, 148–9
  treatment, 149
induced hypothermia, 25
infant botulism, 203–6

diagnosis, 205
epidemiology, 204
pathophysiology, 204
presentation, 205
treatment, 205
infant feeding guidelines, 172
informed consent, 262, 263
inguinal hernia, 255–7
  diagnosis, 256
  disposition, 257
  epidemiology, 256
  pathophysiology, 256
  presentation, 256
  treatment, 256
insect bites, 288–91
intoxication, 215–18
  diagnosis, 217
  disposition, 218
  epidemiology, 216
  pathophysiology, 216
  presentation, 216
  treatment, 217
intracranial mass, 160–3. See also
    medulloblastoma
  diagnosis, 162
  epidemiology, 161
  pathophysiology, 161
  presentation, 161
  treatment, 162
intracranial pressure, 232
intrathoracic injury, 5
intubation
  anaphylaxis, 39
  aspirin overdose, 87
  drowning, 23
  epidural hematoma, 232
  multiple trauma, 5
  respiratory failure, 34, 35
  subarachnoid hemorrhage, 251
intussusception, 155–7, 219–20,
    255
  diagnosis, 156–7, 220
  epidemiology, 156, 219
  pathophysiology, 156, 219
  presentation, 156, 220
  treatment, 157, 220
ipratropium, 54
iron supplements, 65, 66
iron toxicity, 152–5
  diagnosis, 153–4
  epidemiology, 153
  pathophysiology, 153
  presentation, 153
  treatment, 154
iron-deficiency anemia, 64–7
irreversible shock, 27
isotonic crystalloids, 210
Ixodes pacificus, 244
Ixodes scapularis, 244

Kawasaki disease, 30
Kesselbach's plexus, 99, 100
Kingella kingae, 127
knee complaints. *See* limb complaints
Kocher criteria, 128

lacerations, 129–32. *See also* skin
    complaints
  diagnosis, 131
  disposition, 132
  epidemiology, 130
  pathophysiology, 130–1
  presentation, 130, 131
  treatment, 131–2
Ladd's procedure, 168
laparoscopy, 257
laparotomy, 198, 220
laryngoscopy, 44
late disease, Lyme, 245
latent phase, iron toxicity, 153
lateral ankle sprains, 124
Lemierre syndrome, 109–11
  diagnosis, 111
  epidemiology, 110
  pathophysiology, 110
  presentation, 110
  treatment, 111
  vaccination and, 110
leukemia. *See* acute lymphoblastic
    leukemia (ALL)
limb complaints, 121–46
  ankle sprain, 123–6
  fractures, 144–6
  lacerations, 129–32
  Lyme arthritis, 133–5
  nursemaid's elbow, 121–2
  osteomyelitis, 135–43
  septic arthritis, 126–9
  shoulder dislocation, 141–3
  supracondylar fracture, 138–40
Listeria monocytogenes, 237
localized rashes, 290
lumbar puncture (LP)
  febrile seizure, 69
  Lyme meningitis, 245
  meningitis, 238
  subarachnoid hemorrhage,
    251
Lund and Browder chart, 21,
    280
Lyme arthritis, 133–5, 244
  diagnosis, 134
  epidemiology, 134
  pathophysiology, 134
  presentation, 133, 134
  treatment, 134
Lyme disease, 243–6
  cases by State in the USA, 244
  diagnosis, 245

epidemiology, 244
pathophysiology, 244
presentation, 244–5
treatment, 246
Lyme meningitis, 239, 245

magnesium sulfate, 54
magnets, ingestion, 186
malignant hypertension, 226–9
malnutrition, hypovolemic shock and,
    28
malrotation, 48, 165–8
  diagnosis, 167
  disposition, 168
  epidemiology, 166
  pathophysiology, 166
  presentation, 167
  treatment, 167
mastoiditis, 104–6
  diagnosis, 105
  epidemiology, 105
  pathophysiology, 105
  presentation, 105
  treatment, 106
maxillofacial fractures, 282–5
mean arterial pressure, 232
medulloblastoma, 234–6
  diagnosis, 235
  epidemiology, 234
  pathophysiology, 235
  presentation, 235
  treatment, 235–6
meningitis, 236–9, 293
  aseptic, 237, 245
  bacterial, 237, 238
  diagnosis, 238–9
  epidemiology, 237
  GERD and, 48
  pathophysiology, 238
  presentation, 238
  treatment, 239
meningitis with bacteremia, 293
meningococcemia, 291–4
  diagnosis, 293
  epidemiology, 292
  pathophysiology, 292
  presentation, 293
  treatment, 294
mental status assessment
  c-spine injury, 12
  multiple trauma, 6
metabolic acidosis, 25, 86, 87
metabolic decompensation, 28
methotrexate, 198
migraine, 240–2
  diagnosis, 241–2
  disposition, 242
  epidemiology, 241
  pathophysiology, 241

presentation, 241
treatment, 242
milk protein allergy, 253–5
miscarriage, 261
motor vehicle accidents
  c-spine injury, 10–14
  statistics, 4
MRI scanning
  brain tumors, 162
  osteomyelitis, 137, 138
  peritonsillar abscess, 113
MRSA, 127, 137, 138, 248
multiple trauma, 4–6
  diagnosis, 5
  epidemiology, 4
  globe rupture in, 103
  pathophysiology, 4
  presentation, 4–5
  treatment, 5–6
myalgias, 293
myocarditis, 30
myringotomy, 106

nasal foreign body, 96, 99
  diagnosis, 96
  presentation, 96
  treatment, 97
nasal packing, 100
nasoethmoid fractures, 107
neck. *See also* head and neck pain
  decreased mobility, 117, 119
Neisseria gonorrhoeae, 127, 188, 189
Neisseria meningitidis, 237, 292,
    293
neonatal fever, 71–3
  diagnosis, 72
  epidemiology, 71
  pathophysiology, 72
  presentation, 72
  treatment, 72
neuroleptic malignant syndrome
    (NMS), 76–8
  diagnosis, 77–8
  disposition, 78
  epidemiology, 77
  pathophysiology, 77
  presentation, 77
  treatment, 78
neurologic disorders
  constipation and, 177, 178
  intoxication and, 217
neurosurgery, 162, 233
neutropenic fever, 73–6, 82
  diagnosis, 75
  disposition, 75
  epidemiology, 74
  pathophysiology, 74
  presentation, 74
  treatment, 75

NEXUS criteria, 12–13
non-accidental trauma, 16–18. *See also*
    child abuse
  BRUE and, 58
  burns and, 20
  diagnosis, 17–18
  disposition, 18
  epidemiology, 17
  persistent crying and, 208
  pregnancy and, 261
  presentation, 17
  red flags, 17
  subarachnoid hemorrhage and, 250,
    251
  treatment, 18
nose complaints. *See* eye, ear, nose, and
    throat
NSAIDs, 93
nucleic acid amplification, 188, 265,
    266
nursemaid's elbow, 121–2
  diagnosis, 122
  disposition, 122
  epidemiology, 121
  pathophysiology, 121
  presentation, 122
  treatment, 122

obesity, 171, 172
oculocardiac reflex, 108
ondansetron, 151
orbital fracture, 106–9
  diagnosis, 108
  disposition, 108
  epidemiology, 107
  pathophysiology, 107–8
  presentation, 108
  treatment, 108
orbital wall fracture, 108, 109
osmolar gap, elevated, 217
osmotic agents, 162, 259
osteomyelitis, 135–43
  diagnosis, 137
  epidemiology, 136
  pathophysiology, 136–7
  presentation, 137
  treatment, 137
otitis media, 114–16
  diagnosis, 115–16
  epidemiology, 115
  mastoiditis and, 104, 105
  pathophysiology, 115
  presentation, 115
  treatment, 116
Ottawa Ankle Rules, 125
ovarian torsion, 193, 194
overfeeding, 170–2
  diagnosis, 172
  pathophysiology, 171–2

presentation, 172
treatment, 172
oxygen, hyperbaric, 226
oxygenation, maintaining, 232

Panayiotopoulos syndrome, 157–60
papilledema, 162, 235, 246
paraphimosis, 257–60
  diagnosis, 258
  disposition, 260
  epidemiology, 258
  pathophysiology, 258
  presentation, 258
  treatment, 258–60
Parkland formula, 21
Pasteurella infections, 283, 284
patent ductus ateriosus, 63
PECARN criteria, 232
  c-spine injury, 13
  head trauma, 8, 9
pediatric severe sepsis, 37
pelvic examination, 262
pelvic inflammatory disease, 188, 189,
    265
pelvic pain, 260, 261
penetrating trauma, globe rupture,
    102–4
pericarditis, 91–4
  diagnosis, 93
  epidemiology, 92
  pathophysiology, 92
  presentation, 93
  treatment, 93
periodic breathing, 45–6
  diagnosis, 46
  epidemiology, 45
  pathophysiology, 46
  presentation, 46
peripheral perfusion, assessing, 6
peritonsillar abscess, 112–14
  diagnosis, 113
  disposition, 113
  epidemiology, 112
  pathophysiology, 112
  presentation, 112
  treatment, 113
pharyngitis, 110, 111
  strep. *See* streptococcal pharyngitis
pheochromocytoma, 226–9
phimosis, 258
physeal fractures, 145
pink CHD, 60, 61, 62
placenta previa, 262
placental abruption, 261
plastic deformity, 144
Pneumocystis jirovecii, 82
pneumonia, 189–91
  diagnosis, 190
  epidemiology, 190

foreign-body aspiration and, 43
GERD and, 48
pathophysiology, 190
presentation, 190
respiratory failure from, 33, 34
transplant-associated CMV infection
    and, 82
treatment, 191
Poison Control Hotline, 218
poisoning. *See also* intoxication
  BRUE and, 58
  carbon monoxide, 224–6
  poisons, and antidotes, 218
polyethylene glycol, 154, 179, 180, 213
polymerase chain reaction (PCR)
    testing, 238
post-transplant lymphoproliferative
    disease (PTLD), 82
potassium levels, abnormal, 182
pregnancy, 260–3
  diagnosis, 262
  disposition, 262–3
  ectopic. *See* ectopic pregnancy
  epidemiology, 196, 261
  pathophysiology, 261
  presentation, 261
  treatment, 262
Pregnancy Mortality Surveillance
    System, 196
pregnancy testing, 196, 261
primary closure of wounds, 284
prostaglandin therapy, 63, 214
psychosis. *See* acute psychosis
pulse oximetry, four-extremity, 213
puncture wounds, 274
  treatment, 284
purpura fulminans, 293, 294
pyloric stenosis, 48

rabies prophylaxis, 284, 285
radial head subluxation. *See*
    nursemaid's elbow
radiation exposure, thyroid cancer
    and, 14
radiography. *See* X-rays
rashes, 288–91
  dangerous-appearing, 290–1
  diagnosis, 290–1
  epidemiology, 289
  pathophysiology, 289
  presentation, 289
  treatment, 291
red blood cells (RBC)
  destruction, 65, 66
  failure to make, 66
  loss of, 65
red flags
  anaphylaxis, 40
  coronary artery anomaly, 208

GERD, 48
headache, 241
non-accidental trauma, 17
reduction
inguinal hernia, 256
intussusception, 157
paraphimosis, 259–60
shoulder dislocation, 143
referred abdominal pain, 190
rehydration
bulimia and anorexia, 164
oral, 90, 151
resection, tumor, 229, 235, 236
respiratory failure, 32–5
diagnosis, 33–4
epidemiology, 33
pathophysiology, 33
presentation, 33
treatment, 34
respiratory rate, taking, 33
respiratory syncytial virus (RSV),
bronchiolitis and, 50, 51
resuscitation, 3–41. See also fluid
resuscitation
anaphylaxis, 38–41
brain tumors, 162
burns, 19–23
cardiogenic shock, 29–32
c-spine injury, 10–14
drowning, 23–6
ectopic pregnancy, 199
head trauma, 7–10
hypovolemic shock, 26–9
multiple trauma, 3–6
non-accidental trauma, 16–18
respiratory failure, 32–5
septic shock, 35–8
retinal hemorrhage, 18
retropharyngeal abscess, 110, 117–20,
247–9
diagnosis, 248
epidemiology, 117, 248
pathophysiology, 119, 248
presentation, 119, 248
treatment, 119, 248
rhesus status, 262
rheumatic fever, 169
rib fractures, 16, 17
RICE, 125
Rome IV criteria, 178
rotavirus, 151
rule of 7s, meningitis, 239, 245
rule of 9s, burns, 21, 280
Russell's sign, 164

salpingectomy, 198
salpingostomy, 198
Salter–Harris fractures, 125, 145, 146
Sandifer syndrome, 48

schizoaffective disorder, 222
schizophrenia, 222
schizophreniform, 222
secondary brain damage, 232
Seidel's sign, 103
seizures, 157–60
diagnosis, 159
drowning and, 25
epidemiology, 158
febrile. See febrile seizure
inborn error of metabolism and, 147,
149
pathophysiology, 158
presentation, 158–9
treatment, 159
tumors, 235
septic arthritis, 126–9
diagnosis, 127–8
epidemiology, 127
pathophysiology, 127
presentation, 127
treatment, 128
septic shock, 35–8
cardiogenic shock and, 36, 213, 214
CHF and, 63
diagnosis, 36–7
epidemiology, 36
neonatal fever and, 72
pathophysiology, 36
presentation, 36
treatment, 37
serotonin syndrome, 78
serum iron levels, 153, 154
serum reference values, xv
serum salicylate levels, 86
sexual abuse, 189, 262, 264, 271
sexually transmitted infections (STIs),
187–9, 263–6
diagnosis, 188, 262, 265
disposition, 189
epidemiology, 188, 264
pathophysiology, 188, 264
presentation, 188, 264–5
treatment, 189, 265
UTIs and, 268
shaken baby syndrome, 287
shock index, 197
shock syndrome, 27
shoulder dislocation, 141–3
diagnosis, 142–3
epidemiology, 142
pathophysiology, 142
presentation, 142
treatment, 143
shunting, 60
sickle cell disease, 78–80
diagnosis, 79
disposition, 80
epidemiology, 79

osteomyelitis and, 137
pathophysiology, 79
presentation, 79
treatment, 80
SIRS criteria, 36
skeletal survey, 287
skin complaints, 273–94. See also
lacerations
ALL. See acute lymphoblastic
leukemia (ALL)
animal bites, 282–5
burns. See burns
child abuse. See child abuse
foreign-body granuloma, 273–6
meningococcemia, 291–4
rashes, 288–91
slit-lamp examination, 103
sore throat, 110, 111, 113
spina bifida, 178
spinal cord injury without
radiographic abnormality
(SCIWORA), 11, 14
spirometry, 54
staphylococcal scalded skin syndrome,
280
Staphylococcus aureus, 127
MRSA, 127, 137, 138, 248
Stevens–Johnson syndrome, 280
streptococcal pharyngitis, 168–70
diagnosis, 170
epidemiology, 169
pathophysiology, 169
presentation, 169
treatment, 170
streptococci, 110
Streptococcus pneumoniae, 115, 237
subarachnoid hemorrhage, 249–52
diagnosis, 251
disposition, 252
epidemiology, 250
pathophysiology, 251
presentation, 251
treatment, 251–2
subdural hematomas, 1
sudden infant death syndrome (SIDS),
49
superficial burns, 20
superficial partial-thickness burns, 20
supracondylar fracture, 138–40
diagnosis, 139–40
disposition, 140
epidemiology, 139
nursemaid's elbow and, 122
pathophysiology, 139
presentation, 139
treatment, 140
sutures, lacerations, 132
sweating, 89
syndesmotic sprain, 124, 126

synovial fluid, assessment, 128, 134, 135
syphilis, 188, 264, 265
systemic toxicity, 153
systolic blood pressure, 232

tension pneumothorax, 5
testicular torsion, 192–5
tetanus, 285
tetanus prophylaxis, 132
Tetralogy of Fallot, 60
THE MISFITS differential diagnosis
  CHD, 62
  febrile seizure, 70
  malrotation, 167
  seizures, 159
thoracotomy, 44
throat complaints. *See* eye, ear, nose, and throat
thyroid cancer, 14
tick bites, 244
tonsillitis, 112
torsion, 192–5
  diagnosis, 193
  epidemiology, 193
  pathophysiology, 193
  presentation, 193
  treatment, 194
torticollis, 119, 247–9
torus fracture, 145
total body surface area (TBSA), burns, 20, 21
toxic epidermal necrolysis, 280
toxidromes, examination findings, 217
transplant-associated CMV infection, 81–4
  diagnosis, 83–4
  epidemiology, 81–2
  pathophysiology, 82
  presentation, 83
  treatment, 84
traumatic brain injury (TBI). *See also* epidural hematoma, head trauma
  epidemiology, 230
  high-risk patients, 9

incidence, 8
intermediate-risk patients, 9
low-risk patients, 9
secondary brain damage from, 232
Trichomonas, 188, 271
triptans, 242
trismus, 113
trisomy 4–5, 165, 183
troponin, 31, 94
type 1 diabetes, 181
type 2 diabetes, 181

ultrasound (U/S), 1
  appendicitis, 174, 175
  ectopic pregnancy, 197, 198
  foreign body, 275
  globe rupture, 103
  intussusception, 156, 157, 220
  malrotation, 167
  septic arthritis, 128
  torsion, 194
  urinary retention, 177, 180
upper GI series, 167, 168
upper respiratory infection (URI)
  febrile seizure and, 69
  peritonsillar abscess, 113
  retropharyngeal abscess and, 119
urethritis, 188
urinalysis, 194, 268
urinary retention, 176–80
urinary tract infection (UTI), 48, 266–9
  diagnosis, 268
  epidemiology, 267
  neonatal fever and, 71–3
  pathophysiology, 267
  presentation, 267–8
  treatment, 268–9
urine pregnancy tests, 197
urine reference values, xvi
uterine rupture, 261

vaginal discharge, 264
vaginitis, 188, 269–72
  diagnosis, 271

epidemiology, 270
pathophysiology, 270
presentation, 270
treatment, 271
ventricular septal defect, 60, 63
viral gastroenteritis, 26–9
viral perimyocarditis. *See* pericarditis
vital signs
  CHD, 208, 213
  migraine, 241
volvulus, 48
  malrotation with, 165–8
vomiting, 147–72
  acute gastroenteritis, 150–2
  bulimia nervosa, 163–5
  diabetic ketoacidosis, 182
  inborn error of metabolism, 147–50
  intracranial mass, 160–3
  intussusception, 155–7, 220
  iron toxicity, 152–5
  malrotation, 165–8
  overfeeding, 170–2
  seizures, 157–60
  strep pharyngitis, 168–70

Wessel's rule of 3s, 207
Western blot, 134, 245
whirlpool sign, 167
white blood cells (WBC)
  reference values, xv
  septic shock, 36
wound irrigation, 131
wounds. *See* lacerations

X-rays. *See also* chest X-ray (CXR)
  ankle sprain, 123, 125
  c-spine injury, 13
  foreign body, 275
  osteomyelitis, 137
  retropharyngeal abscess, 118, 119
  septic arthritis, 128
  shoulder dislocation, 142
  supracondylar fracture, 139, 140

zygomatic complex, 108